Arteriovenous Access Surgery

Hans Scholz

Arteriovenous Access Surgery

Ensuring Adequate Vascular Access for Hemodialysis

In collaboration with
U. Krüger, K. Petzold, and M. Wunsch
With extra chapters by
J. Janzen and U. Krüger

Springer

Hans Scholz, MD, PhD
Evangelisches Krankenhaus Königin
Elisabeth Herzberge
Department of Vascular Surgery
Berlin
Germany

Translated from the original German edition by M. Wunsch

ISBN 978-3-642-41138-0 ISBN 978-3-642-41139-7 (eBook)
DOI 10.1007/978-3-642-41139-7
Springer Heidelberg New York Dordrecht London

Library of Congress Control Number: 2014944307

Printed on acid-free paper

Springer is part of Springer Science+Business Media (www.springer.com)

Preface to the English Edition

The response to the German edition of our textbook, including requests from abroad, has encouraged us to prepare an English language edition for the international audience as well. We hope that it will be met with as much interest as the original version.

Berlin, Germany
2013

H. Scholz

Preface to the German Edition

Due to demographic change and medical progress, the number of patients suffering from terminal renal insufficiency has been increasing steadily. A longer patient survival on dialysis means that surgeons as well as dialysis units have to face ever more complex situations that call for extensive care. This constitutes a challenge which requires profound knowledge in order to find the best durable solutions to either maintain a pre-existing hemodialysis access or to create a new one, while dealing with an already altered vascular state that offers limited choices.

Here we present a practical textbook which results from looking back at more than 17,000 hemodialysis access operations in the last few decades. It is based on the relevant principles of anatomy, pathophysiology, hemodynamics, and pathology. We are aware of the fact that not everybody will approve of all our concepts. Different strategies may well prove successful too. We intend to present our own ideas regarding pertinent questions in as much detail as necessary. We explicitly do not attempt to give a survey of the entire literature.

For us, hemodynamics is a main focus of interest. I developed, designed, and built the circular flow model, have posed the clinical questions from which I have derived research projects, and have participated in the investigations. I – frequently along with students who prepared their theses – also built the transparent silicone models.

This book project could not have been realized without the support of my coauthors. I have been working with some of them for several decades.

For more than 20 years, Dr. K. Petzold MD and I have been collaborating closely as far as vascular surgery and research are concerned.

Dr. U. Krueger PhD developed the electronic control module for the circular flow system. He also conducted most of the experiments, analyzed and published results, and carried out all computational fluid dynamics investigations.

Dr. M. Wunsch's MD major contributions to the book also comprise his decisive sharp-witted critique and his search of the literature.

Dr. J. Janzen MD, MPhil, whose special interest has included the histopathology of arteriovenous accesses for more than two decades, wrote the respective chapter.

I would also like to thank Dr. H. Petrov MD, head of the Department of Nephrology, for the longstanding cooperation as well as for her advice concerning the chapters on central venous catheters and puncture techniques. Furthermore, I am grateful to the board of directors of our hospital, as they maintain an environment which facilitates scientific research.

Berlin, Germany H. Scholz
2012

Contents

1 Introduction 1
1.1 Introductory Principles. 1
1.2 Vascular Access for Hemodialysis 2
1.3 Requirements for a Permanent Vascular Hemodialysis Access 2
1.4 Choice of the Vascular Access 2
1.5 Preoperative Assessment 3
1.6 Basics of Vascular Access Surgery 3
1.7 Practical Requirements. 5

2 Central Venous Catheters for Hemodialysis 7
2.1 Temporary Catheters 7
2.2 Permanent Catheters. 8
2.3 Handling of Catheters. 9
Literature 10

3 AV Fistulas 11
3.1 Basics 11
3.1.1 Types of Arteriovenous Anastomoses. 11
3.1.2 Pathophysiology of the AV Fistula 12
3.1.3 Special Surgical Aspects of AV Fistulas. 12
3.2 AV Fistula of the Forearm 15
3.2.1 AV Fistulas of the Cephalic Vein 16
3.2.2 AV Fistulas of the Basilic Vein 19
3.2.3 AV Fistula of the Median Antebrachial Vein 21
3.2.4 Repair of AV Fistulas in the Forearm 22
3.3 AV Fistulas in the Cubital Fossa and in the Upper Arm . . . 35
3.3.1 Vascular Anatomy in the Cubital Fossa 35
3.3.2 Technical Hints 37
3.3.3 Arterialization of the Cephalic Vein 38
3.3.4 Arterialization of the Basilic Vein. 45
3.3.5 Arterialization of the Cephalic and Basilic Veins in the Cubital Fossa. 50
3.3.6 Arterialization of the Deep Vein in the Cubital Fossa. 51
3.3.7 Aneurysms in the Cubital Fossa After AV Anastomoses. 51
3.3.8 Great Saphenous Vein as AV Access 52
Literature 54

4 AV Shunts 57
4.1 Pathophysiology 57
4.1.1 Arterial Anastomosis 57
4.1.2 Puncturable Segment 57
4.1.3 Venous Anastomosis 58
4.1.4 Tissue Proliferation Inside the AV Shunt 58
4.2 Hemodynamics of Arteriovenous Grafts 59
4.2.1 Pressure Curves Within an AV Interposition Graft 61
4.2.2 Influence of the Sudden Change of Diameter Between a Narrow Artery and a 7-mm Prosthesis on Blood Flow 61
4.2.3 Influence of the Design and Length of a Graft on Flow Rate 62
4.2.4 Venous Anastomosis 63
4.2.5 Evaluation of the Results 73
4.2.6 Hemodynamics and Shunt Thrombosis 74
4.3 Principles for the Implantation of Prosthetic Shunt Grafts 76
4.3.1 Preoperative Vascular Diagnostics 76
4.3.2 Anesthesia 76
4.3.3 Prevention of Infections 76
4.3.4 Isolation of the Vessels 77
4.3.5 Tunnel for the Prosthetic Graft 77
4.3.6 Fibrin Sealing of ePTFE Graft 77
4.3.7 Placing the Prosthetic Graft in the Subcutaneous Tunnel 78
4.3.8 Position of the Venous Anastomosis 81
4.3.9 Creating an Anastomosis 81
4.4 AV Grafts in the Forearm 85
4.4.1 Straight Graft 85
4.4.2 Loop Graft 86
4.4.3 Repair of Forearm Interposition Grafts 86
4.5 AV Grafts in the Upper Arm 86
4.5.1 Anatomy of the Infraaxillary Veins 86
4.5.2 Straight Graft 88
4.5.3 Loop Graft 90
4.5.4 Repair of Upper Arm Grafts 90
4.6 Infraclavicular Graft 93
4.6.1 Access and Technical Advice 93
4.6.2 Repair of Infraclavicular AV Grafts 98
4.7 Subclavianjugular AV Grafts 99

4.8 Femoral AV Graft . . . 100
4.8.1 Femoral Loop . . . 101
4.8.2 Femorofemoral Crossover Shunt . . . 102
4.8.3 Repair of Femoral Grafts . . . 102
4.9 Other AV Shunts . . . 103
4.10 First Puncture of AV Grafts . . . 103
References . . . 103

5 Arterioarterial Grafts . . . 107
5.1 Physiology of Arterioarterial Grafts . . . 107
5.2 Infraclavicular Arterioarterial Graft . . . 108
5.3 Femoral Arterioarterial Graft . . . 108
5.4 Repair of Arterioarterial Grafts . . . 109
5.5 Clinical Observations . . . 110
5.6 Hints for Handling Arterioarterial Interposition Grafts . . . 110
Literature . . . 110

6 Redo Surgery with Prosthetic Grafts . . . 111
6.1 Thromboses . . . 111
6.1.1 Finding the Cause of Thrombosis . . . 111
6.1.2 Choice of the Thrombectomy Site . . . 112
6.1.3 Incision . . . 113
6.1.4 Technique for Thrombectomy . . . 113
6.1.5 Closure of the Graft . . . 114
6.1.6 Wound Closure . . . 114
6.2 Repair of Graft Aneurysms . . . 114
6.2.1 False Aneurysm . . . 114
6.2.2 Puncture Site Aneurysms . . . 115
6.3 Repair of Graft Stenoses . . . 118

7 Infections . . . 121
7.1 Prevention of Infections . . . 121
7.1.1 Prevention of Perioperative Infections when Creating a Vascular Access . . . 121
7.1.2 Prevention of Perioperative Infections in Redo Surgery . . . 122
7.2 Therapy of Infections of AV Fistulas . . . 122
7.2.1 Early Postoperative Infections . . . 122
7.2.2 Late Postoperative Infections . . . 122
7.2.3 Infections of Thrombosed AV Fistulas . . . 123
7.3 Infections of Prosthetic AV Grafts . . . 125
7.3.1 Early Postoperative Infections . . . 125
7.3.2 Late Infections . . . 127
Literature . . . 130

8 Venous Congestion After the Creation of AV Accesses 131
8.1 Venous Congestive Syndrome 131
8.1.1 Pathophysiology 131
8.1.2 Occlusions/Stenoses of the Forearm Cephalic Veins with Distal AV Anastomoses 132
8.1.3 Occlusions/Stenoses of the Cubital Veins with Distal AV Anastomoses 133
8.1.4 Occlusions/Stenoses of the Axillary Veins with Infraaxillary AV Anastomoses 133
8.1.5 Occlusions/Stenoses of the Axillary Veins or Subclavian Veins with Infraclavicular AV Anastomoses 134
8.1.6 Occlusions/Stenoses of the Brachiocephalic Vein with Peripheral AV Anastomosis and Occlusions/Stenoses of the Contralateral Internal Jugular Vein 134
8.1.7 Occlusions/Stenoses of the Femoral or Iliac Veins with Femoral AV Anastomoses 134
8.1.8 Clinical Symptoms After Curing Venous Congestion 135
8.2 Syndrome of Retrograde Venous Arterialization 136
8.2.1 Pathophysiology 136
8.2.2 Clinical Signs 136
Literature 136

9 Stenoses and Occlusions of the Central Veins 137
9.1 Pathophysiology 137
9.2 Clinical Signs and Investigations 138
9.3 Therapy 138
Literature 139

10 Leakage of ePTFE Grafts (Perigraft Seroma) 141
10.1 Pathophysiology 141
10.2 Clinical Presentation and Therapy 141
10.2.1 Type I 141
10.2.2 Type II 141
10.2.3 Type III 142
10.2.4 Type IV 143
10.2.5 Type V 143
Literature 144

11 Insufficient Peripheral Perfusion and Cardiac Strain After AV Access Creation 145
11.1 Insufficient Peripheral Perfusion 145
11.1.1 Pathophysiology and Stages of Insufficient Perfusion 145
11.1.2 Vascular Investigations 146
11.1.3 Indications for Treatment 148
11.2 Therapy of Insufficient Peripheral Perfusion 148
11.2.1 Flow Reduction 148
11.2.2 Proximalization of the Arterial Inflow 159

11.2.3 Proximalization of the Arterial Inflow into the Distal Arterial Stump ... 171
11.2.4 Comparison of Both Methods for Proximalization ... 171
11.3 Cardiac Strain Caused by AV Accesses ... 171
11.4 Prevention of Insufficient Peripheral Perfusion ... 172
Literature ... 172

12 Arterial Reconstructions of AV Accesses ... 175
12.1 Clinical Presentation and Investigations ... 175
12.1.1 Reduced Arterial Inflow into the AV Access ... 175
12.1.2 Insufficient Peripheral Perfusion ... 176
12.1.3 Indications for Arterial Reconstructions ... 176
12.2 Reconstruction of Upper Extremity Arteries ... 176
12.2.1 Segment I: Stenoses/Occlusions of the Central Subclavian Artery (Aortovertebral Segment) ... 176
12.2.2 Segment II: Peripheral Subclavian Artery (Vertebroaxillary Segment) ... 179
12.2.3 Segment III: Axillary Artery ... 179
12.2.4 Segment IV: Proximal (Infraaxillary) Brachial Artery ... 180
12.2.5 Segment V: Middle Brachial Artery ... 181
12.2.6 Segment VI: Peripheral Brachial Artery ... 181
12.2.7 Segment VII: Forearm Arteries ... 181
12.2.8 Long Occlusions ... 181
12.3 Extreme Dilatation of the Feeding Artery ... 182
Literature ... 183

13 Lymph Edema of the Arm After AV Access Surgery ... 185
13.1 Pathophysiology ... 185
13.2 Postoperative Lymph Edemas ... 185
13.2.1 Local Lymph Edema ... 185
13.2.2 Lymph Edema Distal to Operated Site ... 185
13.3 Chronic Postoperative Lymph Edema ... 186
13.3.1 Lymph Edema with Venous Congestion ... 186
13.3.2 Lymph Edema Without Venous Congestion ... 186
13.4 Prevention of Lymph Edema After AV Access Surgery ... 186
Literature ... 186

14 Nerve Lesions After AV Access Surgery ... 187
14.1 Concerned Nerves ... 187
14.1.1 Distal Cephalic Fistula ... 187
14.1.2 Distal Basilic Fistula ... 187
14.1.3 Elbow Fistula ... 187
14.1.4 Superficialization of the Basilic Vein in the Upper Arm ... 187
14.1.5 Anastomosis Central to the Elbow ... 187
14.1.6 Axillary Anastomosis ... 188
14.1.7 Infraclavicular Anastomosis ... 188

14.1.8 Jugular Anastomosis (Internal Jugular Vein) ... 188
14.1.9 Supraclavicular Approach to the Subclavian Artery ... 188
14.2 Prevention of Nerve Lesions ... 188

15 Special Patient Groups ... 189
15.1 Renal Transplant Recipients ... 189
15.1.1 Creation of a New Vascular Access ... 189
15.1.2 Request for the Closure of an AV Access ... 189
15.2 Patients Who Require Extra Attention ... 190
15.2.1 Diabetics ... 191
15.2.2 Obesity ... 191
15.2.3 Heart Failure ... 191
15.2.4 Hypotension ... 192
15.2.5 Malignancy ... 192
15.2.6 Hypercoagulability ... 192
15.2.7 Amputees ... 192
15.2.8 Pareses ... 192
15.2.9 Dermatologic Diseases ... 192
15.2.10 Septic Disease ... 192
15.2.11 IV Drug Abuse ... 193

16 Anticoagulation with AV Accesses ... 195
Literature ... 196

17 Puncture Techniques ... 197
17.1 Pathophysiology of the Punctured Vessel Wall ... 197
17.1.1 Vein ... 197
17.1.2 ePTFE Prosthesis ... 197
17.2 Puncture Site Selection ... 198
17.2.1 Rope Ladder Puncture ... 198
17.2.2 Area Puncture ... 198
17.2.3 Buttonhole Puncture ... 198
17.3 Puncture Technique ... 199
17.3.1 Angle of Insertion ... 199
17.3.2 Position of the Cannula's Aperture ... 200
17.3.3 Vascular Puncture ... 200
17.3.4 Puncture Direction with Regard to Flow Direction ... 200
17.4 Removal of the Cannula ... 200
17.5 Influence of Single-Needle Dialysis on the Hemodynamics of the Venous Anastomosis ... 201
17.5.1 Investigations in the Circular Flow System ... 201
17.5.2 Numerical Simulation ... 202
17.5.3 Results and Conclusions ... 204
Literature ... 204

18 Monitoring of Vascular Accesses 207
18.1 History 207
18.2 Inspection 207
18.3 Palpation 207
18.3.1 Findings on Palpation for Flow Evaluation 208
18.3.2 Clinical Tests Using Palpation 208
18.3.3 Evaluation of Vascular Morphology 209
18.4 Auscultation 210
18.5 Tests During Dialysis 210
18.5.1 Pressure Surveillance During Dialysis 211
18.5.2 Elimination of Urea 211
18.5.3 Determination of Recirculation 211
18.6 Further Investigations 211
18.6.1 Duplex Sonography 211
18.6.2 Angiography 212
18.7 Documentation 212
Literature 212

19 Histopathology of AV Vascular Accesses 213
19.1 Introduction 213
19.2 Stenosis 213
19.3 Aneurysmatic Dilatation 217
19.4 Atherosclerosis 220
19.5 Calcification/Ossification 221
Literature 223

20 Short Introduction to Fluid Dynamics: Relevant Aspects for Hemodynamics 225
20.1 Principles of Fluid Mechanics 225
20.2 Continuity Equation 227
20.3 Bernoulli's Equation 227
20.4 Flow Separation and Secondary Flow 228
20.5 Viscosity, Shear Rate, and Shear Stress 231
20.6 Hagen–Poiseuille's law and Peripheral Resistance 231
20.7 Blood Viscosity 233
Literature 233

21 Our Methods 235
21.1 Experimental Flow Investigations 235
21.1.1 Creation of the Anastomotic Models for Flow Visualization 235
21.1.2 Pulsatile Flow System 235
21.1.3 Visualization of the Flow Patterns 237
21.2 Computational Fluid Dynamics 237
Literature 240

Appendix 241

Glossary 242

Index 247

Contributors

Jan Janzen, MD, MPhil VascPath Schweiz, Bern, Switzerland

Ulf Krüger, PhD Department of Vascular Surgery, Evangelisches Krankenhaus Königin Elisabeth Herzberge, Berlin, Germany

Karen Petzold, MD Department of Vascular Surgery, Evangelisches Krankenhaus Königin Elisabeth Herzberge, Berlin, Germany

Hans Scholz, MD, PhD Department of Vascular Surgery, Evangelisches Krankenhaus Königin Elisabeth Herzberge, Berlin, Germany

Matthias Wunsch, MD Department of Vascular Surgery, Evangelisches Krankenhaus Königin Elisabeth Herzberge, Berlin, Germany

1 Introduction

1.1 Introductory Principles

In order to provide satisfactory care for a vascular hemodialysis access, it is important to be familiar with some basic principles.

- The hemodialysis patient's survival depends on the vascular access.
- Efficiency of dialysis, quality of life, and life expectancy also depend on the vascular access.
- Each vascular access alters the former physiological state. Consequently, its creation triggers various physiological and pathophysiological reactions.
- Thus the life span of every vascular access is limited. A new access frequently entails the loss of native vessels.
- The maturation of a vascular access and its life span are based on biological reactions, the surgical procedure, and puncture techniques. Therefore they are not entirely predictable.
- Vascular access puncture can only be as good as the prior surgical procedure permits.
- Apart from functionality, the option for a large number of potential future vascular accesses is a crucial criterion when deciding which access to create.
- There are almost always multiple options for creating a permanent hemodialysis access.
- A vascular surgeon needs to know about hemodynamics just as an architect needs to know about structural analysis.
- The selection of the type of access that is most suitable at a given stage requires profound knowledge. This knowledge is of the utmost importance before embarking on any vascular access surgery.
- From a pathophysiological point of view, there are major differences between an arteriovenous (AV) vascular access and an arterial bypass. They cannot be compared to each other.
- Responsible vascular access surgery can only be performed if the surgeon can deal intensively with a large number of patients over a long period of time.
- Before a novel method is adopted, it should be examined with regard to its physiological suitability and theoretical advantages over existing methods.

> The best vascular access is not necessarily that which primarily promises the longest life span. Preference should be given to that which allows for the longest complication-free hemodialysis therapy when taking into account possible future procedures.

> Except for extremely rare constellations, which we have not observed so far, a permanent vascular access for hemodialysis is always feasible.

H. Scholz, *Arteriovenous Access Surgery*,
DOI 10.1007/978-3-642-41139-7_1, © Springer-Verlag Berlin Heidelberg New York 2015

1.2 Vascular Access for Hemodialysis

For hemodialysis there has been a plethora of historic developments which have partly been abandoned (such as Scribner and Buselmaier shunts). A whole variety of graft materials has also been developed. An early major step in AV access surgery was the creation of an arteriovenous anastomosis by Cimino and Brescia.

Basically there are three different options for connecting patients to the hemodialysis machine:

1. Central venous catheters (temporary, permanent)
2. Two variants of arteriovenous access
   - Arterialization of a vein (in situ, superficial transposition)
   - Implantation of a prosthetic arteriovenous interposition graft
3. Arterioarterial interposition grafts

Arteriovenous access and arterioarterial interposition grafts will be referred to as *permanent vascular accesses*.

> In order to prevent misunderstandings, in this book the terms mentioned below are used as follows:
>
> ***AV fistula*** *for an arterialized native vein*
> ***AV shunt*** *for an arteriovenous prosthetic graft*

1.3 Requirements for a Permanent Vascular Hemodialysis Access

Apart from lasting as long as possible, a permanent vascular access should fulfill the following requirements:

- Minimum blood flow for dialysis of at least 300 mL/min
- Puncturability with two needles
- Segment suitable for puncture as long as possible
- Subcutaneous position as close to the surface as possible
- Decrease in flow distal to the AV anastomosis as low as possible
- Cardiac strain as low as possible

1.4 Choice of the Vascular Access

When selecting a vascular access the following criteria should be considered among others:

- State of veins and arteries
- Perfusion distal to the planned anastomosis
- Body weight (obesity)
- Main diagnosis and comorbidity
- Possibly impaired range of motion of extremities (paretic, traumatic)
- Coagulation disorders
- Blood pressure
- Septic foci (e.g., acute osteomyelitis)
- Location and condition of wounds
- Urgency

In view of these numerous criteria, the detailed medical history and a clinical examination of every patient are required before any further evaluation.

The following guidelines can provide help in almost all patients when selecting a vascular access:

> 1. Except for extremely rare constellations, central venous catheters are only used for bridging before a permanent vascular access can be created and used.
> 2. Preexisting central venous catheters as well as the imminent need for hemodialysis mostly call for the rapid creation of a different permanent vascular access.
> 3. If possible, the arterialization of a subcutaneous vein left in situ should always be preferred.
> 4. When creating an AV fistula, the most distal location which is suitable should be chosen.
> 5. Prosthetic material should only be used if there is no suitable vein or if the existing vein does not promise to mature in time for urgent hemodialysis treatment.
> 6. When using prosthetic material, the most distal site that is suitable from a hemodynamic perspective should be selected.

7. If the range of motion of one arm is impaired (e.g., paresis), this extremity should be used.
8. If there is only one arm, another location should be used.
9. If there are chronic septic foci, alloplastic materials should be avoided if possible.
10. Patients in whom arterioarterial (interposition) grafts are indicated are extremely rare.

1.5 Preoperative Assessment

The preoperative assessment is necessary so as to find the most adequate vascular access while taking multiple aspects into account. When taking a patient's *medical history*, main diagnoses such as diabetes mellitus, lupus erythematosus, sclerodermia, plasmocytoma, other neoplasms, irregular arterial blood pressure, and chronic bacterial infections should be explicitly asked for. Furthermore, knowledge of previous AV access surgery and former sites of central venous catheters as well as procedures scheduled in the future (cf. expected lower blood pressure after a planned nephrectomy), coagulation disorders, and symptoms which are due to an insufficient peripheral perfusion is important.

While *examining* the patient, visible edema of the extremities and torso, prominent veins, and scars after surgery and punctures should be looked for.

As far as the veins are concerned, special attention should be paid to the cephalic vein, the basilic vein, and the veins in the cubital fossa. Evaluation is best done after central compression while lightly tapping the veins. If, due to their deep position, a clinical assessment of the veins is not satisfactory, additional duplex sonography is necessary. If there are signs of an obstruction at the upper arm level (increased venous filling, increased pressure when emptying), it is also necessary to investigate there. Even if duplex sonography shows respiration-dependent flow, we expect phlebography to provide additional information if collaterals of the torso are present. Care should be taken to make sure that the respective arm is properly abducted as otherwise axillary stenoses may erroneously be suspected on contrast medium studies.

Arterial examination is relevant in order to see whether the arterialization of a previously selected vein should really be undertaken. It primarily comprises the bilateral palpation of the radial and ulnar arteries, the brachial artery in the cubital fossa and the upper arm. Suspicion of stenosis (weak or absent pulses) should lead to additional color-coded duplex sonography. If this suspicion is confirmed, we perform arterial angiography with percutaneous transluminal angioplasty (PTA) if appropriate. General atherosclerosis (e.g., in diabetic patients) or multiple arterial occlusions may decisively influence the indication for the type of surgery.

1.6 Basics of Vascular Access Surgery

Characteristics of vascular access surgery are:

- Small size of the operative field
- Frequently superficial location of the operative site
- Frequently immunocompromised patients
- Vital importance of the vascular access

Measures to prevent infections include:

- Thorough shave
- Incise film
- Intraoperative administration of antibiotics if alloplastic implants are used
- Meticulous hemostasis before wound closure
- Exact adaptation of the subcutaneous tissue to prevent wound cavities

Under certain circumstances even a small subcutaneous hematoma, which becomes infected, or a perforating subcutaneous suture, whose ends are too long, may cause a fistula, which leads to potentially life-threatening vascular graft infections. We usually do without wound drainage systems but then make sure that there is really no more bleeding at all. As for the upper extremities, only bipolar coagulation should be used. Making the right incision is also important. As all blood vessels of the extremities and the other structures

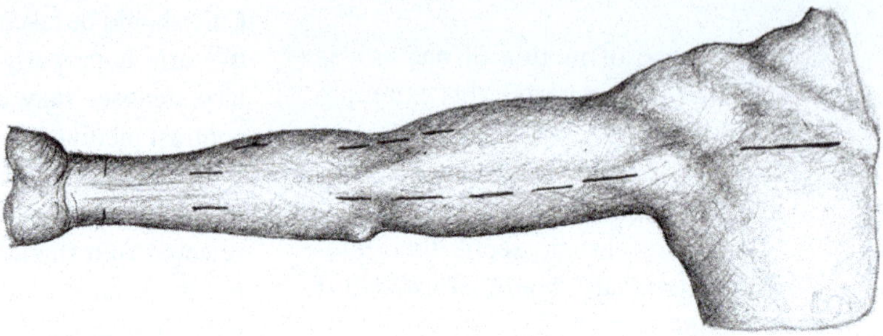

Fig. 1.1 Recommended incisions

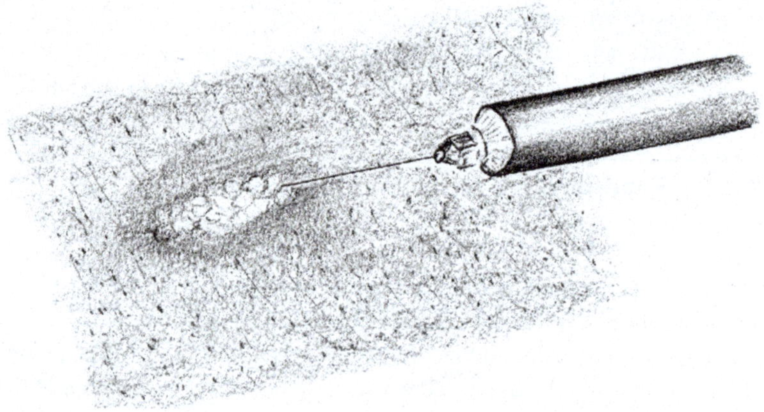

Fig. 1.2 Intracutaneous infiltration with local anesthetics. Immediate incision is possible as instant absence of pain can be achieved

which have to be preserved (including lymphatic vessels) tend to run longitudinally, longitudinal incisions should be preferred (Fig. 1.1). These incisions also allow for the shortest approach and thus leave smaller wounds than other incisions. The only exception is the access for a distal cephalic fistula, if there is a short distance between artery and vein.

In principle all suitable operations of the arm may be carried out using infiltration anesthesia as long as the patient is able and willing to cooperate. The following course of action has proven successful:

- Intracutaneous infiltration with a fine canula in the direction of the planned skin incision (Fig. 1.2)
- Infiltration of the subcutaneous tissue in the direction of the planned incision (Fig. 1.3)
- Infiltration of the subfascial space prior to opening the fascia (Fig. 1.4).

With this technique, the operation may start almost without any delay and mostly without any pain. Should it prove necessary to anesthetize larger nerves in the surgical field, infiltration of the perineurium is recommended (Fig. 1.5).

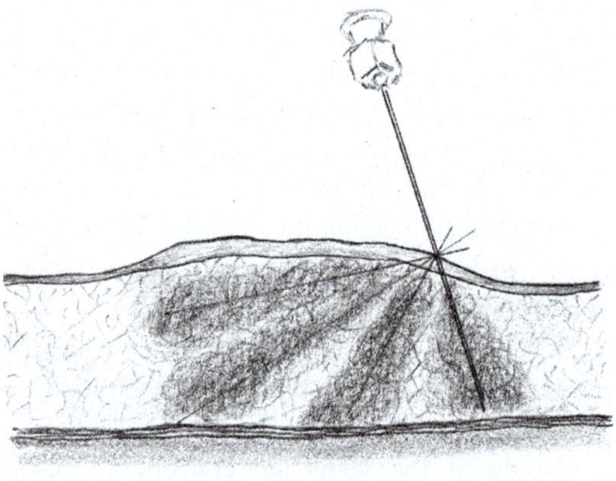

Fig. 1.3 Cross section of the skin during infiltration

For wound dressings we only use loosely-fitting pads. The temporary partial *postoperative immobilization* of an arm is advantageous with some patients. For this purpose we use hook-and-loop fastener –fitted rubber foam splints (Fig. 1.6).

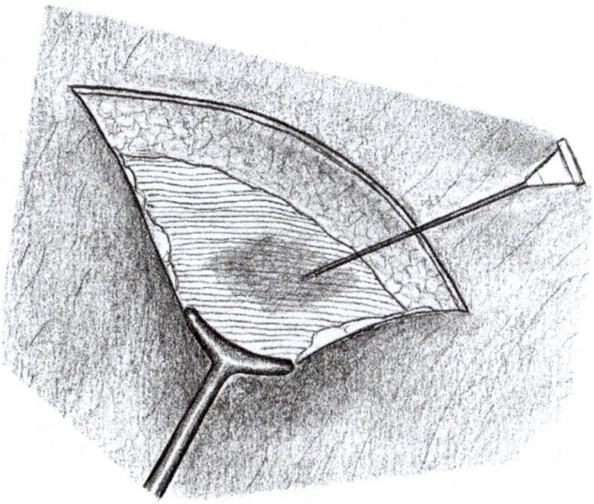

Fig. 1.4 Subfascial infiltration before opening the fascia (e.g., before dissecting the radial or cubital brachial arteries)

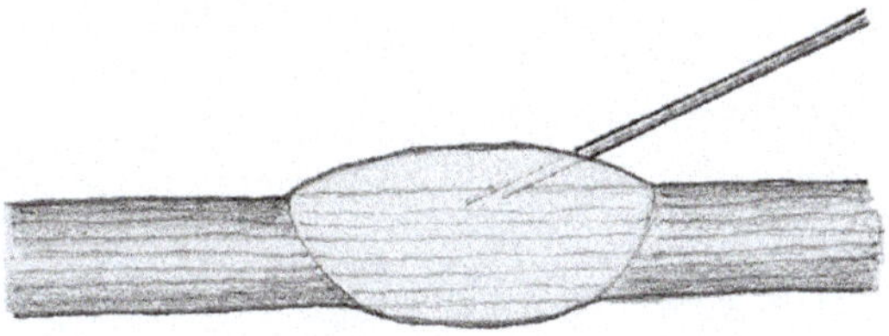

Fig. 1.5 Infiltration of the perineurium to deactivate a nerve

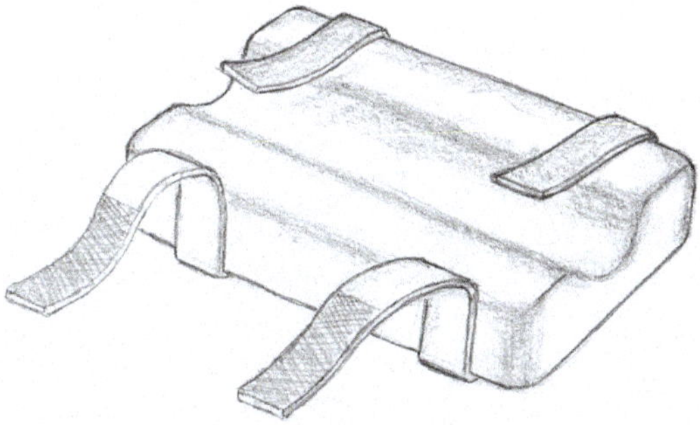

Fig. 1.6 Rubber foam splint for postoperative positioning of the arm

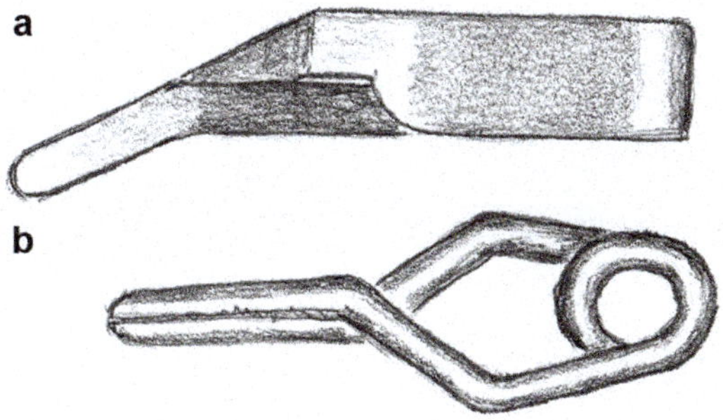

Fig. 1.7 Atraumatic vascular clamps. (**a**) Schwartz clamp. (**b**) Yasargil clamp

1.7 Practical Requirements

Apart from the instruments generally used for vascular surgery procedures, including micro instruments, special atraumatic vascular clamps are important. Soft Yasargil clips (Fig. 1.7) are particularly suited as well as special Schwartz clamps (e.g., Fehling company) with different specifications whose roughened surface areas prevent sliding. Even without presbyopia we recommend the use of magnifying glasses as they encourage more precision when operating. For the complete diagnostic armamentarium, color-coded duplex sonography should be there. Intraoperative angiography should be available, especially for redo surgery. To correct insufficient distal arterial perfusion, intraoperative flow monitoring is required. For a specialized surgical unit there should be at least two surgeons experienced in vascular access surgery.

2 Central Venous Catheters for Hemodialysis

Apart from meeting the diverse biomechanical standards, a catheter should also guarantee a blood flow of at least 250–300 mL/min.

There is a definite distinction between temporary and permanent catheters.

2.1 Temporary Catheters

Indication

- Access for a limited period of time (3–4 weeks at most) until a permanent vascular access or access for peritoneal dialysis can be used, or until dialysis is no longer necessary.

Location

Every catheter may cause venous thrombosis. The risk for thrombosis depends on the:

- Anatomical position of the vein
- Period of time for which the catheter has been used
- Length of the intraluminal segment of the catheter
- Diameter of the catheter
- Thrombogenicity of the material
- Possible coagulation disorders
- Bacterial colonisation of the catheter

Intimal irritation and the risk of thrombosis are much lower in the internal jugular vein than in the subclavian or femoral veins. Criteria for the selection of a suitable vein include the:

- Patency of the vein
- Local conditions (e.g., infections, scar tissue)
- Risk of thrombosis
- Clinical sequelae of a previous thrombosis (e.g., AV access of the ipsilateral arm no longer feasible after thrombotic occlusion of the subclavian vein)

The analysis of the last 1,000 AV access procedures in our patients has shown that in 96.4 % the subclavian veins were used as the venous runoff (Fig. 2.1a). Therefore the protection of these veins is quite important. The following recommendations regarding the sequence for temporary catheter placement are based on this experience (Fig. 2.1b):

1. Right internal jugular vein (shortest intraluminal segment of catheter)
2. Left internal jugular vein (if right internal jugular vein not available)
3. Common femoral vein (to preserve the subclavian veins if internal jugular veins not suited)
4. Right subclavian vein (if jugular and femoral veins not available)
5. Left subclavian vein (if jugular, femoral, and right subclavian veins not available)

A thrombosis of the left subclavian vein often coincides with a thrombosis of the left brachiocephalic vein. On the right side this co-occurrence is extremely rare.

H. Scholz, *Arteriovenous Access Surgery*,
DOI 10.1007/978-3-642-41139-7_2, © Springer-Verlag Berlin Heidelberg New York 2015

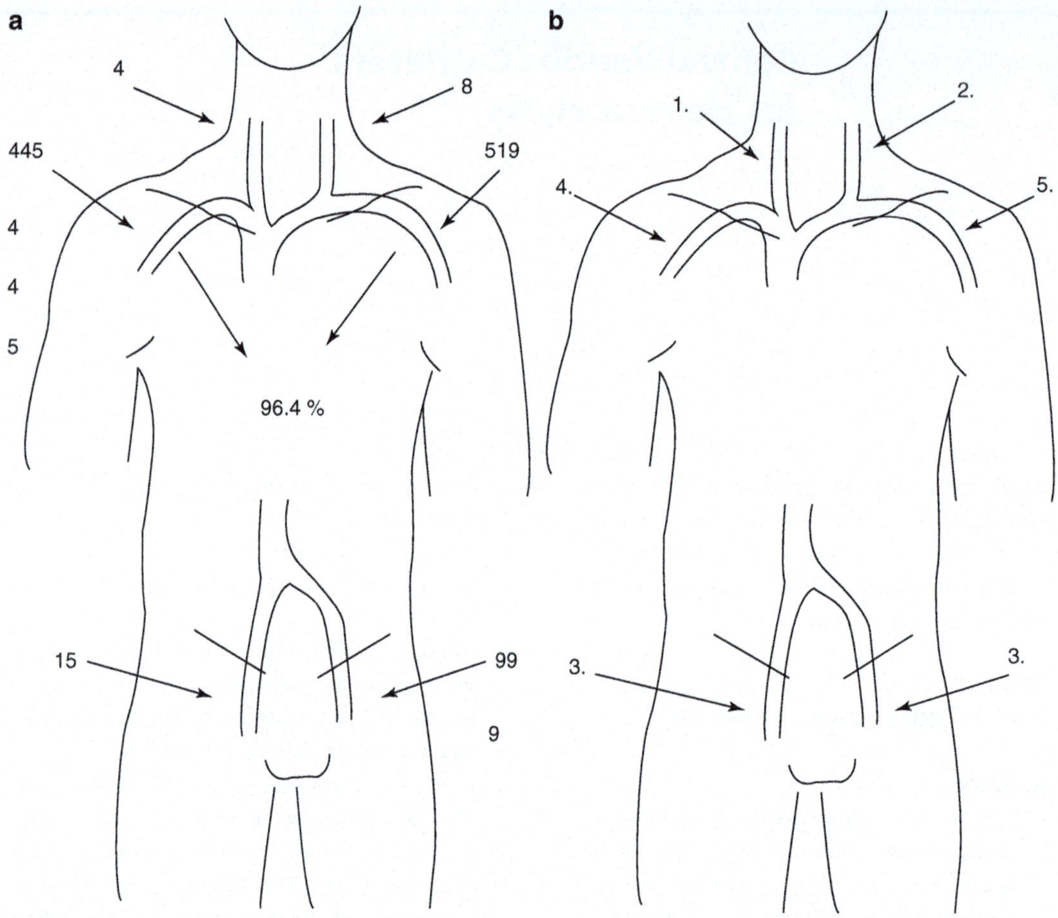

Fig. 2.1 (**a**) Total numbers of patients treated by that specific way out of 1,000. (**b**) Recommended sequence for placement of central venous catheters

Types of Catheters
The higher mean flow (250–300 mL/min) of double lumen catheters (external diameter 11–12 Ch) constitutes an advantage over single lumen catheters (external diameter 8 Ch) with flow volumes of around 200 mL/min. There are also high flow catheters with external diameters of 13 Ch, which grant even higher flows (around 400 mL/min). Polyurethane and silicone are common catheter materials.

Advice for Placement
Sterile conditions (with sterile gown, face mask, and cap) should be maintained when placing a dialysis catheter. Complications will be lower if ultrasound is used to locate the vein. X-Ray *documentation* helps verify the correct final position of the catheter.

2.2 Permanent Catheters

Principle
Characteristics with permanent catheters are:
- Long subcutaneous tunnels
- Felt cuffs which are placed subcutaneously to serve as entrance barriers against microbial invasion

Indication
The indications for permanent catheters vary according to local conditions (vascular surgery unit present?) and preferences of the respective dialysis units. Permanent catheters offer a fast and initially mostly carefree option. Their high medium- and long-term complication rates caused by infections and thromboses, however, can be found in the literature.

We apply strict criteria before placing permanent catheters. From our point of view, permanent catheters should only be placed in patients with a limited life expectancy (weeks to months), in whom creating a vascular access would constitute an exaggerated effort, and who also wish to receive a permanent catheter. Should life expectancy prove longer than predicted, it is still possible to switch to a different vascular access later. Because of the unnecessary tissue trauma, we disapprove of permanent catheters merely to bridge the time before an AV access can be punctured. We plead for the strictly aseptic handling of temporary catheters. We favour placement at new sites if old catheters become infected. Less than 0.2 % of our patients receive permanent catheters.

Site

Criteria similar to those for temporary catheters are valid. With our strict selection criteria (e.g., short life expectancy), it is possible that we are not confronted with the long-term sequelae of venous thromboses. If the jugular veins are not available, the subclavian veins will do as well.

Variants

Different types are on the market. There are double lumen as well as single lumen catheters varying in length. Single lumen catheters are placed in separate subcutaneous tunnels.

Advice for Placement in the Internal Jugular Vein

A permanent catheter should be placed in the operation room using fluoroscopy. After puncturing the internal jugular vein, the guide wire is advanced. A skin incision is made at its exit site. Then the catheter is advanced under fluoroscopic control. The catheter is marked (e.g., where it touches the platysma) when its desired position is reached to prevent its dislocation while pulling it through the subcutaneous tunnel. To prevent kinking, a wide trajectory should be chosen. After creating a subcutaneous tunnel, making a skin incision at the prospective exit site, and pulling the catheter through the tunnel (felt cuff caudad to the clavicula), the final fixation and wound closure take place.

2.3 Handling of Catheters

Asepsis

The potential duration of use is adversely affected by bacterial contamination. Sterile techniques should be used when handling a catheter (exit site and connectors).

Connecting the Catheter

- Spray disinfection of the connectors.
- Face masks for patients and staff and sterile gloves and caps for staff.

Catheter Site Dressing

After each dialysis session the catheter is disinfected. A sterile dressing is applied. Special attention is paid to the exit site. Non-alcoholic disinfectants should be used if required so as not to damage the catheter material. A transparent chlorhexidingluconate dressing, which has to be changed only once per week, has proven useful. Abundant growth of (facial) hair may require more frequent dressing changes.

Prevention of Thrombosis

After finishing a dialysis session, the catheter is flushed with normal saline and then filled with a heparin solution.

Outpatient vs Inpatient Status

Permanent Catheters Patients with permanent catheters can be treated as outpatients. They and possibly also their next of kin should be instructed to observe necessary hygiene rules.

Temporary Catheters We proceed as follows with catheters in the jugular (or subclavian) vein:

- Patients who are not living alone and are able to cooperate are treated as outpatients (written informed consent required).
- With patients who are noncompliant or live by themselves we discourage outpatient status.

With a catheter in a femoral vein, we insist on bed rest and safe thrombosis prophylaxis. These patients are not discharged.

Literature

Astor BC, Eustace JA, Powe NR, Klag MJ, Fink NE, Coresh J (2005) Type of vascular access and survival among incident hemodialysis patients: CHOICE Study. J Am Soc Nephrol 16:1449–1455

Hecking C, Aschwanden M, Dickenmann M, Thalhammer C, Blum B, Bilecen D, Jaeger KA (2006) Efficient haemodialysis despite complete central venous thrombosis. Vasa 35:243–244

Jean G, Vanel T, Chazot C, Charra B, Terrat JC, Hurot JM (2001) Prevalence of stenosis and thrombosis of central veins in hemodialysis after a tunneled jugular catheter. Nephrologie 22:501–504

Saxena AK, Panhotra BR, Sundaram DS, Al-Hafiz A, Naguib M, Venkateshappa CK, Abu-Oun BA, Hussain SM, Al-Ghamdi AA (2006) Tunneled catheters' outcome optimization among diabetics on dialysis through antibiotic-lock placement. Kidney Int 70:1629–1635

Schlieps K, Erley C (2010) Prävention hämodialysekatheterassoziierter Infektionen. Nephrologe 5:535–544

Shaldon S, Chiandussi L, Higgs B (1961) Hemodialysis by percutaneous catheterization of the femoral artery and vein with regional heparinization. Lancet 2:857

Weijmer MC, van den Dorpel MA, Van de Ven PJ, ter Wee PM, van Geelen JA, Groeneveld JO, van Jaarsveld BC, Koopmans MG, le Poole CY, Schrander-Van der Meer AM, Siegert CE, Stas KJ (2005) Randomized, clinical trial comparison of trisodium citrate 30% and heparin as catheter-locking solution in hemodialysis patients. J Am Soc Nephrol 16:2769–2777

AV Fistulas

3

In this book all direct anastomoses between an artery and a vein are called AV fistulas even if the vein has been transposed from its original position either as part of the first operation or at a later stage (e.g., transposed brachiobasilic fistula).

3.1 Basics

3.1.1 Types of Arteriovenous Anastomoses

Basically there are three types of arteriovenous anastomoses (Fig. 3.1):

- Laterolateral
- Terminoterminal
- Lateroterminal

A *laterolateral anastomosis* (Fig. 3.1a) lets blood flow in both directions. With functioning venous valves there is no distally-directed retrograde venous flow. Then the situation is the same as with a lateroterminal anastomosis. Insufficient valves, however, allow for the retrograde arterialization of the venous tree with subsequent venous stasis, edema of the respective extremity, and trophic disturbances. Therefore we disapprove of this type of anastomosis.

A *terminoterminal anastomosis* (Fig. 3.1b) requires the distal ligation of the artery. Thus an occlusion of the AV-anastomosis simultaneously also

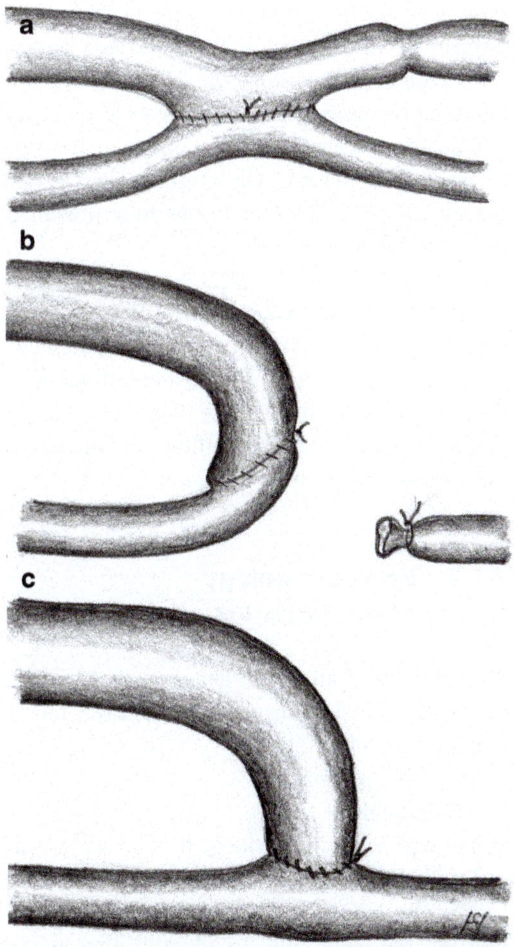

Fig. 3.1 Possible variants of AV anastomoses: (**a**) laterolateral, (**b**) terminoterminal, (**c**) lateroterminal

H. Scholz, *Arteriovenous Access Surgery*,
DOI 10.1007/978-3-642-41139-7_3, © Springer-Verlag Berlin Heidelberg New York 2015

results in the proximal occlusion of the artery. Therefore we disapprove of this type of anastomosis, too.

With a *lateroterminal anastomosis* (Fig. 3.1c) the patency of the vein is preserved even if the feeding artery becomes occluded.

> A lateroterminal anastomosis is the only reasonable option for AV fistulas.

Anastomotic Angle Most frequently arteriovenous anastomoses are placed in the distal forearm or near the cubital fossa. In both positions we prefer perpendicular anastomoses. Near the wrist the anastomosed vein is fed both from the proximal and the distal arterial segments due to its low outflow resistance. That is why a right angle is advantageous. Similar flow conditions may prevail in the cubital fossa.

Diameter of the Anastomosis Despite commonly held views, even an anastomotic diameter of more than 3–4 mm has almost no influence on the flow in the AV fistula. The flow rate is mainly determined by the arterial inflow resistance and the venous outflow resistance.

3.1.2 Pathophysiology of the AV Fistula

The palpable thrill in the anastomotic region is caused by pressure changes. The arterial inflow into the vein leads to:

- Increased pressure
- Pulsating thrill
- Increased shear near the wall
- Oscillations (changes of flow direction)

Morphologic alterations result in the dilation of the vein and frequently also in its elongation.

The extent of these changes depends on:

- Hemodynamic conditions
- The site of the arterialized vein
- Other individual factors

The dilation of the vein decreases its outflow resistance. Consequently its flow increases. Furthermore the feeding artery undergoes changes. The increased outflow into the AV anastomosis raises its wall shear. The physiological adaptation to this stress also leads to the dilation of the artery. The resulting diminished arterial resistance further increases the flow rate in the fistula.

Owing to the manifold interdependent factors which influence changes of both artery and vein, different final states may occur (Fig. 3.2).

Ideally the arterialized vein becomes a large-diameter vessel with a sufficient flow, which may be punctured easily (Fig. 3.2a).

Quite often, elongation leads to stenoses caused by kinking (Fig. 3.2b). Upstream from there, aneurysmatic dilatations of the vein may develop due to the increased intraluminal pressure. Stenoses near the anastomosis frequently cause thrombosis in the postoperative weeks and months (Fig. 3.2c). Intraoperative tissue trauma and the particular mechanical strain of the curved path of the vein near the anastomosis are the most likely causes for these stenoses. General sclerosis of the entire arterialized vein, which leads to stenoses and occlusions, is relatively rare (Fig. 3.2d). This outcome is mainly observed with previously damaged veins (e.g., after chemotherapy, intravenous drug abuse). Likewise, an extreme dilatation of the feeding artery is relatively rare (Fig. 3.2e). Puncturing a fistula leads to alterations of the vein. These are described in detail in Chap. 17.

3.1.3 Special Surgical Aspects of AV Fistulas

Paying attention to numerous technical details when creating an AV fistula determines its early and late success rate.

Spasm of the Vein

Mainly in children and adolescents, the vein may become spastic after surgical exposure and dissection. This spasm can effectively be overcome by hydraulic dilatation using heparin solution.

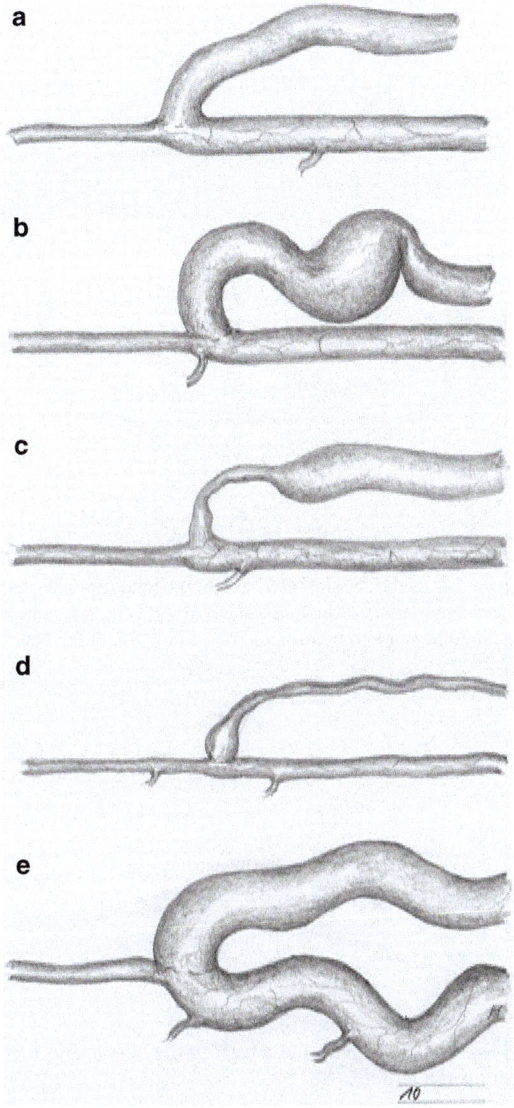

Fig. 3.2 Potential development of an AV fistula: (**a**) optimal outcome (even dilation of the vein), (**b**) dilation of the vein with kinking and aneurysm formation, (**c**) venous stenosis close to the anastomosis, (**d**) long high grade venous stenosis, (**e**) extreme dilation of the proximal artery

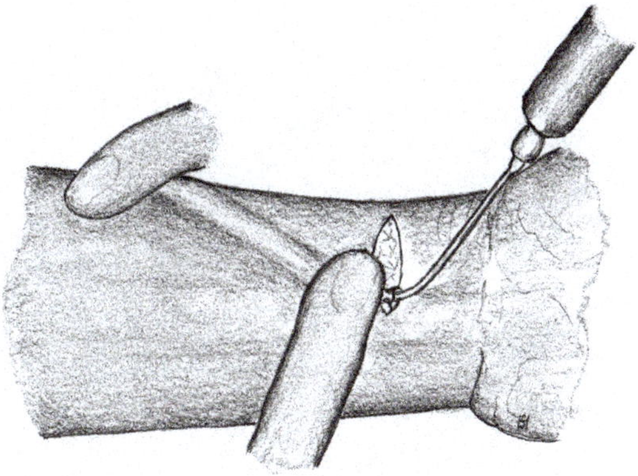

Fig. 3.3 Hydraulic dilation of the fistula's vein

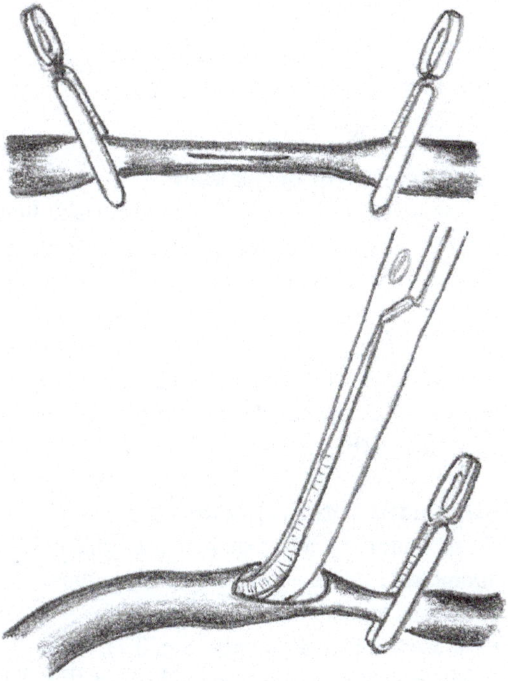

Fig. 3.4 Mechanical dilation of a small caliber artery using a microdissector

For this purpose a blunt canula is inserted into the vein, which is then gently dilated to its maximum diameter. The surgeon uses his gloved fingers to seal the canula and to empty the syringe. The assistant percutaneously compresses the vein. Thus the entire length of the vein (e.g., cephalic vein of forearm or upper arm) can be dilated step by step (Fig. 3.3).

Spasm of the Feeding Artery

The artery may also become spastic during surgical exposure, especially in young patients. Anastomosing a spastic artery may lead to a narrow anastomosis with a diminished flow and subsequent thrombosis. Gentle spreading with a microdissector may solve this problem (Fig. 3.4).

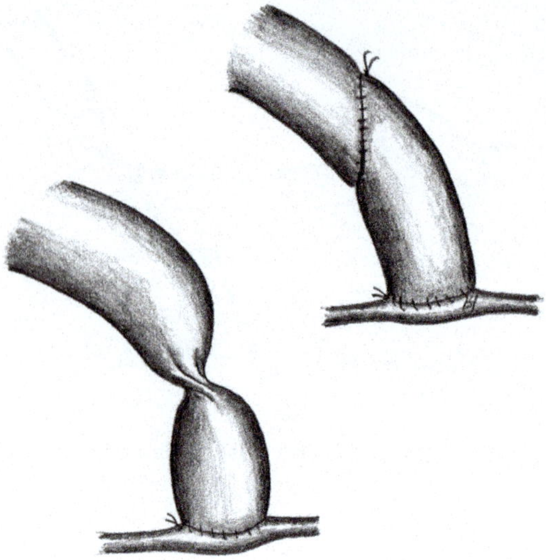

Fig. 3.5 Repair of a venous torsion which causes a stenosis by suturing a new anastomosis

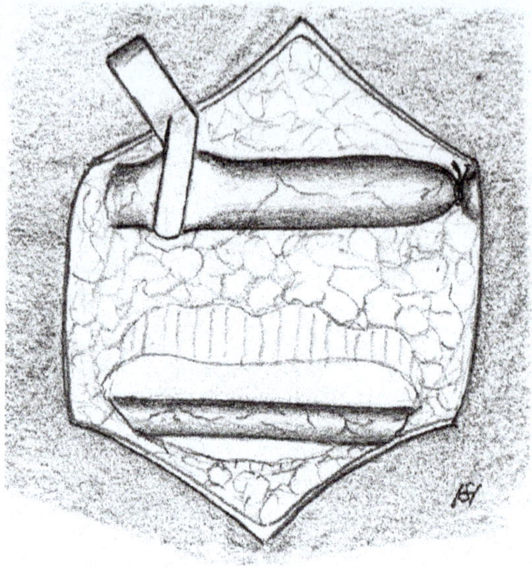

Fig. 3.6 Surgical site after isolation of the cephalic vein and radial artery. To avoid torsion of the vein, its position should be marked by a standardized position of the clamp

Rotational Error of the Vein

A venous torsion of only 30° may cause a high grade stenosis or occlusion (Fig. 3.5). Redoing the anastomosis is the only way to repair this situation. This technical mistake can be avoided if the correct rotation of the tightly-filled vein is marked (e.g., using a vascular clamp at its entry into the subcutaneous tissue) before creating the anastomosis (Fig. 3.6).

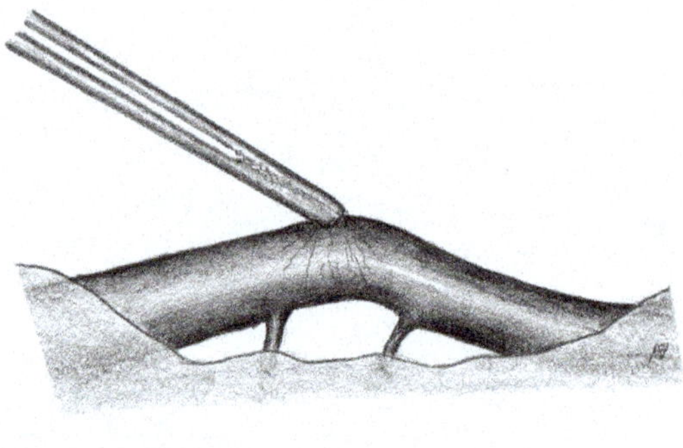

Fig. 3.7 Grasp only the adventitia for atraumatic handling of a vessel

Atraumatic Suturing Technique

Every trauma to a vessel increases the risk of thrombosis. The following guidelines for atraumatic surgery should be observed:

- Grasp the adventitia only (Fig. 3.7)
- Lift the vessel carefully using a dissector (Fig. 3.8)
- Use a fine pointed blade to open the clamped, tightly-filled artery (Fig. 3.9)
- Use closed forceps gently to keep the vascular aperture open (Fig. 3.10)
- Begin suturing at the less accessible side (Fig. 3.11)

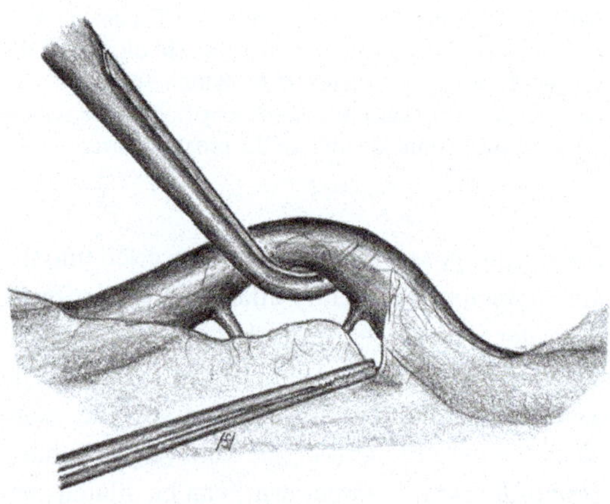

Fig. 3.8 Atraumatic manipulation of a vessel using a dissector

Kinking of the Anastomosed Vein

Near the anastomosis, a curved path of the vein which avoids sharp turns is important. After declamping, the path of the vein has to be verified (lid retractor). If there is kinking, the strangulating subcutaneous tissue has to be removed

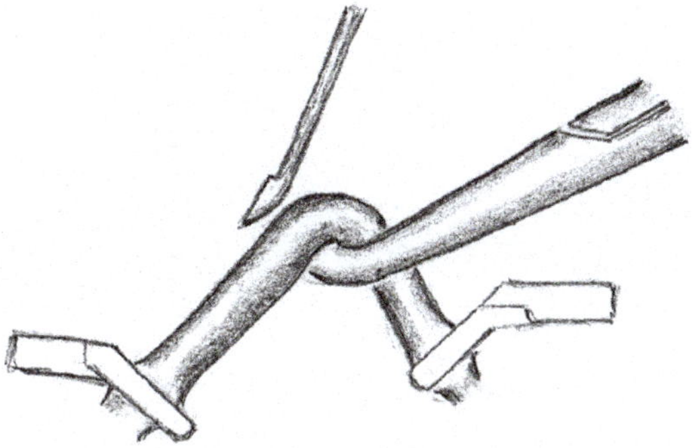

Fig. 3.9 Arteriotomy of a small artery. It is important to lift the tightly-filled artery to avoid injury to the posterior vessel wall

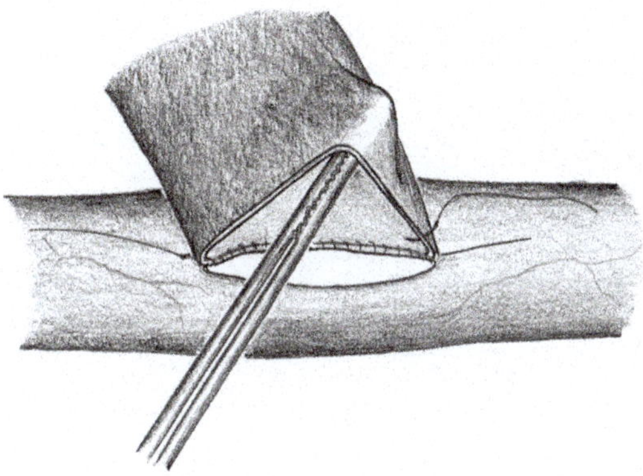

Fig. 3.10 Keep the vein open with closed forceps

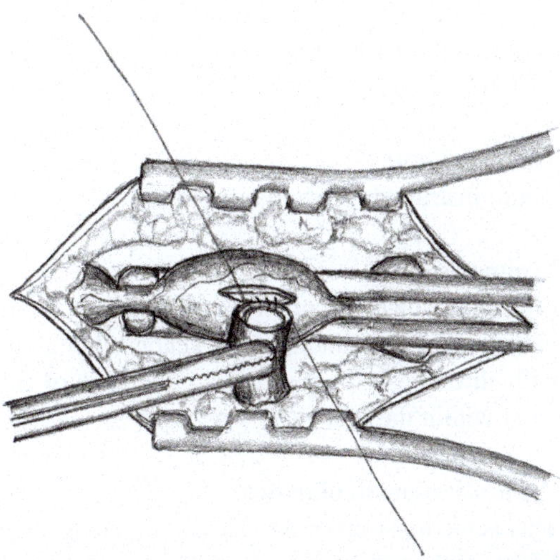

Fig. 3.11 Begin the suture at the most inaccessible side

(Fig. 3.12) unless the kinking is due to excess length (Fig. 3.13) of the vein. Then the vein should be shortened.

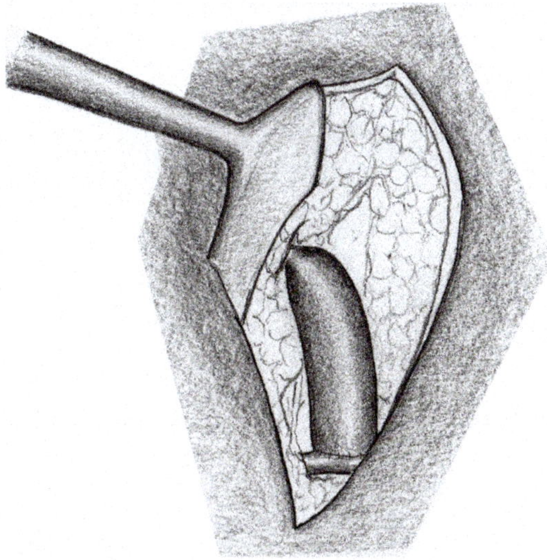

Fig. 3.12 Kinking of the vein due to strangulation of surrounding tissue

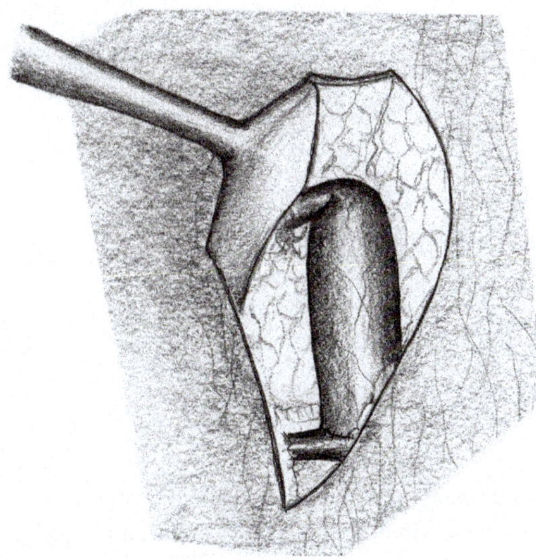

Fig. 3.13 Kinking of a vein which is too long

Intraoperative Prevention of Thrombosis

We flush the artery and the vein with heparinized saline before clamping.

3.2 AV Fistula of the Forearm

There are usually two or rarely three veins of the forearm which are suited for the creation of AV fistulas. Most often the cephalic vein can be used,

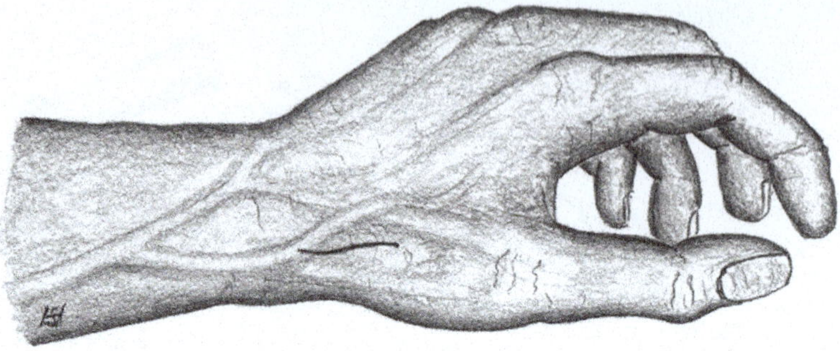

Fig. 3.14 Incision for snuff box fistula

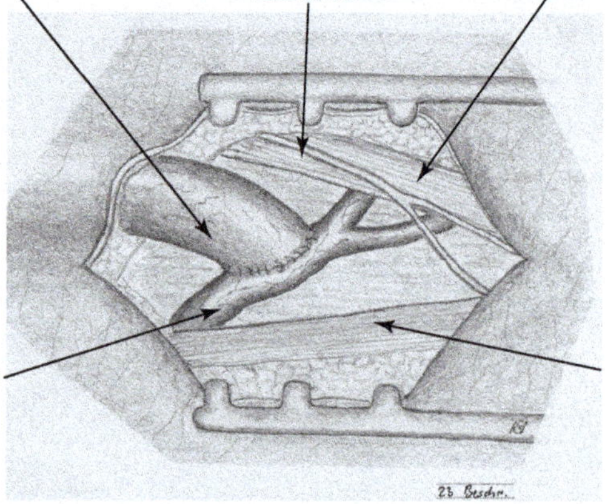

Fig. 3.15 Anatomy of snuff box fistula

and less frequently the basilic and median antebrachial veins.

3.2.1 AV Fistulas of the Cephalic Vein

Depending on an indivual's cephalic vein, its arterialization may be undertaken at different levels.

Snuff Box Fistula

Indication/prerequisites

First access if suitable cephalic vein and strong pulse of the radial artery in the anatomical snuff box.

Contraindication

Expressed sclerosis of the radial artery in the forearm, as the flow will then remain insufficient.

Approach

- Longitudinal incision in the snuff box between the tendons of the extensor pollicis and abductor pollicis longus muscles (Fig. 3.14).
- Watch out for the superficial branch of the radial nerve during the exposure of the cephalic vein in the subcutaneous tissue.
- Lateroterminal anastomosis (Figs. 3.15 and 3.16).

Technical note

Micro instruments recommended.

Prognosis

From our own experience, around 15 % of patients develop inflammatory venous alterations with thrombosis in the motion segment of the wrist within the first year.

Evaluation/particularities

This is the most distal AV fistula. It increases the length of the venous segment that is available for puncture by around 4 cm as compared to the distal radiocephalic fistula. If thrombosis occurs, the dilated cephalic vein and the radial artery will usually still be well-suited for the creation of a distal forearm fistula.

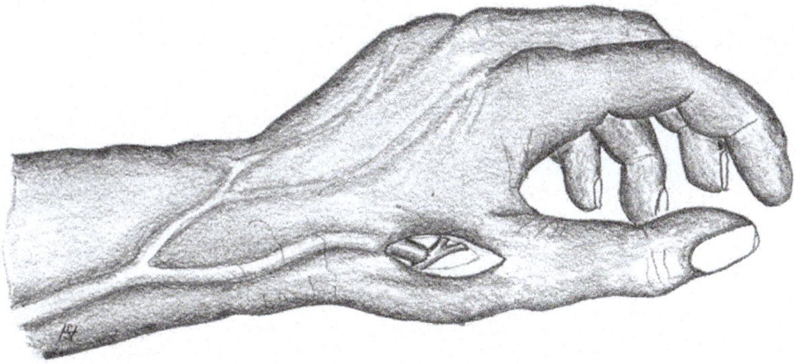

Fig. 3.16 Surgical site of a snuff box fistula

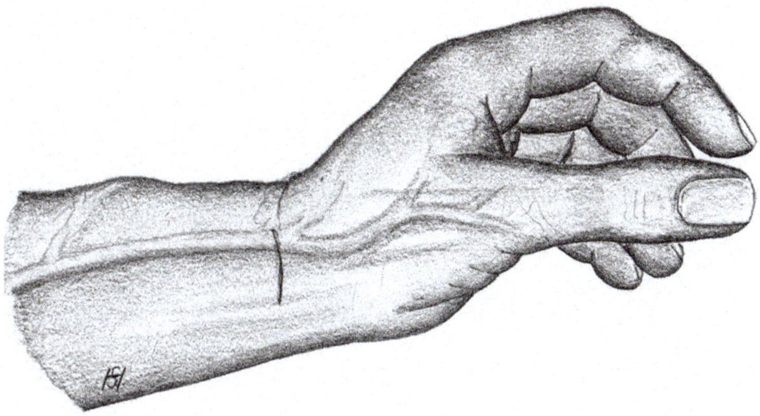

Fig. 3.17 Incision for distal cephalic fistula if radial artery and cephalic vein are close to each other (radiovolar transverse incision)

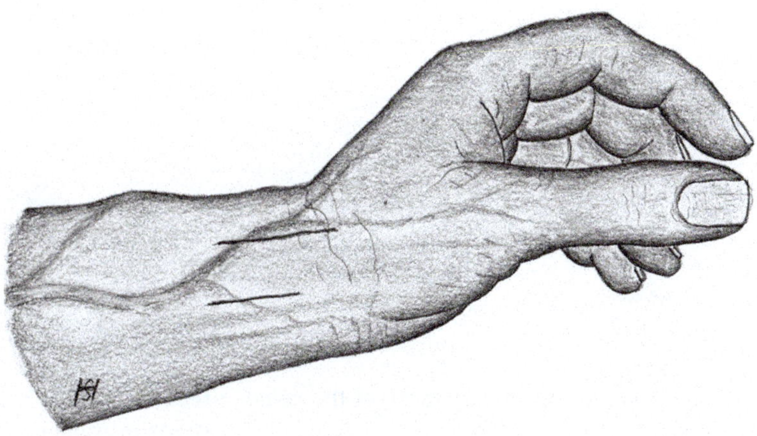

Fig. 3.18 Incisions for distal cephalic fistula if radial artery and cephalic vein are not close to each other (two longitudinal incisions)

Distal Radiocephalic Fistula of the Forearm

Indication/prerequisites

Well-developed cephalic vein up to the forearm and strong pulse of the radial artery at the wrist.

Contraindication

Expressed sclerosis of the radial artery in the forearm, as then the flow is and will remain insufficient.

Approach

- The choice of incision depends on the distance between artery and vein. If they lie close to each other, we suggest a 2–3 cm transverse incision (Fig. 3.17). If there is a longer distance between the vessels, two separate longitudinal incisions are recommended (Fig. 3.18).
- Sufficient exposure of a venous segment while preserving the radial cutaneous antebrachial

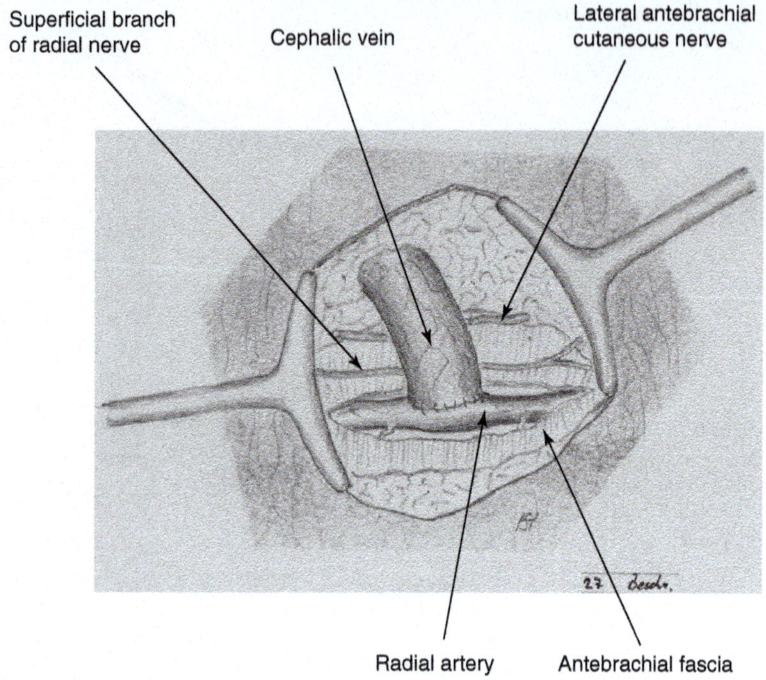

Fig. 3.19 Anatomy of distal cephalic fistula

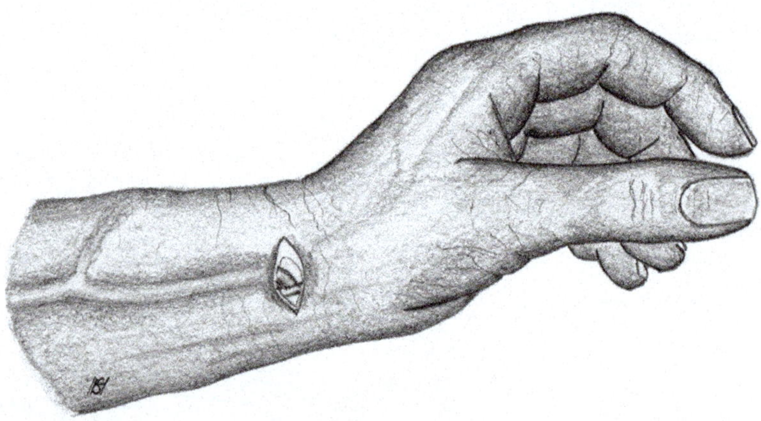

Fig. 3.20 Distal cephalic fistula

nerve and the superficial branch of the radial nerve.

- Longitudinal incision of the antebrachial fascia and exposure of the radial artery medial to the flexor carpi radialis muscle.
- Distal dissection of the vein and shifting of the venous stump to the artery for anastomosis (Figs. 3.19 and 3.20).

Technical note

Micro instruments are recommended for small size vessels.

Prognosis

This is the AV fistula with the best long term function. Under favorable circumstances it may be used for more than 25 years.

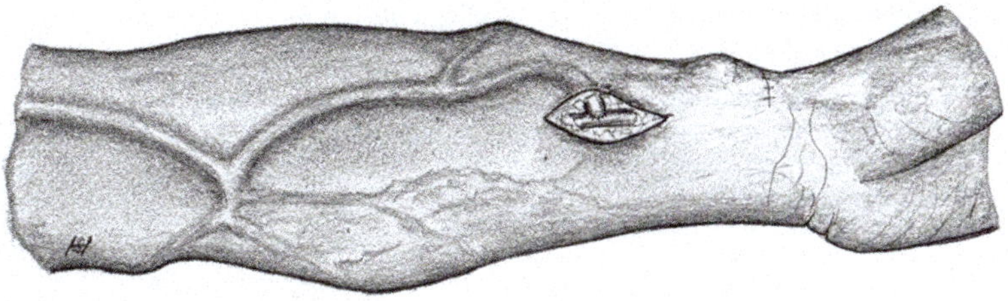

Fig. 3.21 Proximalization of distal cephalic fistula

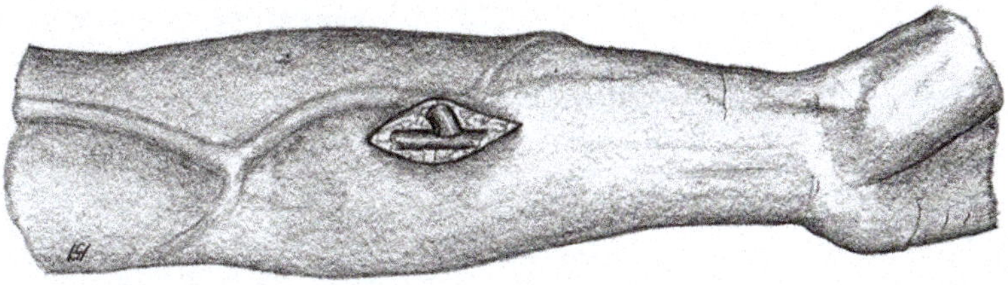

Fig. 3.22 Proximal cephalic fistula in the forearm

Evaluation/particularities
Most important native AV vascular access. To be preferred as first access.

Proximal Cephalic Fistula

Indication/prerequisites
Frequent secondary procedure after distal cephalic fistula has failed. Possible with unsuitable distal segment of the vein but suitable cephalic vein in the proximal forearm.

Approach

- Longitudinal incision down to the fascia at the medial margin of the brachioradial muscle in the proximal forearm.
- Exposure of the vein from a separate longitudinal incision. (Please note that the artery lies relatively far beneath the surface. Thus the distance between artery and vein may also be quite long.)
- Longitudinal incision of the antebrachial fascia at the medial margin of the brachioradial muscle while preserving the superficial branch of the radial nerve.
- Distal ligation of the vein and shifting of its proximal stump to the artery.
- Trimming of the vein for correct length.
- Anastomosis (Figs. 3.21 and 3.22).

Prognosis
Good long term results.

Evaluation/particularities
Decisively shorter segment for puncture at the forearm, but making good use of still suitable vein segments there.

3.2.2 AV Fistulas of the Basilic Vein

Distal Basilic Fistula

Indication/prerequisites
Unsuitable cephalic vein in the forearm but suitable basilic vein and ulnar artery in the forearm.

Approach
Close to the wrist the distance between the basilic vein and the ulnar artery tends to be relatively long. Therefore two separate longitudinal incisions are made.

- Isolation of the basilic vein before deciding on a more proximal incision for the ulnar artery.
- Exposure of the ulnar artery medial to the tendon of the flexor carpi ulnaris muscle while taking care not to injure the ulnar nerve (Fig. 3.23).
- Pulling the proximal end of the distally ligated basilic vein through a subcuticular tunnel to

Fig. 3.23 Anatomy of ulnar artery in the distal forearm

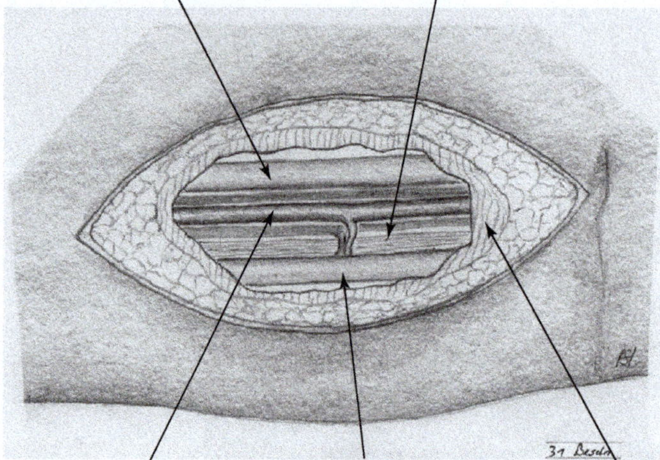

Fig. 3.24 Distal basilic fistula

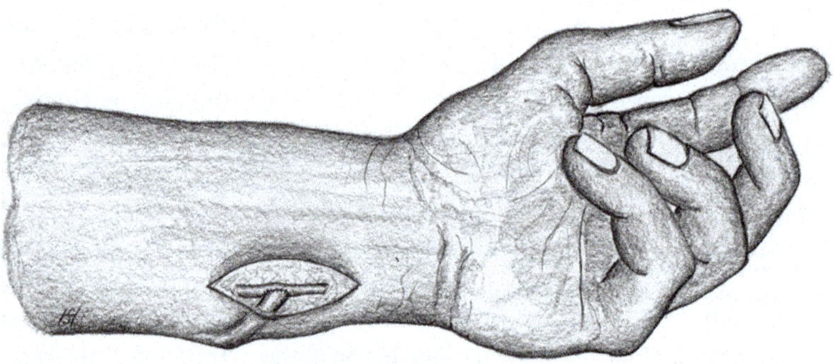

the ulnar artery while preserving the integrity of the dorsalis manus branch of the ulnar nerve.
- Trimming of the vein for correct length.
- Anastomosis (Fig. 3.24).

Prognosis

Good long term results despite expressed tendency of the basilic vein to dilate more than desired.

Evaluation/particularities

Frequently neglected access due to "rolling" veins, difficult puncturability, and difficult positioning of the arm during dialysis. The fistula is punctured while flexing the elbow. It is easier when the skin is stretched. Correct positioning of the arm is facilitated by using cushions or folded towels.

Proximal Basilic Fistula

Indication/prerequisites

Unsuitable cephalic vein but suitable basilic vein and suitable ulnar artery in the forearm.

Approach (Fig. 3.25)

Same procedure as with the distal basilic fistula. It is important to note the considerably deeper and more medial position of the ulnar artery between the two heads of the flexor carpi ulnaris muscle. In rare cases the radial artery can be used to feed the basilic vein (Fig. 3.26). This may be realized in the case of a small diameter ulnar artery and a large diameter radial artery (e.g., after a previous cephalic fistula). However, the longer distance to the radial artery is a disadvantage.

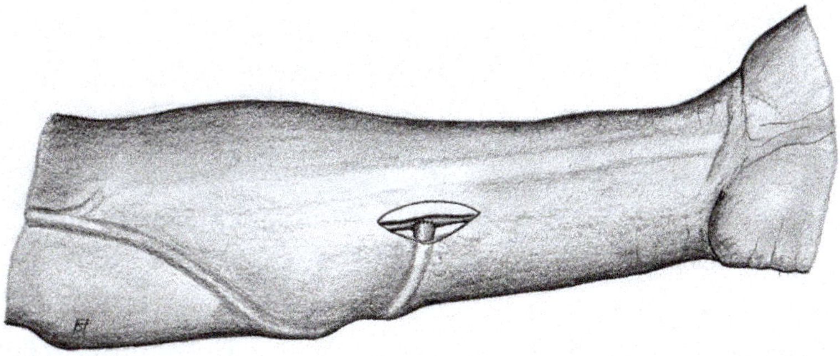

Fig. 3.25 Proximal basilic fistula in the forearm

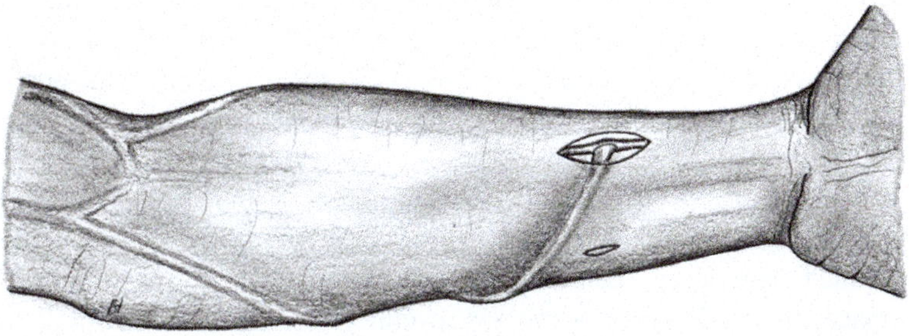

Fig. 3.26 Arterialization of the basilic vein via the radial artery

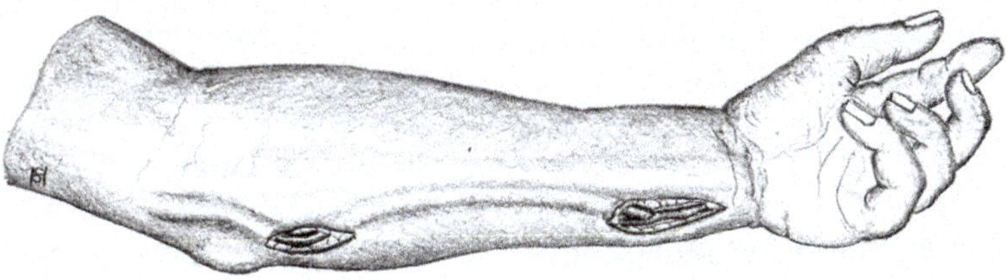

Fig. 3.27 Superficialization of the arterialized basilic vein in the forearm

Prognosis and evaluation
Similar to distal basilic fistula, but definitely shorter venous segment that can be punctured.

Transposition of Basilic Vein in the Forearm (Fig. 3.27) In our opinion the superficialization of a brachiobasilic fistula in the forearm should preferably be delayed so as first to wait and see how it matures.

Indication
Fixation of an extremely mobile, and/or deeply-imbedded, and well-dilated basilic vein to facilitate puncturing.

Approach
- Isolation of the arterial anastomosis and of the basilic vein near the cubital fossa beginning with volar longitudinal incisions.
- Ulnar incisions to free the entire vein in the forearm.
- Dissection of the vein near the anastomosis, and removal of the vein from its natural bed.
- Creation of a volar, subcutaneous tunnel, passage of the vein, and reestablishment of the vascular continuity.

Prognosis and evaluation
Very rare indication. Good long term results.

3.2.3 AV Fistula of the Median Antebrachial Vein (Fig. 3.28)

Indication/prerequisites
Unsuitable cephalic and basilic veins in the forearm but suitable median antebrachial vein.

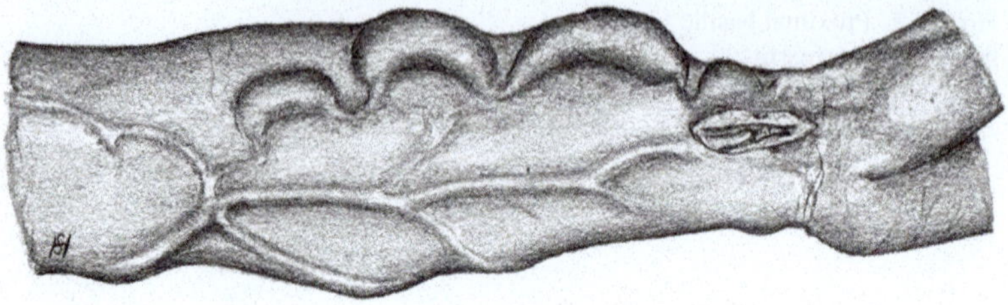

Fig. 3.28 Arterialization of the antebrachial vein

Approach
The median antebrachial vein should be anastomosed either to the ulnar or to the radial artery, as due to its anatomical varieties either one might be better suited than the other. Depending on the anatomy, one or two longitudinal incisions are necessary.

Prognosis
Limited experience. Under particular circumstances this access may serve for several years but tends to develop scarred stenoses.

Prognosis and evaluation
Rare indication mostly after previous forearm AV fistulas.

3.2.4 Repair of AV Fistulas in the Forearm

In the long run, various (morphologic) changes occur that impair the function of a vascular access. These encompass:

- Thromboses
- Venous stenoses due to tissue proliferation or kinking
- Venous aneurysms
- Runoff mainly through side branches
- Difficult puncture due to deep path of the vein
- Retrograde venous perfusion of the forearm due to central venous stenosis or occlusion
- Reduced arterial perfusion of the hand
- Infections
- Stenoses of the feeding artery

Frequently several mutually influencing pathologic changes coexist. When correcting these changes, care should be taken to preserve the venous segments suitable for puncture.

Thrombosis of Forearm AV Fistulas

Any operation should:

- Find the underlying cause of a thrombosis.
- Remedy the cause.
- Restore the previous function (thrombectomy).

A thrombectomy is a demanding procedure which requires extensive experience. Based on the presentation and the pathogenesis of a thrombosis, we distinguish between three forms: perioperative thrombosis, early thrombosis, and late thrombosis.

Perioperative Thrombosis

Definition
Thrombosis within the first 48 h after surgery.

Causes

- Morphologic alterations of the vein.
- Stenoses of the artery, the anastomosis, or the vein possibly caused by surgical mistakes or compression (hematoma).
- Hypercoagulability.
- Altered vessels (traumatic surgical technique, previous chemotherapy, IV drug abuse).
- External compression (dressing).

Therapy
The wound should be reopened as soon as possible to correct potential morphologic causes. If a stenosis results from a rotational error, kinking, or an anastomosis which is simply too narrow, a new anastomosis should be created after thrombectomy. If these causes can be excluded, a transverse venotomy close to the anastomosis is followed by thrombectomy and examination of the thrombi.

- Should mainly white thrombi prevail, most likely hypercoagulability exists. Then laboratory tests for coagulation disorders should be ordered. After a successful thrombectomy,

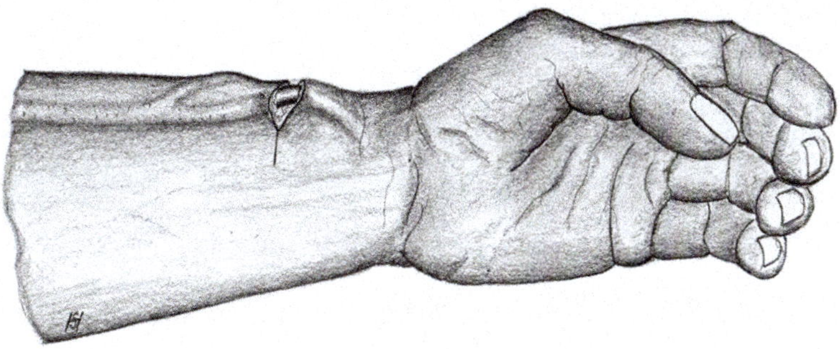

Fig. 3.29 Incision for thrombectomy of distal cephalic fistula (short distance between artery and vein)

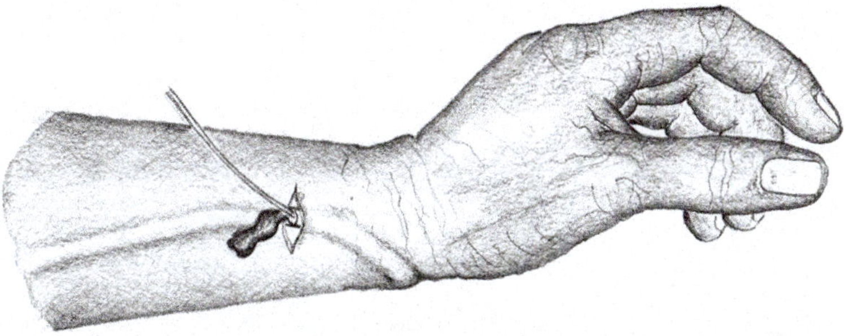

Fig. 3.30 Thrombectomy via the incision chosen in Fig. 3.29

temporary systemic heparinization is subsequently switched to oral anticoagulation.

- Should red thrombi prevail, an increased thrombogenicity of the vessels is likely. Then the postoperative administration of heparin for 3–5 days should be sufficient for the fistula to remain patent. Should chronic vascular damage have been caused by previous injections (chemotherapy, IV drug abuse), continuous use of anticoagulants is recommended.

Early Thrombosis

Definition

Thrombosis occurring between 2 days and 2 weeks after surgery.

Causes

Early thrombosis is frequently observed with previously damaged veins (chemotherapy, IV drug abuse). Sometimes the vein can be palpated as a thin and fibrous strand.

Therapy

Thrombectomy should always be attempted. If no morphologic cause close to the anastomosis is suspected, we recommend approaching the vein proximal to the previous incision (for the anastomosis) because of almost certain scarring.

Late Thrombosis

Definition

Thrombosis after the second week post surgery.

Causes

History taking and clinical examination mostly suffice to discover the probable cause. Stenoses of the anastomoses, stenoses of the vein, aneurysm, and infections are likely. Likewise, an abacterial inflammation of the venous segment close to the anastomosis is a possible cause. Erythema and an increased sensitivity to touch can frequently be found.

Therapy

Thrombectomy is performed via an incision proximal to the distal venous segment. If the suspected morphologic cause is situated close to the anastomosis, the site of the skin incision should be selected based on the distance between artery and vein in view of a potential proximalization of the anastomosis.

Approach for a short distance between artery and vein

The vein is exposed from a transverse incision proximal to the anastomosis followed by thrombectomy (Figs. 3.29 and 3.30). If this

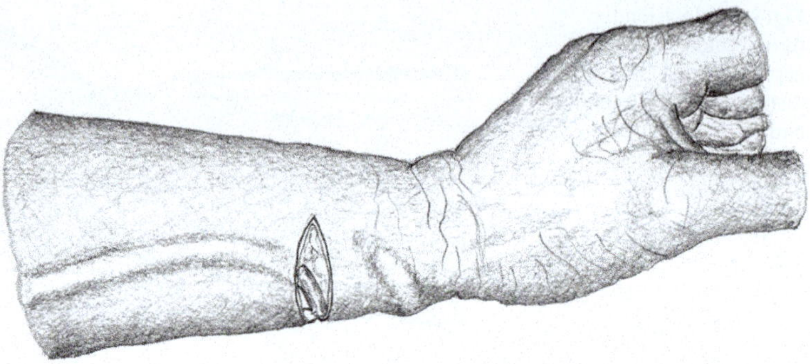

Fig. 3.31 Extension of the transverse incision and proximalization of the anastomosis if thrombectomy fails (cf. Fig. 3.29)

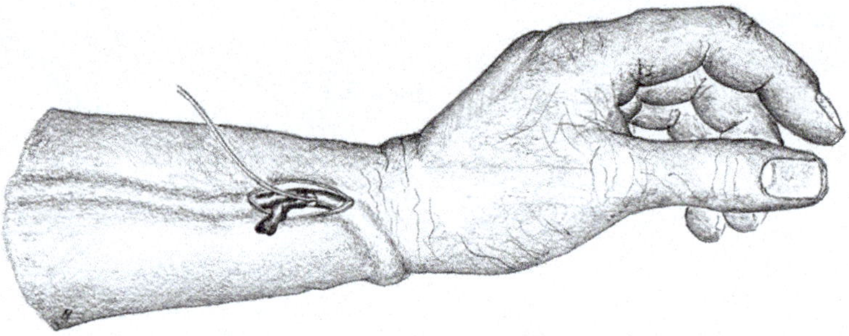

Fig. 3.32 Incision (longitudinal) for thrombectomy of distal cephalic fistula with far distance between artery and vein

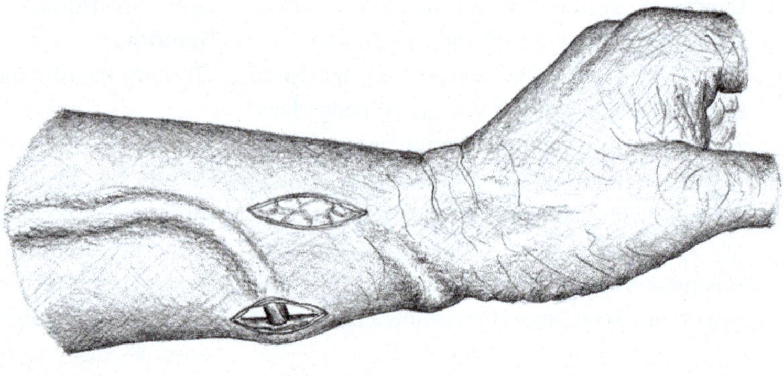

Fig. 3.33 Isolation of the vein and creation of a new proximal anastomosis (two incisions) if thrombectomy (one incision) fails (cf. Fig. 3.32)

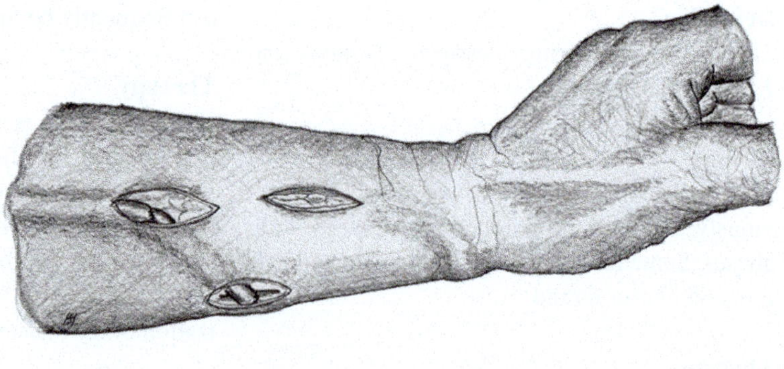

Fig. 3.34 Arterial feeding of the vein via a short interposition graft if thrombectomy fails (cf. Fig. 3.33)

thrombectomy maneuver is futile, the transverse incision is extended volarly towards the artery so as to create a new proximal anastomosis (Fig. 3.31).

Approach for a long distance between artery and vein

The vein is exposed via a longitudinal incision proximal to the anastomosis (Fig. 3.32).

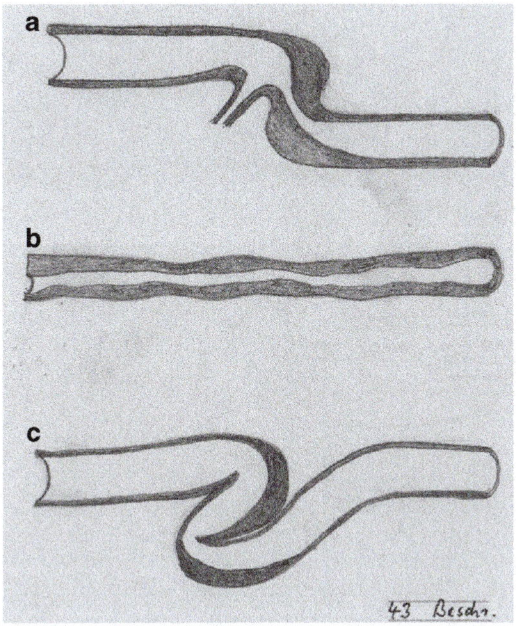

Fig. 3.35 Possible venous stenoses: (**a**) close to a side branch, (**b**) long "inflammatory" stenosis, (**c**) kinking

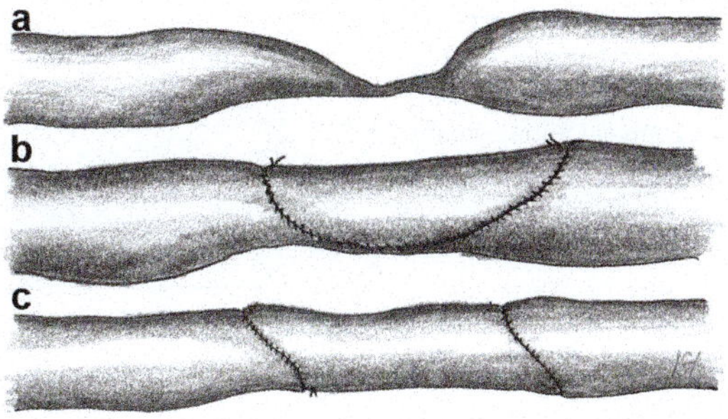

Fig. 3.36 Repair of a venous stenosis (**a**) using a patch (**b**) or a graft (**c**)

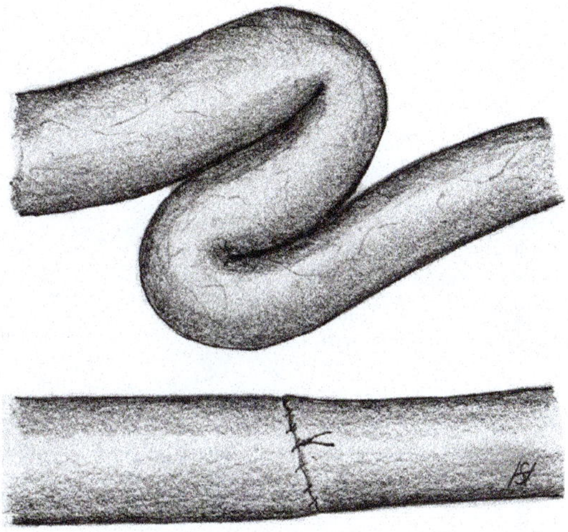

Fig. 3.37 Resection of a kinking venous segment

If an attempt at thrombectomy is futile, the artery is exposed via an additional longitudinal incision. Depending on the distance between artery and vein and the state of the remaining vein, either the shortened vein is reanastomosed to the proximal artery (Fig. 3.33), or a graft is implanted to re-establish vascular continuity (Fig. 3.34).

Venous Stenosis of Forearm AV Fistula

Possible causes are intraluminal tissue proliferation resulting from hemodynamic changes, inflammatory shrinking of the lumen (frequently after chemotherapy or IV drug abuse), or kinking (Fig. 3.35). The latter goes together with the (desired) dilation of the vein.

Diagnosis

To palpate a superficially-running vein over its entire length is frequently sufficient for its evaluation. This proves more difficult if the vein runs further beneath the surface. In addition to routine color-coded duplex sonography we advocate phlebography before complex reconstructive surgery. Placing the needle into the vein also allows for retrograde imaging of the artery.

Therapy

Unless caused by kinking, short stenoses should primarily be treated by percutaneous transluminal angioplasty (PTA). Recurrent restenoses or stenoses refractory to PTA are amenable to surgery. Both patch plasty and interposition grafts are feasible options (Fig. 3.36). Stenoses due to kinking usually require surgery. It is almost always possible to resect the elongated, kinking segment and to create an end-to-end anastomosis (Fig. 3.37). A long highly-stenosed or occluded segment of the vein, however, should

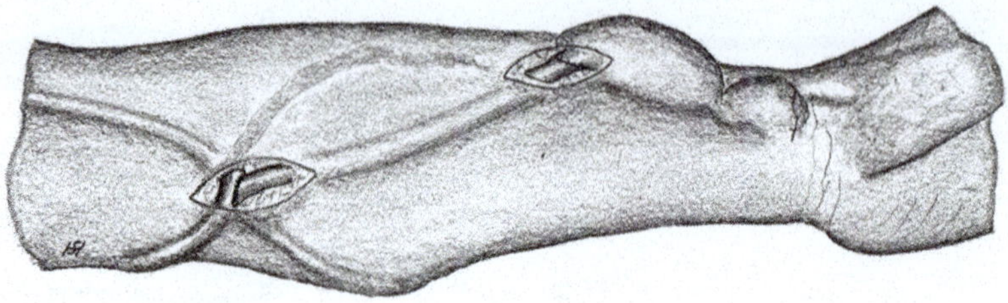
Fig. 3.38 Using a prosthetic bypass (diameter of at least 7 mm recommended) to circumvent a long stenosis of a distal cephalic fistula

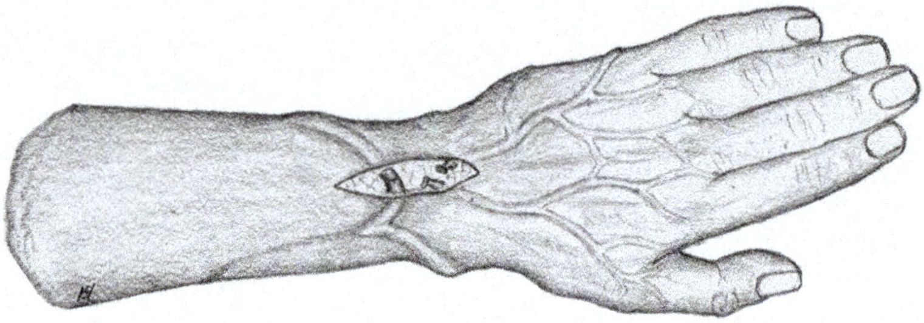
Fig. 3.39 Proximal occlusion of a distal radiocephalic fistula. Creation of a new runoff via a side branch to the basilic vein

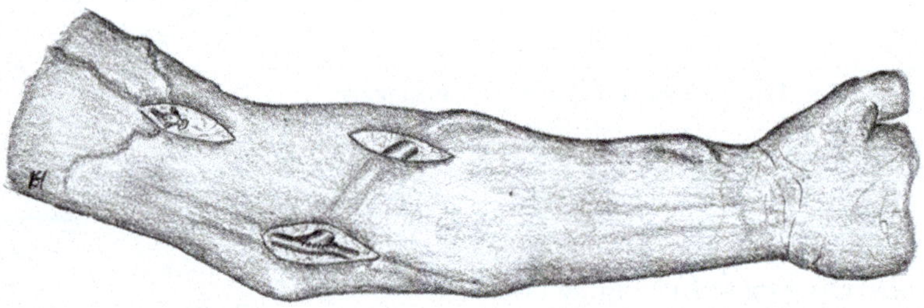
Fig. 3.40 Proximal venous occlusion of a distal cephalic fistula. Salvage of the fistula by transposing the cephalic vein into the basilic vein

be replaced by a graft for future punctures (Fig. 3.38). It is also possible to mobilize and transpose the distal stump of a proximally occluded cephalic vein to a suitable side branch which drains into the basilic vein in the forearm so as to preserve puncturability (Fig. 3.39). Likewise, a distal brachiocephalic fistula which is occluded proximal to the cubital fossa can be preserved if it is anastomosed to the basilic vein there (Fig. 3.40).

Aneurysms

Aneurysms occur because the venous walls are rather thin. Nearly all aneurysms develop at frequent puncture sites with the already frail scar tissue of the venous wall being submitted to repetitive extra strain. Furthermore, the intraluminal pressure can also be too elevated for the thin vessel wall as the result of a high arterial influx or a venous outflow that is impaired by stenoses (Figs. 3.41 and 3.42).

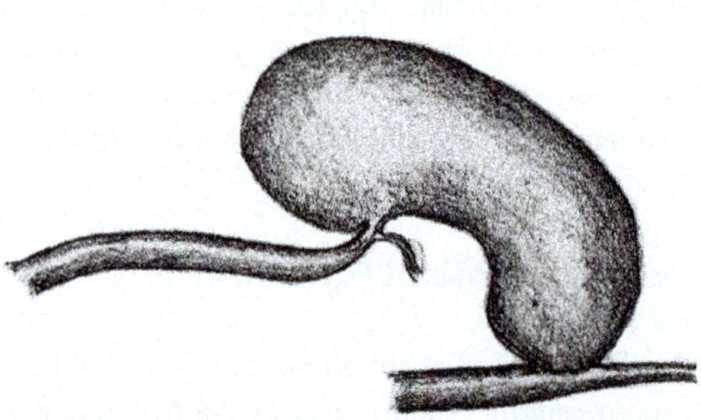
Fig. 3.41 Kinking of the arterialized vein caused by an upstream aneurysm

Diagnostics

Morphologic and clinical findings (inspection and palpation) as well as other (compounding) factors influence the indication for surgery. Duplex sonography and angiography via venipuncture with retrograde arterial imaging can add extra useful information preoperatively. Diagnostic interests concern:

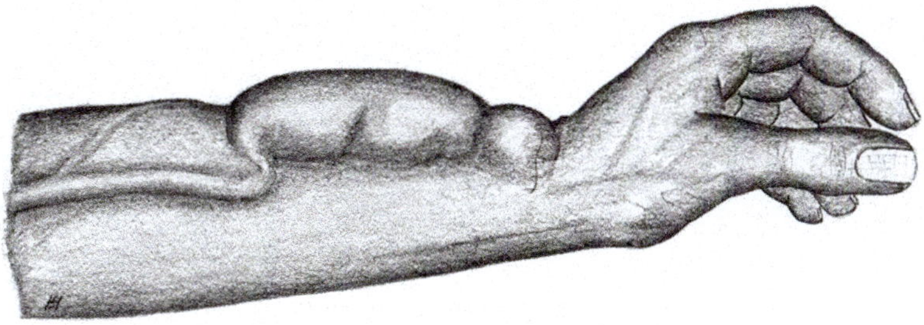

Fig. 3.42 Aneurysm of a distal radiocephalic fistula

- The morphology of the vein including its central runoff
- Flow volume

Indications for surgery
Important criteria are:

- Aneurysm size
- Risk of rupture
- (Partial) thrombosis
- Functional restrictions
- Combination with stenosis
- Cosmetics

These morphologic and functional aspects have to be weighed against:

- Risk for septic complications when using prosthetic grafts
- Complexity of the operation
- Life expectancy of the patient
- Feasibilty of future AV access surgery

Therapy
There are basically four different surgical options:

1. Resection of the aneurysm with direct end-to-end anastomosis.
2. Partial resection of the aneurysm wall and closure with (running) suture either leaving the vein in situ or creating a new extra tunnel for the vein.
3. Resection of the aneurysm and interposition of an alloplastic graft.
4. Creation of a new AV access with (delayed) ligation of the pre-existing aneurysmatic vascular access.

Resection of the Aneurysm with Direct end-to-end Anastomosis

Indication/prerequisites
Short aneurysm, end-to-end anastomosis feasible.

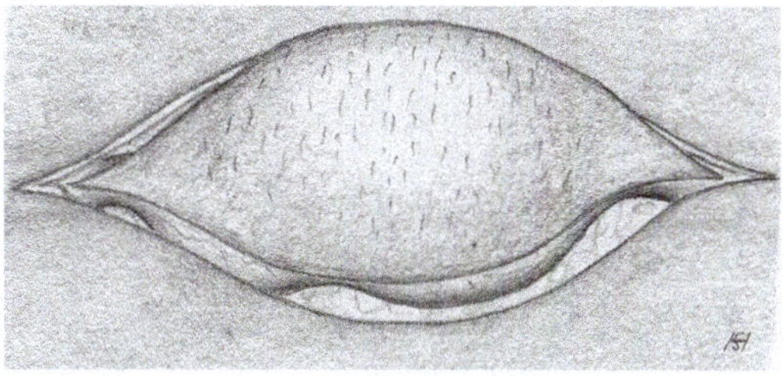

Fig. 3.43 Elliptical skin excision over the aneurysm

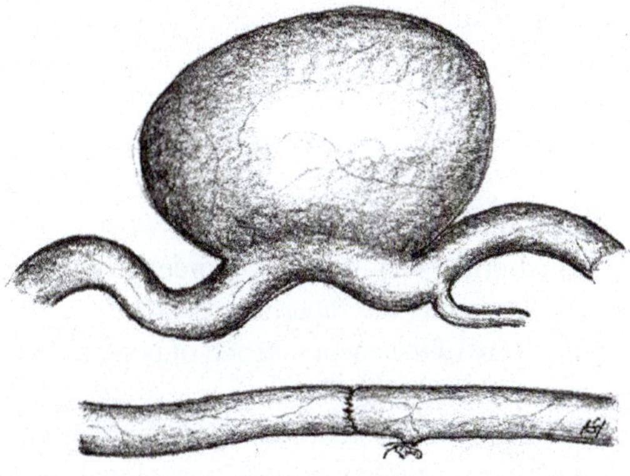

Fig. 3.44 Repair of an aneurysm via excision and direct suture

Contraindication
(Local skin conditions).

Approach
Longitudinal incision over the aneurysm.

Technical notes

- Appropriate incision to resect the superfluous skin (Fig. 3.43) if applicable.
- Exposure of the aneurysm.
- Exposure of the afferent and efferent venous segments.
- Resection of the aneurysm with end-to-end anastomosis (Fig. 3.44).

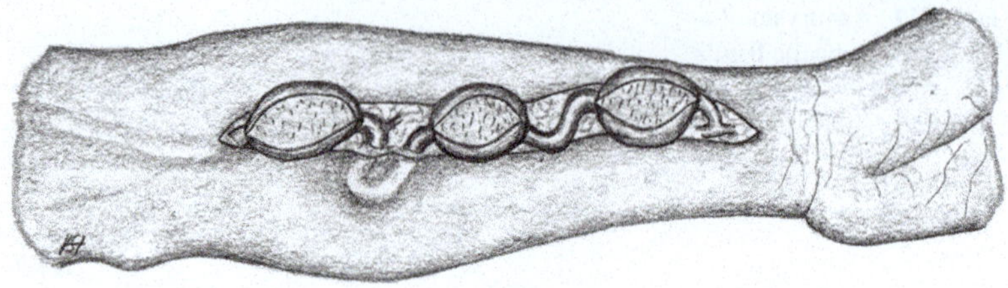

Fig. 3.45 Long circular exposure of the aneurysmatically-altered vein

Prognosis
Good long term results.

Distinctive feature
The fistula runs directly through the scarred area.

Partial Resection of the Aneurysm Wall and Closure with Direct Suture

Indication/prerequisites
AV access worth preserving.

Contraindications
- Extremely thin skin.
- Lack of subcutaneous cover.

Approach
Longitudinal incision over the aneurysm.

Technical notes
- Appropriate skin incision in order to simultaneously resect the superfluous skin.
- Exposure of the aneurysm and of potential stenoses (Fig. 3.45).
- Resection of the stenosed segment and partial longitudinal resection of the vessel wall leaving behind enough tissue to create a new lumen (Fig. 3.46).
- In some cases we recommend complete excision of the aneurysm and formation of a new vessel ex situ. Suturing the neovessel over a (Foley) catheter facilitates the creation of an even lumen (Fig. 3.47).

Depending on the length of the vein there are two options for placement:

1. With *long aneurysms* in the forearm, the vein is severed near the anastomosis with subsequent reconstruction (Fig. 3.48) and transposed into a new extraanatomic subcutaneous tunnel before being reanastomosed (possibly combined with flow reduction) (Fig. 3.49).

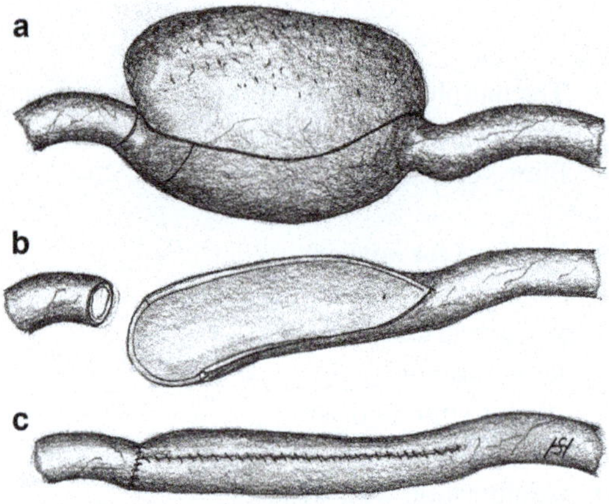

Fig. 3.46 Example for the surgical salvage of the venous wall after resection of an aneurysm: (**a**) resection line, (**b**) after resection, (**c**) after completion

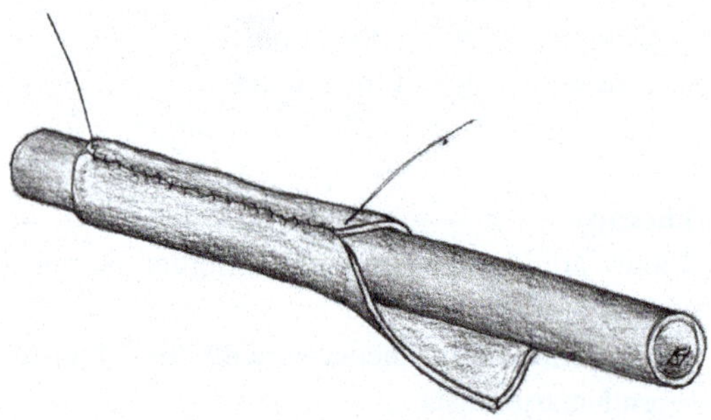

Fig. 3.47 Creation of a new venous lumen using remaining wall portions of an aneurysm which are united over a catheter

2. With *short aneurysms* it may suffice to leave the vein in situ before wound closure (Fig. 3.50).

Prognosis
Good long-term results if increased pressure due to stenoses and/or unnecessarily high inflow is excluded.

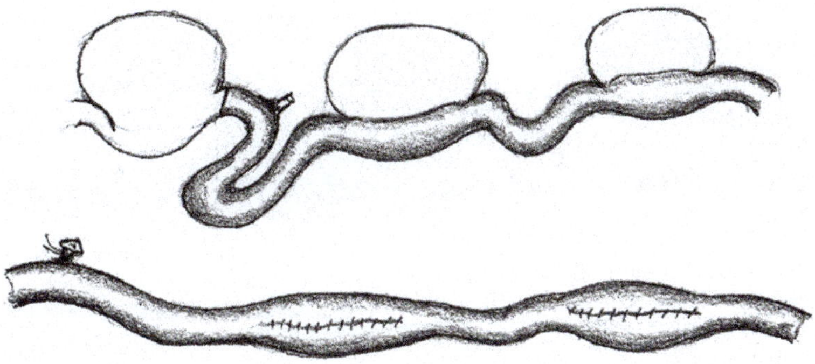

Fig. 3.48 Example for the salvage of an aneurysmatic fistula vein

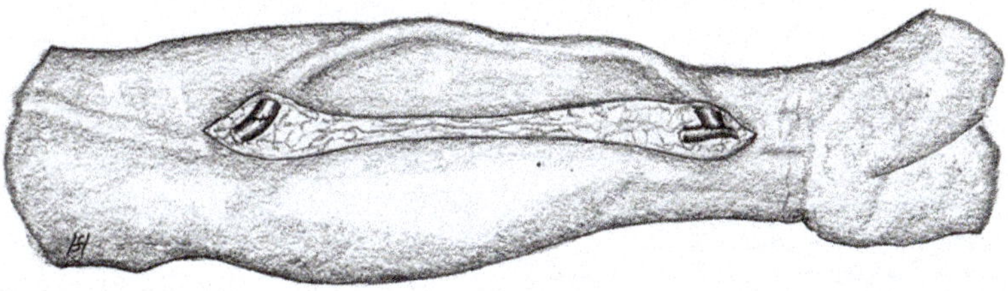

Fig. 3.49 Transposition of the vein (cf. Fig. 3.48) into a new subcutaneous tunnel

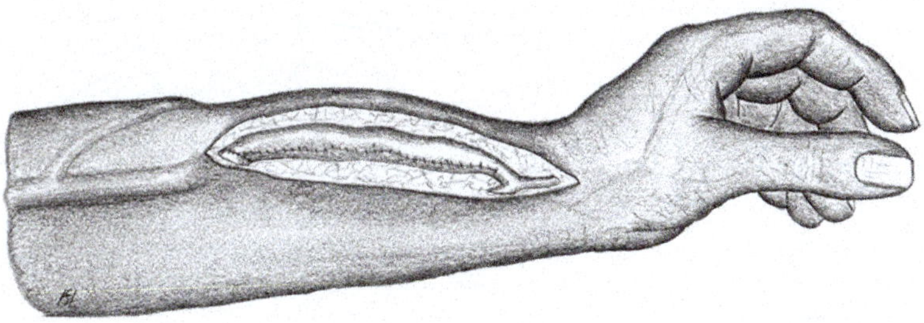

Fig. 3.50 Long segment isolation of the aneurysm and creation of a new lumen

Evaluation/particularities

With long segmental reconstructions, placement of the vein in a separate tunnel with a new anastomosis should be aimed for. The time required for such a complex procedure may well exceed 2 h.

Resection of an Aneurysm and Interposition of an Alloplastic Graft

Indications

Aneurysmatic wall not suited for puncture due to:

- Calcifications
- Inflammatory changes
- Structural weakness

Contraindication

Chronic septic foci with risk for hematogenous infection of the graft material.

Approach

Longitudinal incision over the aneurysm as described above (Fig. 3.51).

Technical notes

- Complete resection of the aneurysmatic vein and interposition of an adequate caliber prosthesis (Fig. 3.52).
- Placement of the prosthesis in a separate extraanatomic subcutaneous tunnel with long grafts.

Prognosis

Good long term results.

Evaluation and particularities

Markedly shorter time required than for reconstruction of the vein. Preserves use of the feeding artery and the efferent vein.

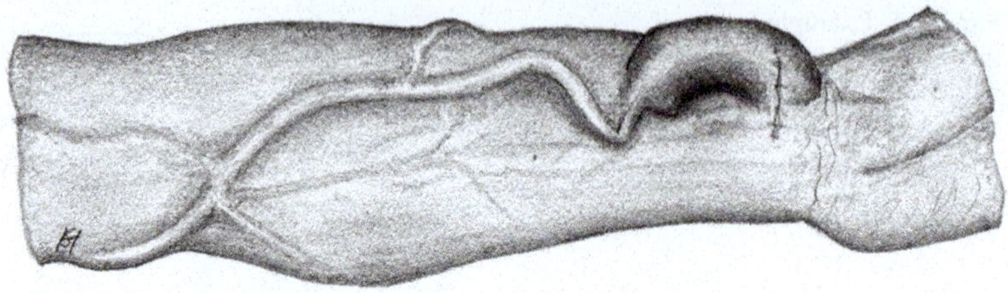

Fig. 3.51 Aneurysm of a distal radiocephalic fistula close to the anastomosis

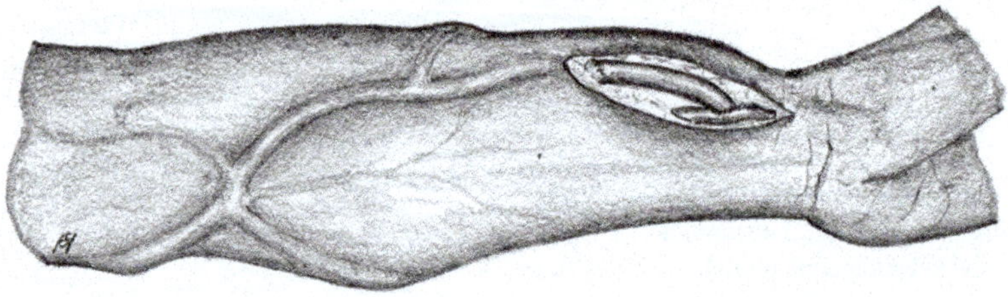

Fig. 3.52 Interposition of a prosthetic graft if aneurysm wall unsuitable

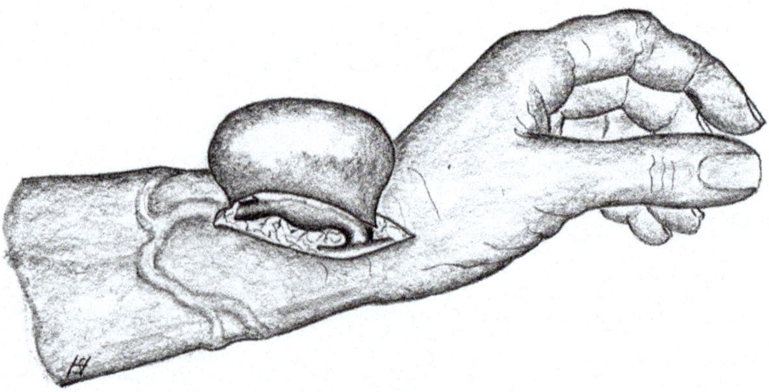

Fig. 3.53 Occlusion of the cephalic vein. Surgical site before planned excision of the aneurysm and ligature of the AV anastomosis

Surgical Ligation of an Aneurysmatic Fistula After Creation of a New Different AV Access

Indications

- Aneurysmatic AV access unsuitable for puncture or too complex to repair.
- Suitable vessels available for the successful creation of a new AV access.

Approach

With a large aneurysm which is close to the anastomosis, both the aneurysm and the anastomosis are exposed via a longitudinal incision if the aneurysm touches the anastomosis (Fig. 3.53).

Technical note

After creating a new AV fistula the time needed for its maturation should pass before it is punctured. Only then should the aneurysm be resected.

Relevant Outflow into Venous Side Branches

The outflow into side branches of an arterialized vein occurs if venous valves are insufficient. This may have existed primarily or develop due to a high intraluminal pressure caused by stenoses obstructing the outflow or by a high arterial inflow.

Diagnostics

A superficial vein may be evaluated by palpation. A deep venous position also requires color-coded duplex sonography of the side branches with respective flow measurements. If a stenosis of the venous outflow is suspected, the vein should be punctured directly for phlebography.

Indications

- Unsatisfactory maturation of the vein of an AV access.

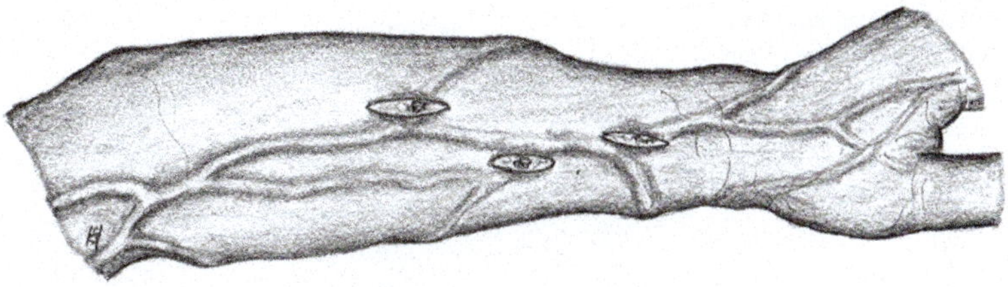

Fig. 3.54 Cephalic vein with insufficient side branches. Ligature of the side branches in order to increase flow in the main vein

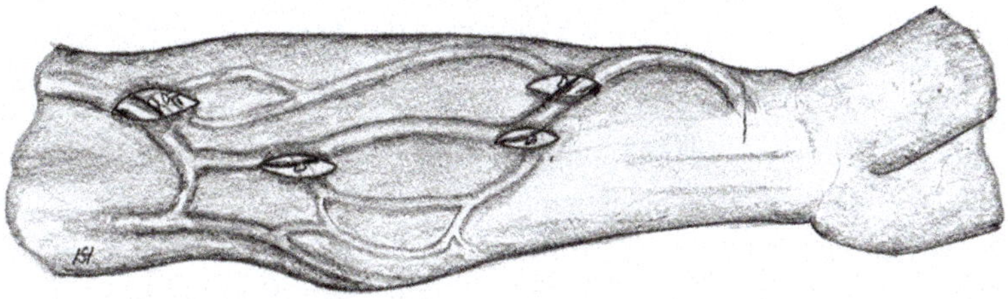

Fig. 3.55 Similar clinical presentation as in Fig. 3.54

- Flow of AV fistula too low.
- Shunt flow too high (excess cardiac strain, reduced peripheral perfusion).

Approach
Longitudinal incision over the take-off of the insufficient side branch (Fig. 3.54).

Technical notes
- Primary treatment of possible stenoses of the runoff.
- It is advisable to sever the side branch. Ligation only might later lead to kinking of the venous trunk by scarring.

Prognosis
Hardly any complications.

Evaluation/particularities
Effective treatment.

Ramification of the Venous Trunk

If the venous trunk ramifies into multiple proximal small side branches, flow and pressure of the single branches may be too low for sufficient dilation of the trunk. Then surgery should aim at increasing flow and pressure in the one branch which seems best by disconnecting all the others. Likewise, a fistula flow which is too high may justify the disconnection of venous sidebranches leading to a subsequent increase of the outflow resistance and consecutive decrease of fistula flow.

Diagnostics
If palpation and duplex sonography yield no satisfactory results, phlebography should be considered.

Indication/prerequisites
- Insufficient venous dilation
- High flow

Approach
Longitudinal incision over the ramification (Fig. 3.55).

Technical note
Severance of the appropriate venous branches.

Prognosis
Good.

Evaluation/particularities
This operation will likely result in an initial decrease of flow as well as in a marked dilatation of the venous trunk followed by a secondary increase in flow.

Vein Situated Deeply Beneath the Surface

A deep position of the vein, which renders puncturing difficult or impossible, can be found in obese patients or in those with anatomical variations with the (superficial) vein (partially) running beneath the fascia. In these cases a transposition of the vein is necessary.

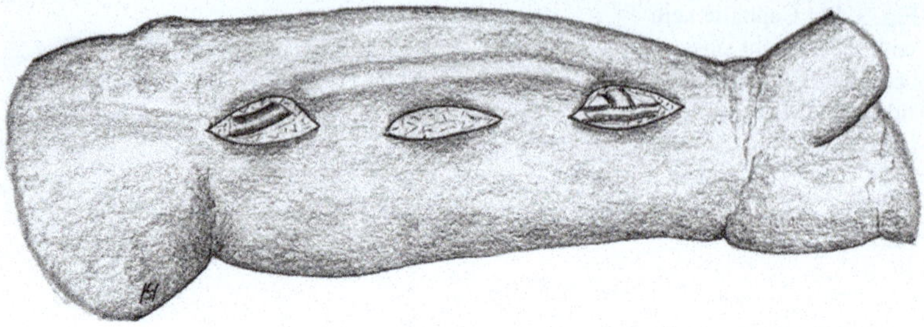

Fig. 3.56 Subcutaneous superficialization of an arterialized cephalic vein in an obese patient

Diagnostics
To evaluate the venous morphology, color-coded duplex sonography and phlebography are recommended if appropriate.

Indication/prerequisites
Difficult puncturability due to a position of the vein far beneath the surface, and also satisfactory venous diameter.

Approach
Total exposure of the vein over its total length in the forearm through mostly two to three skin incisions.

Technical notes
- Create a separate, extraanatomic, and subcutaneous tunnel.
- Sever the vein near its anastomosis.
- Pull the tightly-filled vein through the new tunnel.
- Create and check new anastomosis (Fig. 3.56).

Prognosis
If the large diameter of the vein allows for sufficient flow, good long-term results can be expected.

Evaluation/particularities
Rare procedure requiring at least 2 h.

Insufficient Arterial Inflow

If the flow is unsatisfactory despite a well-developed cephalic vein, an underlying diminished arterial inflow may be due to:
- A stenosis of the anastomosis.
- An isolated stenosis of the feeding artery.
- A long atherosclerotic stenosis of the artery (as frequently observed with the radial arteries of diabetics).
- A relative stenosis over a long segment of the not yet fully-developed feeding artery.

Diagnostics
Duplex ultrasonography can mostly help find the cause. Should this not be the case, we perform an additional arteriography.

Indication
For us the indication for a reconstruction is based on the cause, urgency, venous flow, and extent of venous dilation.

Stenoses of and/or Close to the AV Anastomosis

Therapy
Creation of a new proximal anastomosis, as a reconstruction of the already existing anastomosis, is mostly too cumbersome because of scarring.

Approach
Longitudinal incision over the anastomosis.

Technical notes
- Exposure of the vein near the anastomosis.
- Proximal mobilization of the vein. and determination of the site for the new anastomosis.
- Exposure of the artery proximal to the original anastomosis.
- Dissection of the artery close to the anastomosis for the new anastomosis.

Prognosis
Very good long term results.

Isolated Stenosis of the Feeding Artery

Therapy
PTA possibly also with stent. Surgical reconstruction if this fails.

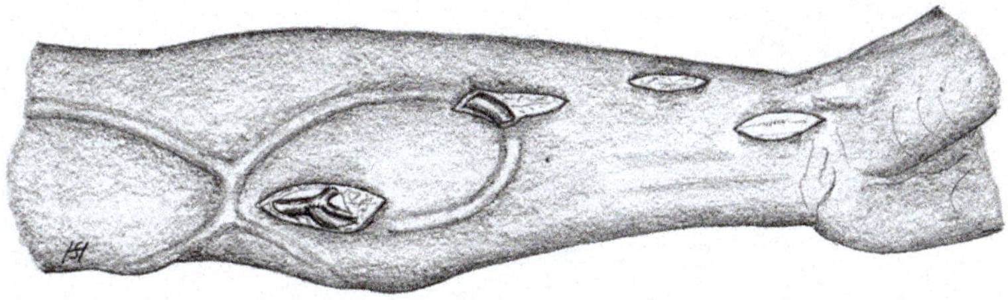

Fig. 3.57 Looped transposition of the distal cephalic vein into the brachial artery if flow in the radial artery is insufficient

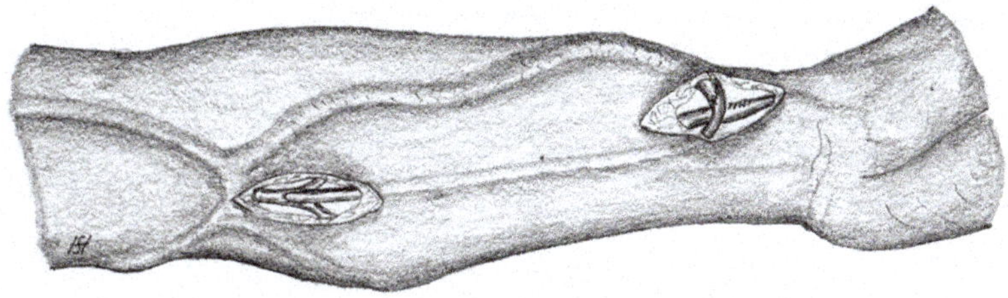

Fig. 3.58 Unsatisfactory flow in the radial artery. Feeding the cephalic vein from the brachial artery via a small lumen prosthesis which is not meant for puncture

Atherosclerotic Stenosis of a Long Segment of the Radial Artery

Therapy

There are three options for reconstruction.

Looped Transposition of the Distal Cephalic Vein for Feeding by the Brachial Artery Near the Elbow

Indication/prerequisites

- Large enough diameter of the vein over the entire length of the forearm.
- Large enough diameter of the brachial artery.

Technical notes

- Exposure of the distal vein through short longitudinal incisions.
- Exposure of the brachial artery through a longitudinal incision distal to the cubital fossa.
- Creation of an arched subcutaneous tunnel for the vein.
- Distal severance of the vein and new anastomosis in the cubital fossa (Fig. 3.57).

Prognosis

Good long term results if vessels are suited.

Feeding the Cephalic Vein Via a Small-Diameter Interposition Graft from the Brachial Artery Close to the Elbow

Indication/prerequisites

- Moderately-developed cephalic vein which seems to be suited for an AV access but not suited for a partial transposition.
- Large diameter of brachial artery.

Contraindication

None in particular.

Technical notes

- Exposure of the brachial artery distal to the cubital fossa through a longitudinal incision.
- Exposure of the AV anastomosis.
- Creation of a distally-curved or crook stick-shaped (crook stick shunt) subcutaneous tunnel for a 4-mm (ePTFE) prosthesis.
- Ligation of the AV anastomosis and severance of the vein.
- Anastomosis between vein and prosthesis.
- Lateroterminal anastomosis between brachial artery and prosthesis (Fig. 3.58).

Prognosis

Good.

Evaluation/particularities

Limited surgical effort leading to the effective feeding of the fistula's vein. Frequent temporary lymph edemas at the volar side of the forearm.

The small diameter graft is not intended for puncture.

Peripheral Feeding of the Cephalic Vein Via a Wide-Diameter Interposition Graft from the Brachial Artery Near the Cubital Fossa

Indication/prerequisites

- Large diameter of cephalic vein, which is embedded in scar tissue that is not suited for partial transposition.
- Wide lumen brachial artery.

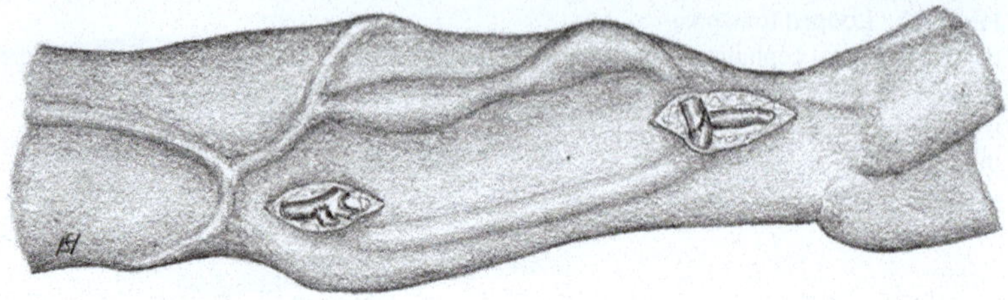

Fig. 3.59 Feeding the cephalic vein from the brachial artery via a wide lumen (7 mm) prosthetic graft. Puncturing of this graft is possible

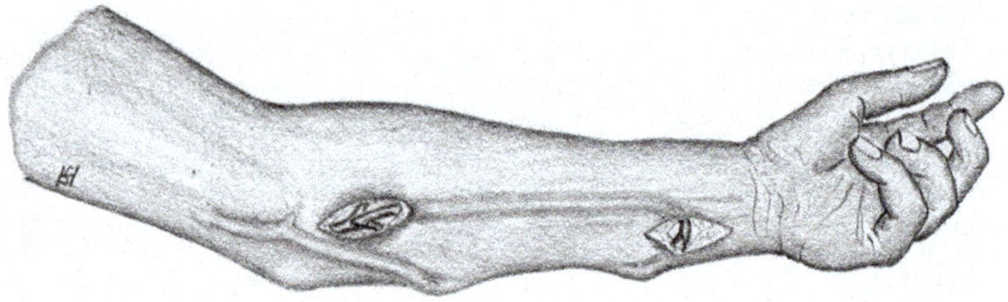

Fig. 3.60 Feeding the basilic vein from the brachial artery via a narrow-lumen graft if flow in the ulnar artery proves insufficient

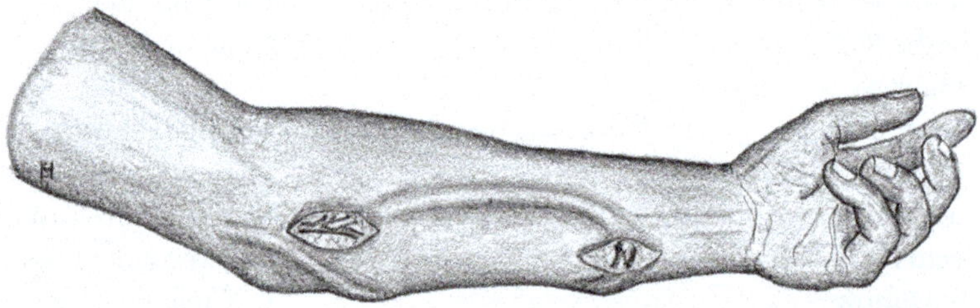

Fig. 3.61 Feeding the basilic vein from the brachial artery via a wide-lumen graft if flow in the ulnar artery proves insufficient

Contraindication
None in particular

Technical note
Same procedure as described for small diameter interposition grafts, but use of a 7-mm (ePTFE) graft (Fig. 3.59).

Prognosis
Good.

Evaluation/particularities
Same as with small diameter grafts. The graft may however also be punctured.

For a distal AV fistula of the basilic vein with a reduced inflow via the ulnar artery, the same options for reconstruction also exist using grafts (Figs. 3.60 and 3.61).

Rare Reconstructions

Apart from the morphologic and functional alterations of forearm AV fistulas mentioned above, there are numerous other rare alterations. Among these we discuss only one because of its clinical importance: the retrograde arterialization of a forearm cephalic fistula with an anastomosis in the cubital fossa. Possible causes include stenoses or occlusions of the proximal venous runoff after a cephalic AV fistula has been created in the cubital fossa, or its primary retrograde arterialization. In order for retrograde flow to occur, the venous valves of the cephalic vein have to be insufficient while the distal outflow is provided via collaterals to the basilic vein. Mostly then there will be a forearm edema with pronounced venous collaterals (Fig. 3.62). In some cases the cephalic vein in the forearm can be used as AV access.

Indication/ prerequisites
Considerable edema of the forearm and/or inefficient vascular access.

Retrogradely-perfused cephalic vein suitable for puncture.

- Suitable distal radial artery.
- Suitable vein in the cubital fossa for proximal runoff.

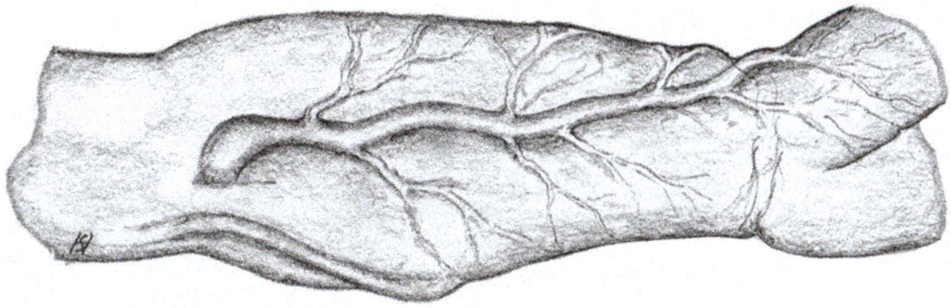

Fig. 3.62 Retrograde arterialization of the cephalic vein in the forearm. Multiple side branches drain the vein

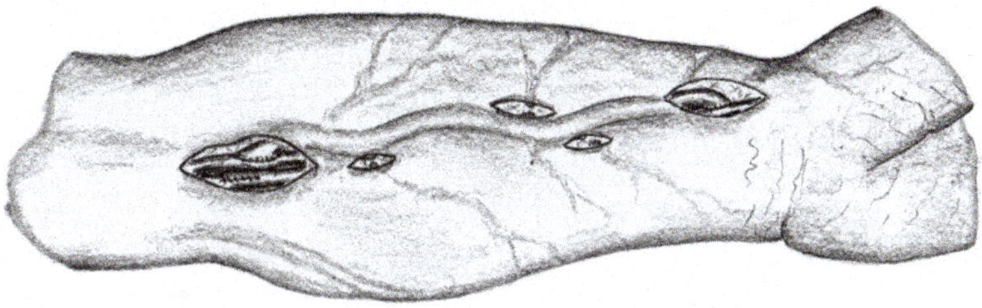

Fig. 3.63 Repair of the situation presented in Fig. 3.62. After ligatures of the side branches, the distal radial artery feeds the vein, and the cubital anastomosis to the deep vein provides the outflow

Technical notes

- Exposure of the arterial anastomosis in the cubital fossa via a longitudinal incision and choice of a suitable (deep) vein for anastomosis.
- Exposure of the radial artery and of the cephalic vein close to the wrist.
- Occlusion of the AV anastomosis in the cubital fossa and dissection of the vein.
- Terminolateral anastomosis of the cephalic vein to a draining vein in the cubital fossa.
- Lateroterminal anastomosis of the radial artery to the cephalic vein close to the wrist.
- Ligation of side branches (Fig. 3.63).

Prognosis

Depending on the quality of the anastomosed vein in the cubital fossa.

Evaluation/particularities

Rare operation which preserves the cephalic vein for puncturing.

3.3 AV Fistulas in the Cubital Fossa and in the Upper Arm

The sheer number of possibilities for AV anastomoses in the cubital fossa entails the danger of multiple complications. A sound anatomical knowledge is essential.

The decision for AV fistulas in the elbow is based on the following conditions:

1. Occluded or definitely unsuitable veins in the forearm.
2. Probably unsuitable veins in the forearm which would need a long maturation period before being ready for puncture while there is an imminent need for dialysis.
3. Definitely unsuitable arteries in the forearm (check if arterialization via an interposition graft from the brachial artery is possible).

3.3.1 Vascular Anatomy in the Cubital Fossa

Subcutaneous Veins (Fig. 3.64)

The cephalic and basilic veins cross the cubital fossa superficial to the fascia. The deep fascia (antebrachial fascia) has to be distinguished from the superficial fascia (superficial antebrachial fascia), which divides the subcutaneous adipose tissue into two layers. The development of this superficial fascia shows many individual variations. Both veins are interconnected via median veins, which also drain the median antebrachial vein. Close to this venous confluence, the median cubital vein establishes the connection to the deep vein. There is a multitude of variations of the described anatomy either as

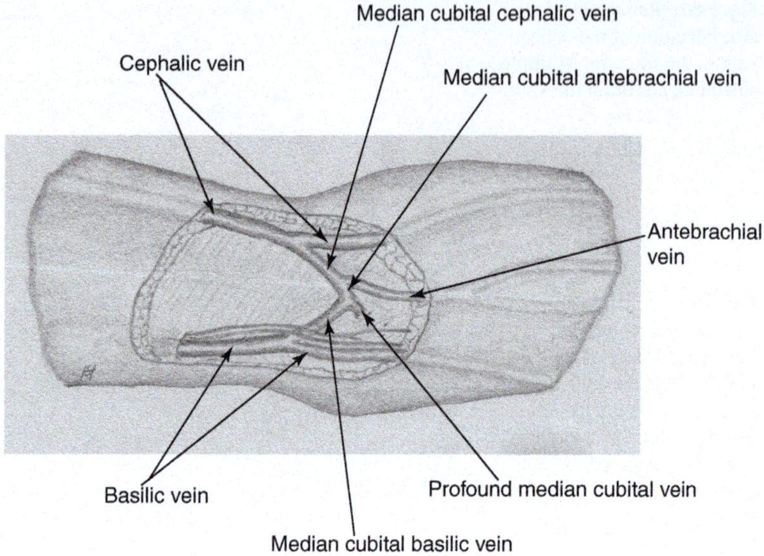

Fig. 3.64 Anatomy of the veins in the cubital fossa

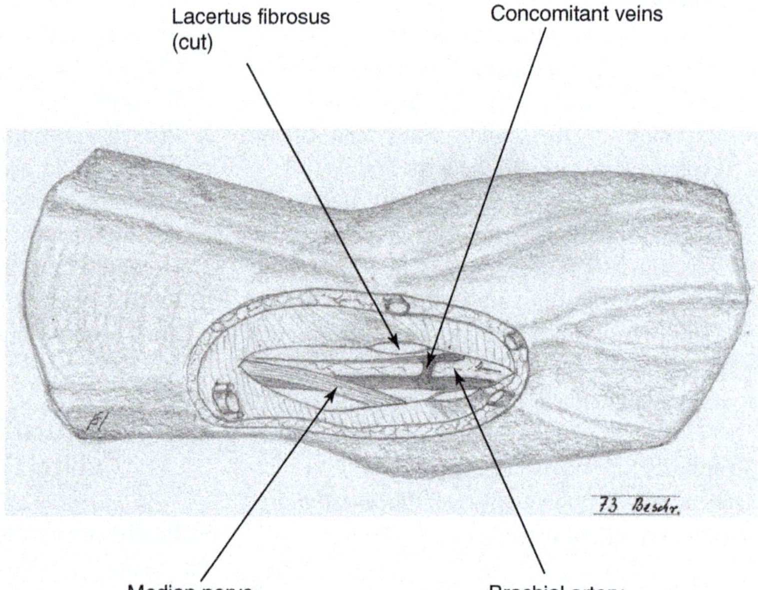

Fig. 3.65 Anatomy of the brachial artery in the cubital fossa

natural variants, or likewise after thrombophlebitis or previous operations. The choice of the most appropriate option constitutes the creative aspect of surgery.

Deep Veins

The brachial veins (often double, rarely single) together with ropeladder-type concomitant veins accompany the brachial artery. The deep vein is hardly ever used for venipuncture.

Arteries

The arterial anatomy varies less than the venous anatomy (Fig. 3.65). The arteries exclusively run beneath the fascia. The brachial artery divides into the ulnar and radial arteries usually 2–5 cm distal to the joint line. The interosseous artery rarely originates from the division. It originates more often from the ulnar artery than from the radial artery. A proximal takeoff of the radial artery in the upper arm is a clinically important variant (around 0.5 % of our patients).

3.3.2 Technical Hints

Preoperative Diagnostics

If veins and arteries can be evaluated clinically, no further examinations are necessary. If the veins cannot thus be evaluated adequately (e.g., in adipose patients), duplex ultrasound of the proximally compressed veins seems necessary. If the situation remains unclear or if there are signs of central venous stenoses or occlusions, we recommend a phlebography. As for the arterial system, arteriography might help clarify findings.

Principles Concerning the Choice of AV Anastomoses

The selection of the right, adequate elbow fistula is difficult because of the multitude of possible anastomoses. Leaving anatomical variants out, there are still eight venous segments in the confined space of the cubital fossa each of which can show three morphologic states (Fig. 3.66a) resulting in 3^8 possible morphologic findings. Keeping in mind this variety the following principles should be observed:

1. The only purpose of such an AV anastomosis is the arterialization of a puncturable vein in the upper arm. Only a lateroterminal anastomosis to the proximal venous stump is permitted. *A laterolateral anastomosis between artery and vein is taboo.*
2. If one of the two puncturable veins of the upper arm (cephalic vein or basilic vein) is better suited than the other, only this vein should be anastomosed. The continuity of the other vein is preserved.
3. If neither of these two veins is definitely suitable alone, both should be arterialized.
4. If both veins are unsuitable or occluded, in rare cases the deep vein may also be arterialized with subsequent transposition (similar to the basilic vein).

Access for AV Fistulas in the Cubital Fossa

It is almost always possible to create elbow fistulas using local infiltration anesthesia. Access to the brachial artery is always the same regardless of which vein is anastomosed in the cubital region. The following principles should be observed:

1. Longitudinal incision distal to the antecubital fold over the palpable brachial artery (Fig. 3.66b) down to the fascia, taking into account traversing nerves. With the exception of the profound median cubital vein, the median cubital veins always lie superficially to the interindividually highly-varying superficial antebrachial fascia.
2. Preparation of the vein suited for anastomosis.
3. Longitudinal incision of the antebrachial fascia/cutting of the lacertus fibrosus, and exposure of the brachial artery.
4. Distal ligation and severance of the vein selected for anastomosing, local heparinization, and clamping (e.g., with Schwartz or Yasargil clamps).
5. Transverse splitting of the longitudinally-opened fascia (Fig. 3.67).
6. Bilateral clamping of the artery (e.g., Schwartz or Yasargil clamps), longitudinal arteriotomy,

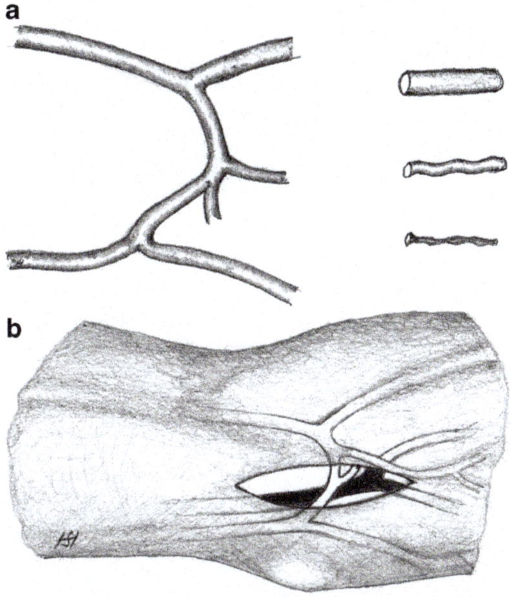

Fig. 3.66 (**a**) Different presentations of the veins which are suitable for anastomoses in the cubital fossa. *Top*: normal lumen, *middle*: narrow lumen, *bottom*: occluded lumen. (**b**) Access to the brachial artery and to the cubital veins via a longitudinal incision distal to the cubital fossa

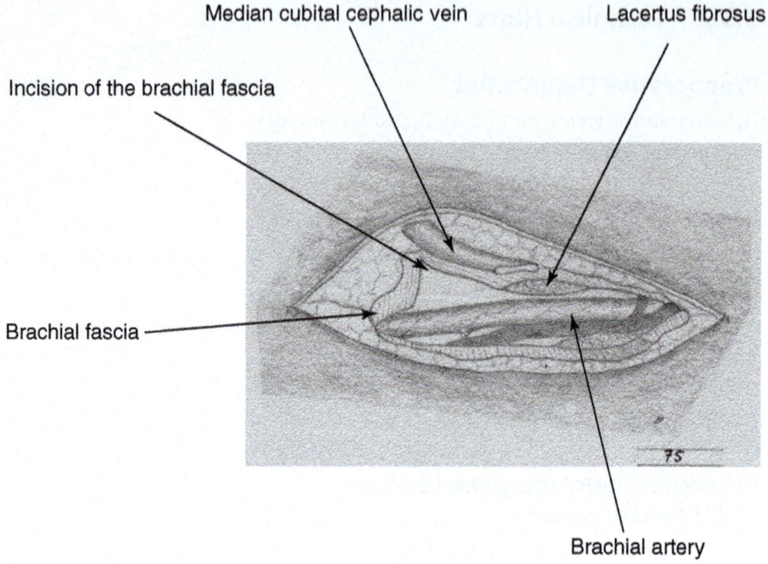

Fig. 3.67 Elbow fistula. Severance of the fascia to prevent kinking of the vein

local heparinization, and lateroterminal anastomosis (running suture 6–0 or 7–0).

7. Wound closure with subcutaneous and epidermal sutures after hemostasis.

3.3.3 Arterialization of the Cephalic Vein

In addition to the cephalic vein in the forearm, the cephalic vein in the upper arm offers the second most important option of an AV vascular access. Frequently it can be used for many years. Therefore the different ways of its arterialization and reconstruction are discussed in detail.

Varieties of Anastomoses

Basically there are eight alternatives for the arterialization of the cephalic vein in the cubital region. Each of these has its own indication.

Arterialization Via the Cephalic Median Cubital Vein

Indication

Suitable trunk and sufficient length of the cephalic median cubital vein (Fig. 3.68a, b)

Technical note

Preserves the interconnections of the veins which are not used.

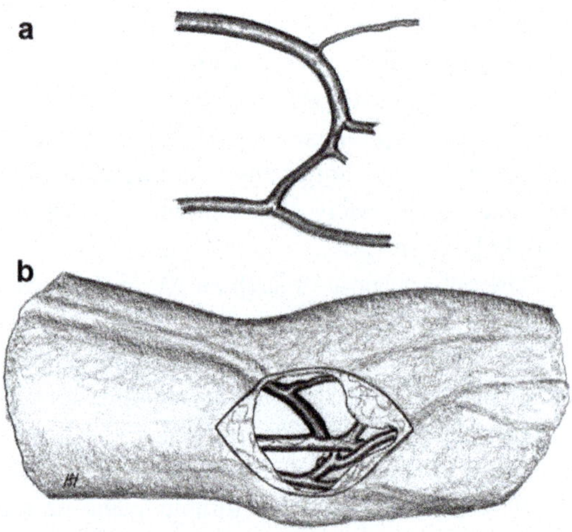

Fig. 3.68 (**a**) Venous anatomy. (**b**) Arterialization of the cephalic vein via the cephalic median cubital vein

Arterialization Via the Cubital Median Antebrachial Vein

Indication

Suitable trunk of the cubital cephalic median vein and the median antebrachial vein, if the added lengths of these veins are required due to the long distance to the brachial artery (Fig. 3.69a, b)

Technical note

Preserves the connection between the median basilic vein and the profound median cubital vein.

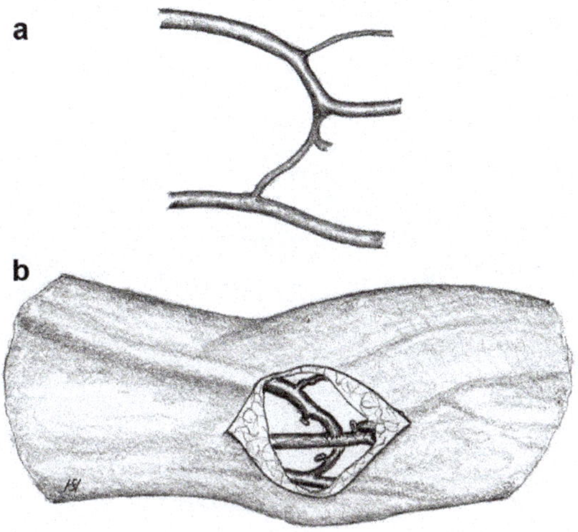

Fig. 3.69 (**a**) Venous anatomy. (**b**) Arterialization of the cephalic vein via the cubital median antebrachial vein

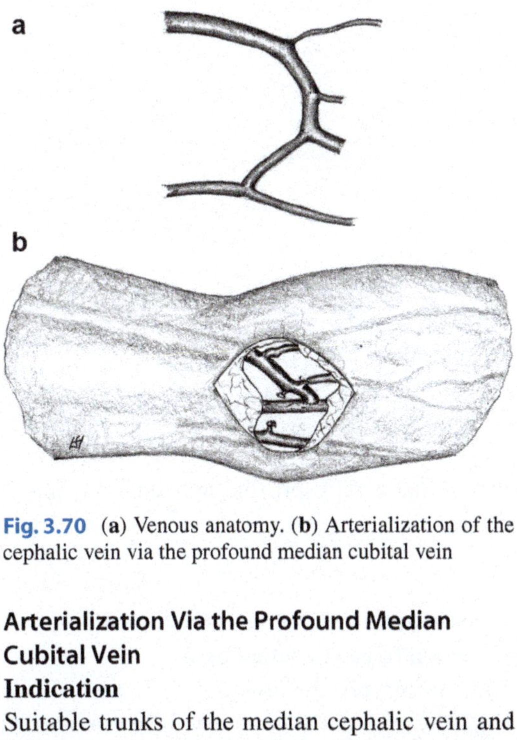

Fig. 3.70 (**a**) Venous anatomy. (**b**) Arterialization of the cephalic vein via the profound median cubital vein

Arterialization Via the Profound Median Cubital Vein

Indication

Suitable trunks of the median cephalic vein and the profound median cubital vein, if the median antebrachial vein is not suited, and the added lengths of the suited veins are insufficient to reach the brachial artery (Fig. 3.70a, b).

Technical note

Ligation and dissection of the median antebrachial vein.

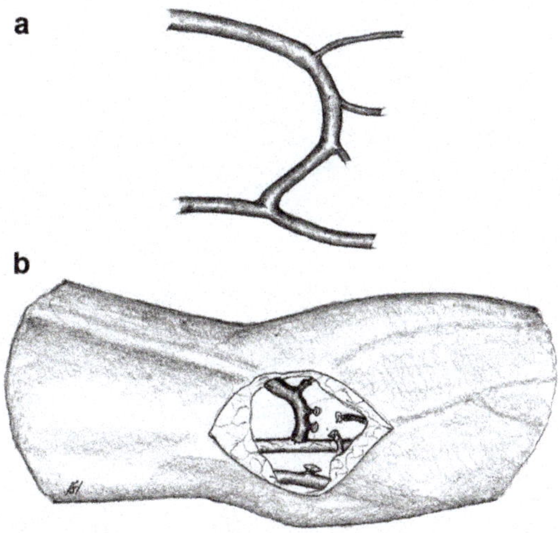

Fig. 3.71 (**a**) Venous anatomy. (**b**) Arterialization of the cephalic vein via the cubital median basilic vein

Arterialization Via the Cubital Median Basilic Vein (Fig. 3.71a, b)

Indication

Suitable median cephalic and basilic veins, if the cubital median antebrachial vein and the profound median cubital vein are suitable and the added lengths of the former veins are sufficient (Fig. 3.71a, b).

Technical note

Dissection of the median antebrachial and the profound median cubital veins.

Arterialization Via the Cephalic Vein in the Proximal Forearm

Indication

Unsuitable median cephalic vein but suitable segment of the cephalic vein near the cubital fossa (Fig. 3.72a, b).

Technical note

The cephalic vein is exposed via a separate longitudinal incision of the proximal forearm.

Arterialization Via an Interposition Graft Originating Distal to the Cubital Fossa

Indication

Unsuitable cubital median cephalic vein but suitable cephalic vein of the proximal forearm distal to the cubital fossa (Fig. 3.73a, b).

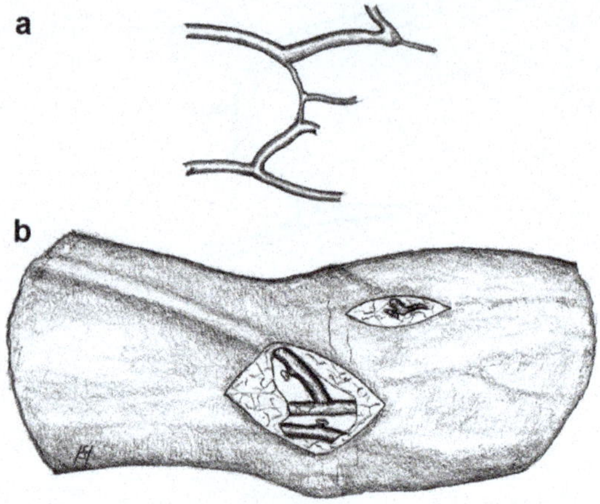

Fig. 3.72 (**a**) Venous anatomy. (**b**) Arterialization of the cephalic vein via the cephalic vein in the proximal forearm

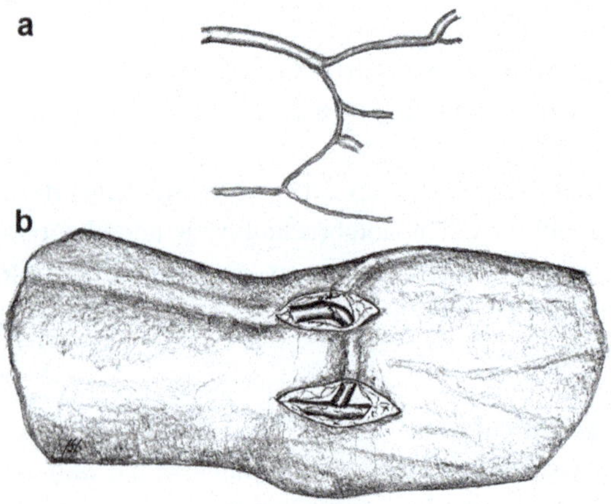

Fig. 3.73 (**a**) Venous anatomy. (**b**) Arterialization of the cephalic vein via an interposition graft originating distal to the cubital fossa

Technical note

Exposure of the artery and vein through separate longitudinal incisions. The preferred diameter of the ePTFE prosthesis is either 4 mm or 5 mm.

Arterialization Via an Interposition Graft Originating Proximal to the Cubital Fossa

Indication

Cephalic vein suited proximal to the elbow only (Fig. 3.74a, b).

Technical note

Exposure of the artery and vein through separate longitudinal incisions. The preferred diameter of the ePTFE prosthesis is either 4 mm or 5 mm.

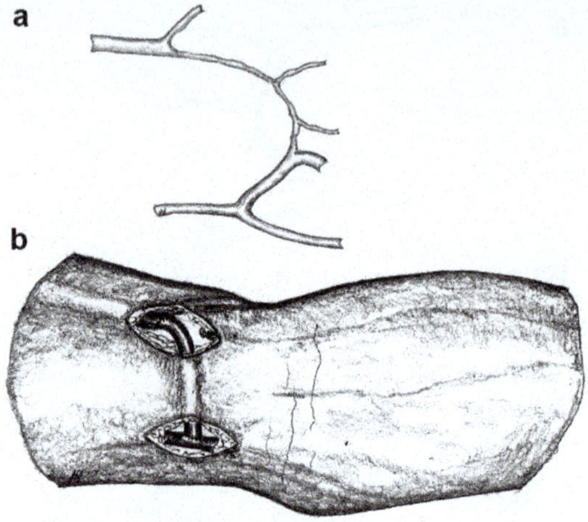

Fig. 3.74 (**a**) Venous anatomy. (**b**) Arterialization of the cephalic vein via an interposition graft originating proximal to the cubital fossa

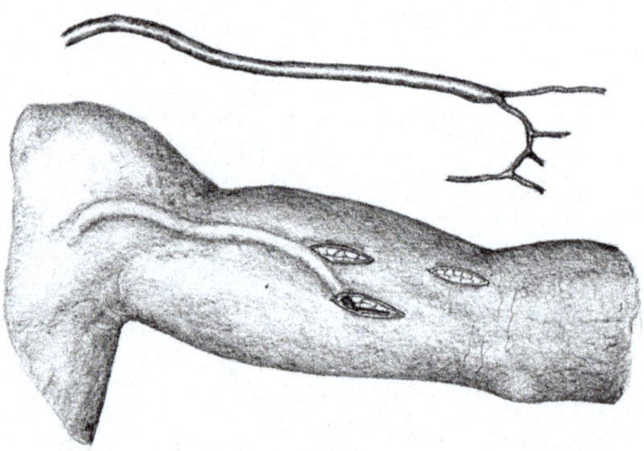

Fig. 3.75 Proximal anastomosis of the cephalic vein in the upper arm

Arterialization Via Direct Anastomosis Proximal to the Cubital Fossa

Indication/prerequisite

Cephalic vein suited proximal to the elbow only; also contraindication against prosthetic material (Fig. 3.75a, b).

Sufficient length of the segment which is suitable for puncture.

Technical note

Exposure of the vein via two longitudinal incisions. Separate longitudinal incision for the artery.

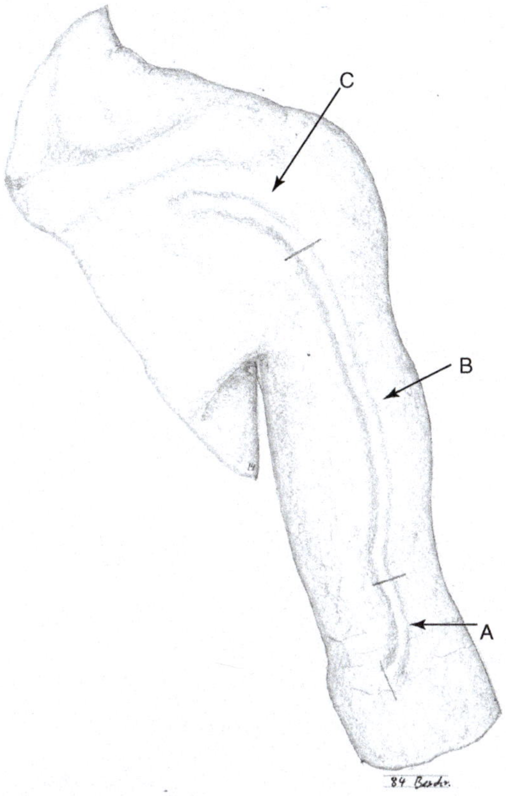

Fig. 3.76 Segments of the cephalic vein after arterialization distal to the cubital fossa: (*A*) cubital segment, (*B*) upper arm segment, (*C*) shoulder segment

Reconstructions of the Arterialized Cephalic Vein of the Forearm

Depending on individual factors such as previous use and puncture traumas, numerous morphologic changes may develop. From a functional and morphologic point of view, the arterialized cephalic vein may be divided into three segments: (*A*) cubital segment, (*B*) upper arm segment, (*C*) shoulder segment (Fig. 3.76).

Reconstruction of the Cephalic Vein in the Cubital Fossa

Stenoses

The primary treatment of a short stenosis near the anastomosis should be PTA. If the result is unsatisfactory or a restenosis develops, a patch plasty is recommended (cf. Fig. 3.36b). A long stenosis near the anastomosis is much more frequent. There are basically two repair options as follows.

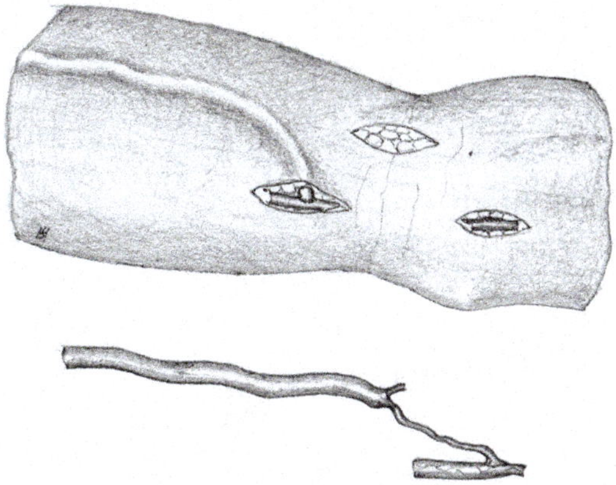

Fig. 3.77 Proximalization of the arterial feeding with a short stenosis of the cubital segment

Anastomosing the Cephalic Vein Proximal to the Cubital Fossa

Indication/prerequisites

With an anastomosis proximal to the cubital fossa, the distal stenosed segment is no longer needed (Fig. 3.77).

Technical note

Ligation of the old anastomosis, exposure of the vein and the brachial artery via separate incisions.

Arterialization of the Cephalic Vein of the Upper Arm Using an Interposition Graft

Indication

- Long distance stenosis or distal occlusion of the vein.
- Suitable large diameter segment of upper arm cephalic vein which is still long enough for puncture (Fig. 3.78).

Technical note

Ligation of the AV anastomosis through a longitudinal incision, exposure of the vein where its diameter is large, and exposure of the brachial arteries via longitudinal incisions. Preferred diameter of ePTFE grafts: 4 or 5 mm.

Aneurysms

Aneurysms close to the anastomosis occur frequently. Indications for reconstruction include size, functional limitations, rapid growth, or cosmetics.

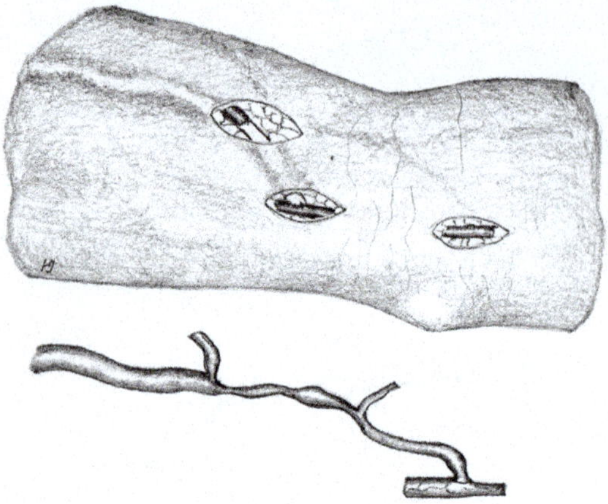

Fig. 3.78 Proximal feeding via an interposition graft with a long stenosis of the cubital segment

Luminal Narrowing by Partial Wall Resection

Indication

Aneurysmatic segment that is not elongated (Fig. 3.79).

Technical note

The aneurysm is exposed via a longitudinal incision over its center from the anastomosis to the normal lumen. Then the aneurysmatic wall is resected and subsequently closed with a continuous suture.

Partial Resection of the Aneurysm and Creation of a New Lumen

Indication

Elongation of the aneurysmatic segment (Fig. 3.80).

Technical note

A longitudinal incision over the aneurysmatic segment facilitates its exposure from the anastomosis to the proximal segment which has to be preserved. Then adequate parts of the aneurysm are resected to allow for the re-establishment of vascular continuity using the remaining vessel to create a new lumen.

Reconstruction of the Upper Arm Cephalic Vein

Stenoses

PTA is an effective treatment for short stenoses. If PTA fails or restenosis occurs, patch plasty or short interposition grafts are used.

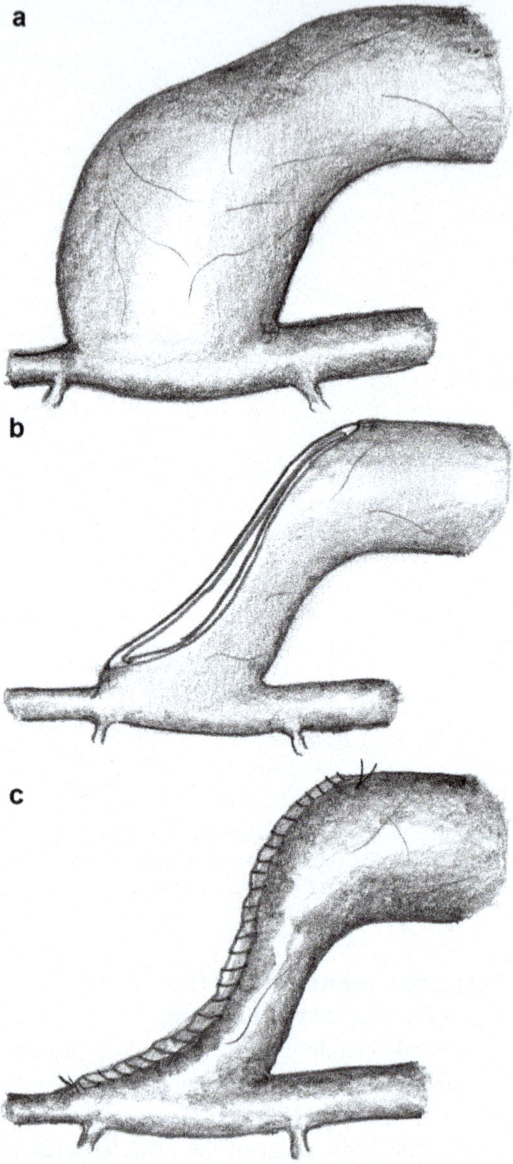

Fig. 3.79 Example for the reconstruction of an aneurysm in the cubital region that is not elongated by wall resection: (**a**) aneurysm, (**b**) elliptical resection, (**c**) closure with continuous suture

With proximal *long segment* stenoses we recommend the implantation of an interposition graft to the proximal (axillary) brachial vein (Fig. 3.81).

Indication/prerequisites

- High grade, long stenosis of the cephalic vein of the upper arm or shoulder.
- Distal venous segment suitable for puncture.

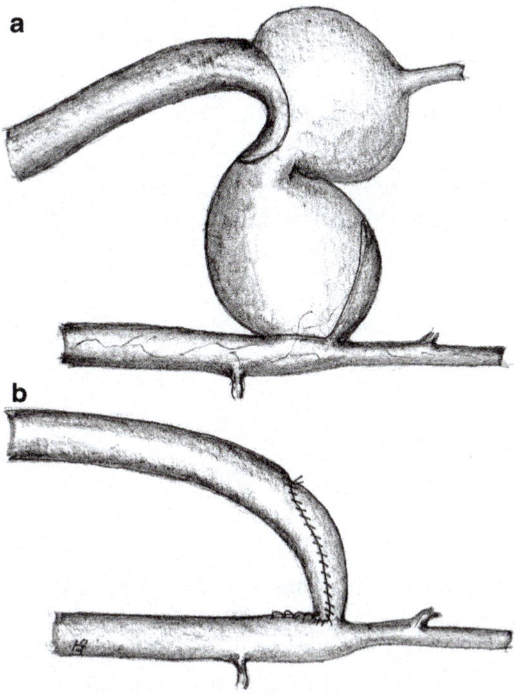

Fig. 3.80 Example for the reconstruction of an elongated aneurysm in the cubital region: (**a**) before reconstruction, (**b**) after reconstruction

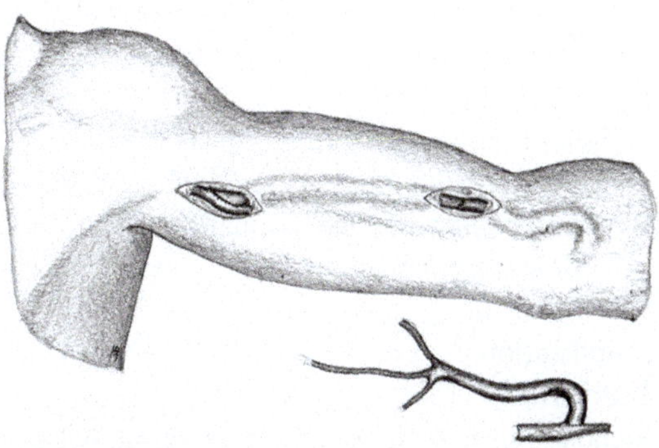

Fig. 3.81 Long stenosis/occlusion of the cephalic vein in the upper arm. Preservation of the patent venous segment by interposing a prosthesis that is anastomosed to the infraaxillary deep vein

Technical note

Exposure via two longitudinal incisions.

Deep Position of the Upper Arm Cephalic Vein

In morbidly obese patients the pathway of the cephalic vein of the upper arm can be so far from the surface that puncturing is hardly possible or not possible at all. Under these circumstances the transposition of the cephalic vein of the upper arm is indicated (Figs. 3.82 and 3.83).

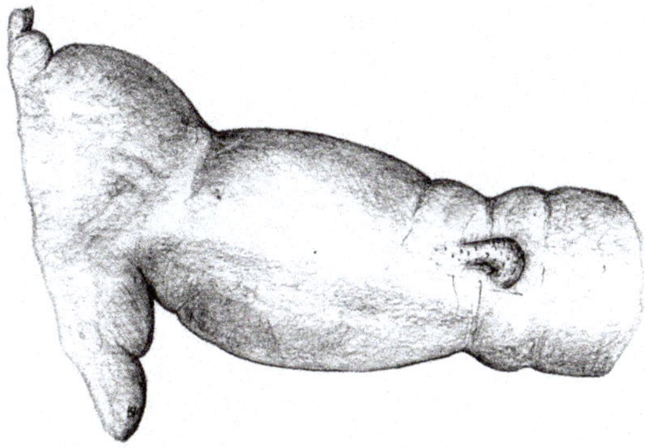

Fig. 3.82 Deep position of the upper arm cephalic vein in an obese patient

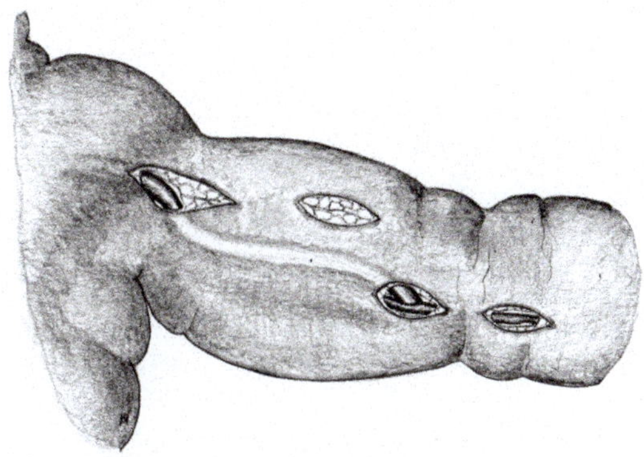

Fig. 3.83 Surgical site after superficialization of the cephalic vein

Indication

Deep position of a suitable upper arm cephalic vein.

Technical note

Exposure of the vein over a long distance mostly via three longitudinal incisions, dissection close to the anastomosis, and placement in a separate subcutaneous tunnel.

Reconstruction of the Cephalic Vein in the Shoulder Region or Close to the Axillary Vein

Most frequently stenoses occur where the cephalic vein joins the axillary vein. Long stenoses in the shoulder region are rare.

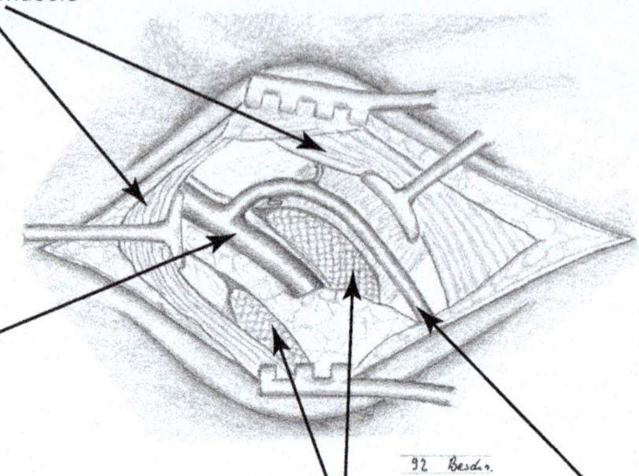

Fig. 3.84 Anatomy of the confluence of the cephalic and axillary veins

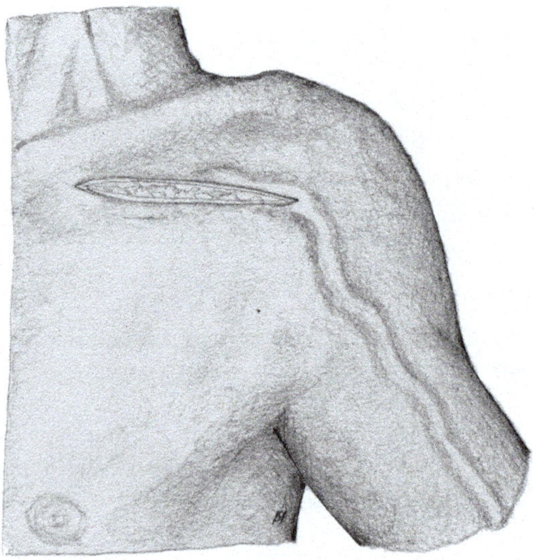

Fig. 3.85 Skin incision to expose the proximal cephalic vein where it joins the axillary vein

Anatomy of the Proximal Cephalic Vein (Fig. 3.84)

In the shoulder region the cephalic vein follows the anterior margin of the deltoid muscle. Centrally it crosses the pectoralis minor muscle and descends through a fascial gap into the adipose tissue of the subpectoral space. Near its junction with the axillary vein there are often tight strands of fibrous connective tissue.

Approach to the Junction of the Cephalic and the Axillary Veins (Fig. 3.85)

The cephalic vein is exposed in the sulcus between the deltoid and the pectoralis major muscles (arm adducted, transverse incision). Then the vein is followed to the axillary vein by dissecting the pectoralis minor muscle and cutting the fibrous strands mentioned above.

As for the reconstruction of a stenosis close to the cephalic/axillary junction, there are four options:

- Mobilization
- Resection with new anastomosis
- Resection with interposition graft
- Transposition of the cephalic vein to the (infraaxillary) brachial vein

Mobilization

Indication

Stenosis due to kinking without fixed luminal narrowing at the entry site into the axillary vein. Can often only be evaluated during surgery (Fig. 3.86).

Technical notes

- Mobilization of cephalic vein up to junction frequently necessary.
- Cutting of strangulating fibrous strands.

Resection and New Anastomosis

Indication

Short intraluminal stenosis at junction (Fig. 3.87).

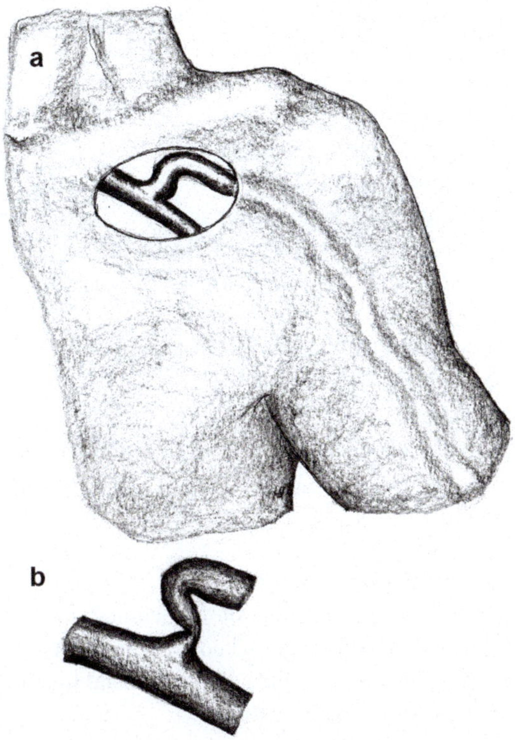

Fig. 3.86 Repair of a stenosis at the junction of the proximal cephalic vein by removing strangulating connective tissue strands

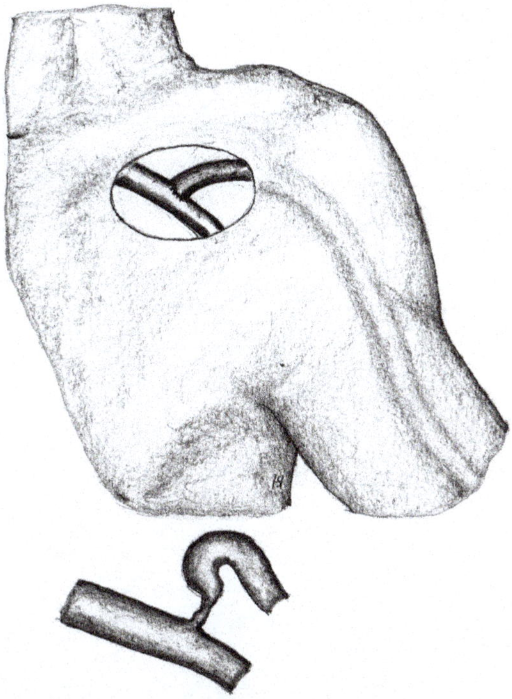

Fig. 3.87 Repair of a short stenosis of the junction of the cephalic vein with the axillary vein by resection and creating a new anastomosis

Technical note

Exposure of cephalic vein up to where it joins the axillary vein.

Resection and Prosthetic Graft

Indication

Long stenosis at cephalic/axillary junction which is not suited for direct anastomosis (Fig. 3.88).

Technical note

Adequate caliber for prosthesis should be 6 or 7 mm.

Transposition of the Cephalic Vein to the (Infraaxillary) Brachial Vein

Indication

Long stenosis in the shoulder region (Fig. 3.89).

Technical notes

- Exposure of the cephalic vein in the proximal upper arm or shoulder region, dissection and ligation of the proximal stump (mostly two longitudinal incisions).
- Exposure of the (infraaxillary) brachial vein (longitudinal incision).
- Creation of a curved subcuticular tunnel for the mobilized cephalic vein.
- Terminolateral anastomosis to the brachial vein.

3.3.4 Arterialization of the Basilic Vein

The basilic vein in the upper arm should only be used if the cephalic vein is unsuitable or occluded. The advantage of the upper arm basilic vein is its early and wide dilation. A definite disadvantage is that it almost always has to be superficialized. The basilic vein enters the subfascial space around 2–4 cm proximal to the cubital space, where it cannot be punctured safely without complications. Therefore almost always its superficialization is necessary. *We plead for a delayed transposition.*

Anastomotic Options

The approach begins with a longitudinal incision over the brachial artery distal to the cubital fossa. Which venous segment is chosen in order to connect the artery to the upper arm basilic vein depends on the venous morphology. It is during surgery that the appropriate vein is selected.

Feasible options include:

- Median cubital basilic vein
- Profound median cubital vein
- Median cubital antebrachial vein
- Basilic vein of the forearm

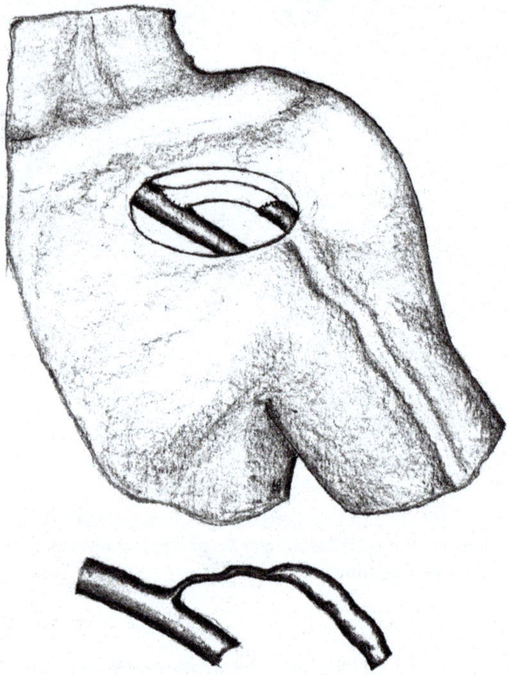

Fig. 3.88 Repair of a long stenosis of the junction of the cephalic vein with the axillary vein by resection and insertion of a prosthetic graft

Arterialization Via the Cubital Median Basilic Vein

Indication

Suitable segment of the cubital median basilic vein which is long and wide enough (Fig. 3.90a, b).

Technical note

Dissection and ligation of the cubital median basilic vein before the takeoff of the profound median cubital vein, and additional distal ligation of the basilic vein if possible.

Arterialization Via the Profound Median Cubital Vein

Indication

Suitable trunks of the median basilic and profound median cubital veins with sufficient added lengths of both veins to cover the distance to the brachial artery (Fig. 3.91).

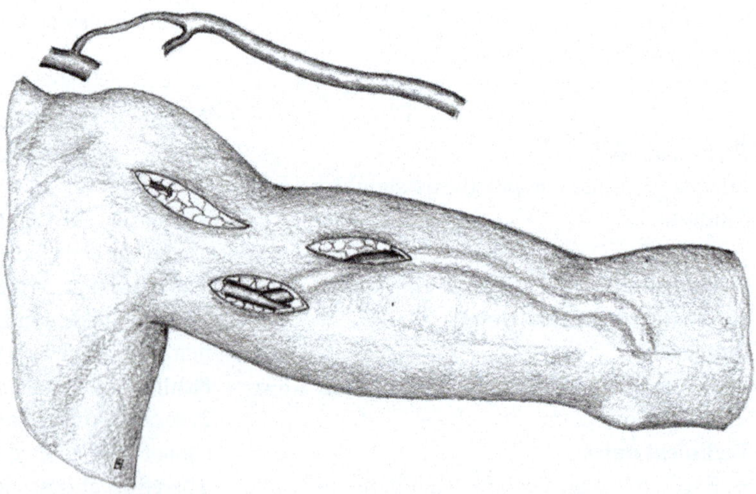

Fig. 3.89 Long stenosis of the cephalic vein in the shoulder region. Transposition to the infraaxillary deep vein

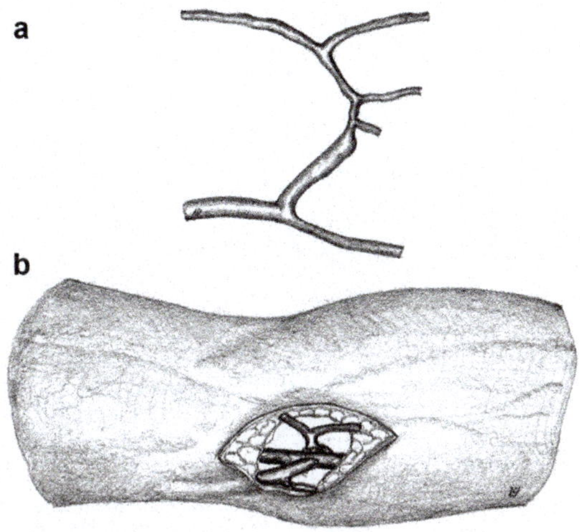

Fig. 3.90 (**a**) Venous anatomy. (**b**) Arterialization of the basilic vein via the median cubital basilic vein

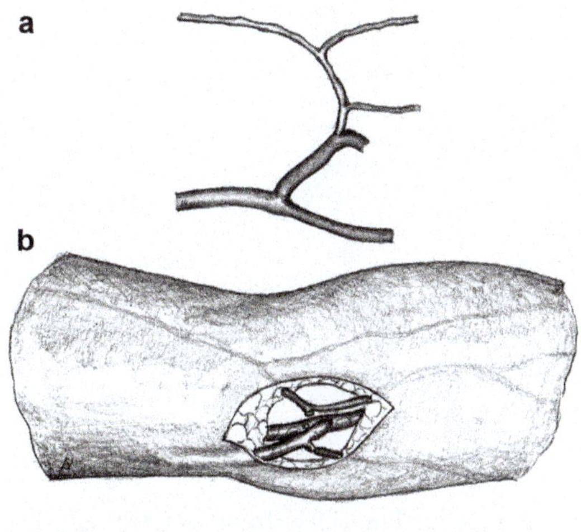

Fig. 3.91 (**a**) Venous anatomy. (**b**) Arterialization of the basilic vein via the profound median cubital vein

Technical note

Preservation of the connection between median antebrachial vein and median cephalic vein. If possible, distal ligation of basilic vein.

Arterialization Via the Cubital Median Antebrachial Vein

Indication

Suitable trunks of the median cubital basilic vein and median cubital antebrachial veins. Sufficient added lengths of both veins because of long distance to brachial artery (Fig. 3.92a, b).

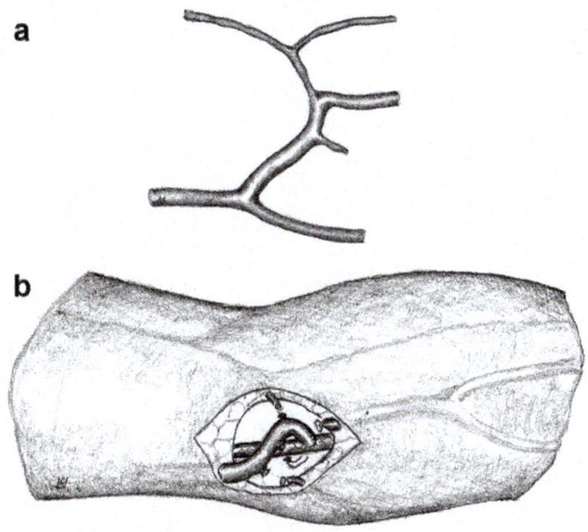

Fig. 3.92 (**a**) Venous anatomy. (**b**) Arterialization via the cubital median antebrachial vein

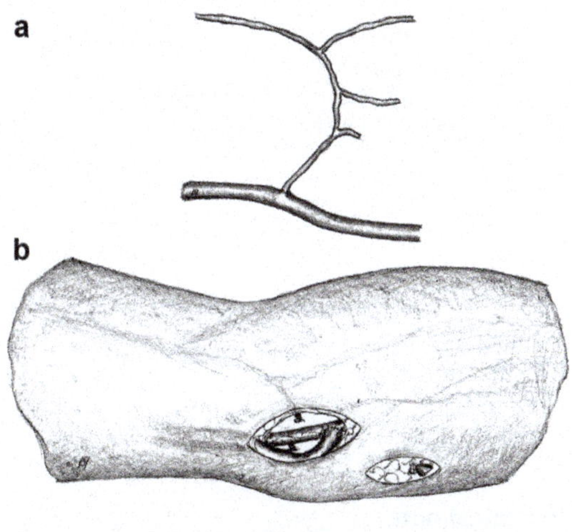

Fig. 3.93 (**a**) Venous anatomy. (**b**) Arterialization of the basilic vein via the basilic vein from the proximal forearm

Technical note

Ligation of the profound median cubital vein and median cephalic vein. If possible perform distal ligation of the basilic vein.

Arterialization Via the Forearm Basilic Vein (Fig. 3.93)

Indications

- Cubital median basilic vein unsuitable.
- Patent basilic vein of the proximal forearm.

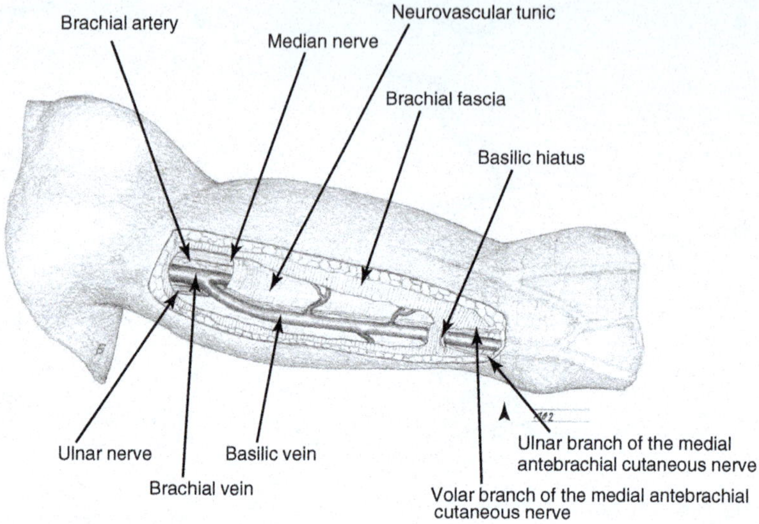

Fig. 3.94 Anatomy of the basilic vein in the upper arm

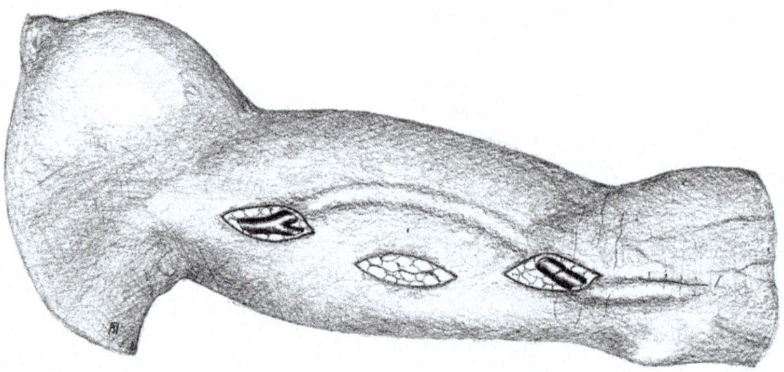

Fig. 3.95 Superficialization of the basilic vein in the upper arm while preserving the anatomosis distal to the cubital fossa

Technical note

Exposure of the basilic vein of the proximal forearm via a separate longitudinal incision.

Superficialization of the Basilic Vein in the Forearm

We always perform a delayed superficialization of the basilic vein (usually after 4–8 weeks). The vein should be sufficiently dilated (duplex control) without stenoses. If uncertainties remain we recommend a phlebography by puncturing the basilic vein in the cubital fossa.

Anatomy

The basilic vein pierces the brachial fascia shortly proximal to the cubital fossa at the basilic hiatus. Beneath the fascia it runs ulnar to the neurovascular bundle (Fig. 3.94) from which it is separated by the neurovascular tunic. Near the axilla, the basilic vein variably joins the (median) brachial veins.

Surgical procedures

Two different procedures have proven successful:

- Superficialization with preservation of the arterial anastomosis.
- Superficialization with new anastomosis proximal to the cubital fossa.

Superficialization with Preservation of the Arterial Anastomosis

Indication

Sufficient length of the vein for a (curved) superficial path (Fig. 3.95).

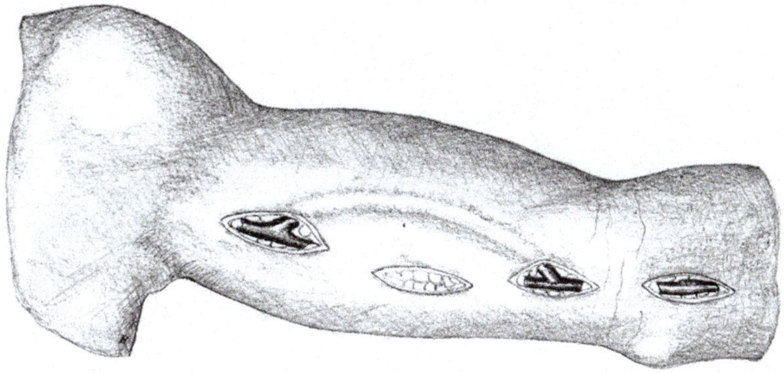

Fig. 3.96 Superficialization with new arterial anastomosis proximal to the cubital fossa

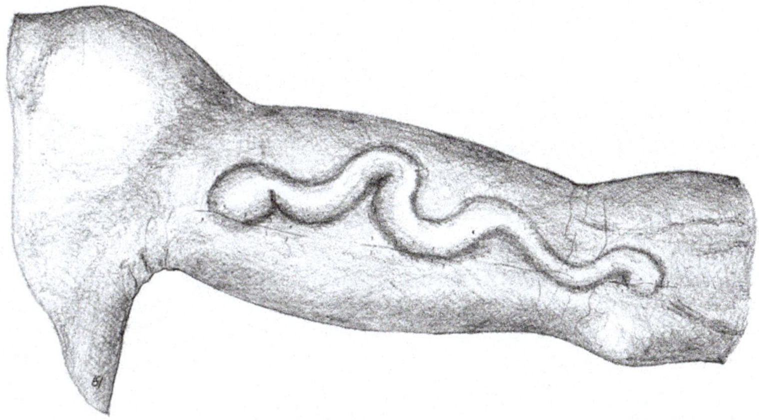

Fig. 3.97 Pronounced dilatation of the basilic vein in the forearm with stenosis where it enters the subfascial space

Technical notes

- Exposure of the basilic vein in the upper arm using (three) short longitudinal incisions.
- Transection of the vein shortly proximal to the cubital fossa, then pulling the vein out of its original bed with proximal exit site at the axillary wound.
- Preparation of a suitable ventral subcutaneous tunnel to the cubital incision and placement of the vein in this tunnel. (For this purpose the vein should be tightly-filled to avoid torsion.)
- Terminoterminal anastomosis of both venous stumps.

Superficialization with New Arterial Anastomosis Proximal to the Cubital Fossa (Fig. 3.96)

Indication

Basilic vein which is too short for a curved superficial path, or unsuitable venous segment close to the arterial anastomosis.

Technical notes

- Exposure of the basilic vein in the upper arm using (three) short longitudinal incisions.
- Exposure of the AV anastomosis via a longitudinal incision distal to the cubital fossa and dissection of the vein.
- Pull distal vein out at the axillary wound.
- Creation of a suitable subcutaneous tunnel between the axillary incision and the incision of the distal upper arm.
- Exposure of the brachial artery, placement of the vein in the tunnel, new arterial anastomosis (proximalization).

Reconstruction of the Transposed Basilic Vein in the Upper Arm

The superficialized basilic vein in the upper arm tends to dilate more than in its original bed. A frequent cause for extreme dilation is a short stenosis close to where the basilic vein joins the brachial vein due to an aperture in the brachial fascia which is too narrow (Fig. 3.97). It is

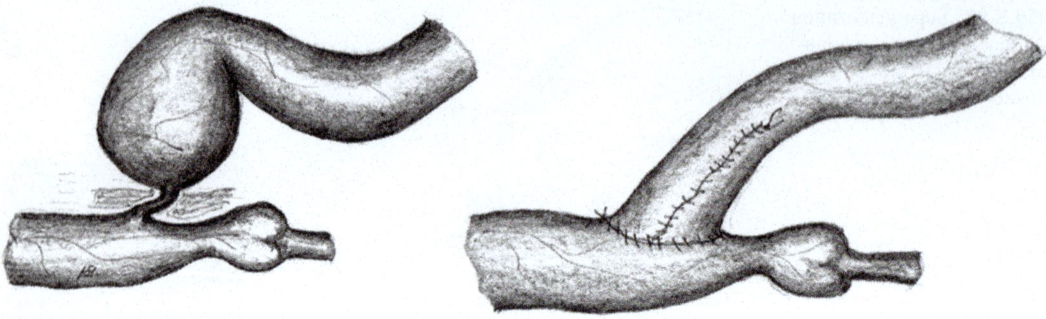

Fig. 3.98 Reconstruction of a stenosis at the entry into the subfascial space

usually possible to correct the situation by resecting the stenotic segment, narrowing the lumen of the dilated vein, and creating a new anastomosis (Fig. 3.98).

3.3.5 Arterialization of the Cephalic and Basilic Veins in the Cubital Fossa

If the suitability of both veins is questionable, the simultaneous arterialization of both veins may be indicated. Depending on the vascular morphology, there are three options using:

- The profound median cubital vein.
- The median antebrachial vein.
- The connection between the median veins.

Arterialization Via the Profound Median Cubital Vein

Indication

If the profound median cubital vein is the best vessel for feeding both veins (Fig. 3.99a, b).

Technical note

Ligation of the median antebrachial vein.

Arterialization Via the Median Antebrachial Vein

Indication

If the median antebrachial vein is the best vessel to feed both veins (Fig. 3.100a, b).

Technical note

Ligation of the profound median cubital vein.

a

b

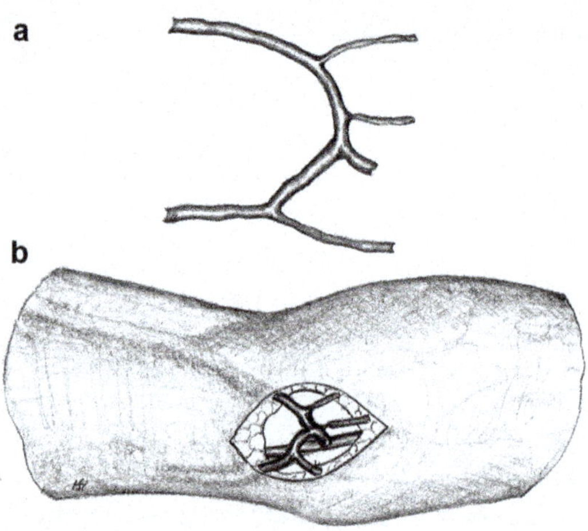

Fig. 3.99 (a) Venous anatomy. (b) Arterialization of the basilic and cephalic veins via the profound median cubital vein

a

b

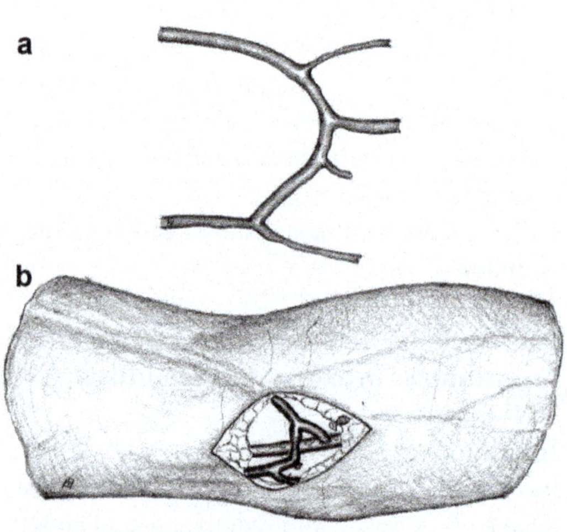

Fig. 3.100 (a) Venous anatomy. (b) Arterialization of the basilic and cephalic veins via the median antebrachial vein

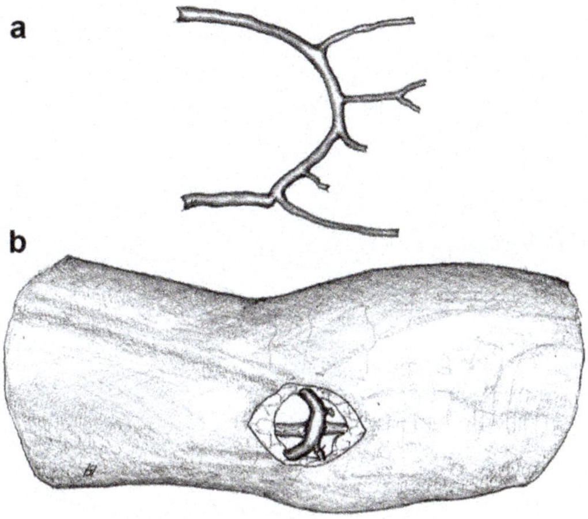

Fig. 3.101 (a) Venous anatomy. (b) Arterialization of the basilic and cephalic veins via a laterolateral anastomosis to the confluence of the median veins

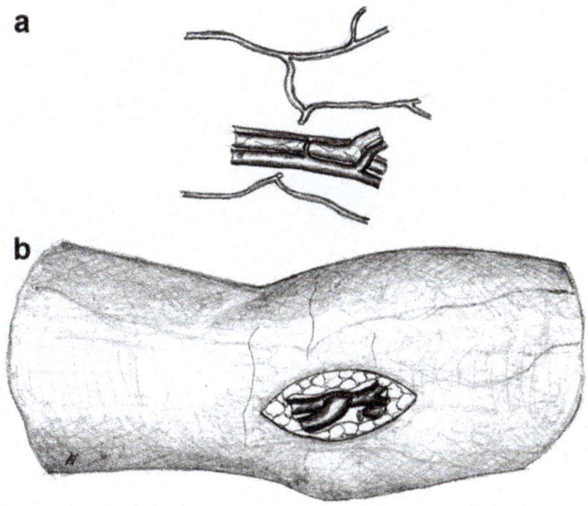

Fig. 3.102 (a) Venous anatomy. (b) Arterialization of the deep brachial vein

Arterialization Via the Confluence of the Median Veins

Indication

If the profound median cubital vein and the median antebrachial vein are not suited (Fig. 3.101a, b).

Technical note

Laterolateral anastomosis between the median vein and the brachial artery. Ligation of side branches.

3.3.6 Arterialization of the Deep Vein in the Cubital Fossa

The arterialization of the deep vein should be reserved for exceptional circumstances, as the necessary transposition requires considerable effort due to numerous side branches and the proximity of nerves.

Indication

No suitable superficial veins, implantation of prosthetic material contraindicated (e.g., persistent septic foci) (Fig. 3.102a, b).

Technical note

Only feasible if the caliber of the deep concomitant vein is sufficient (at least 3–4 mm).

Superficialization of the Deep Vein in the Upper Arm

Indication/prerequisites

Certain knowledge that the deep vein has dilated sufficiently (Figs. 3.103 and 3.104).

Technical note

The superficialization of the deep vein demands an even more careful and atraumatic approach than usual.

- Exposure of the vein via (mostly three) longitudinal incisions in the upper arm.
- Exposure of the AV anastomosis via a longitudinal incision distal to the cubital fossa and dissection of the vein.
- Taking the distal vein out via the proximal incision.
- Creation of a subcutaneous tunnel between the axillary incision and the incision of the distal upper arm, passage of the vein through the tunnel.
- Lateroterminal anastomosis of the vein and the brachial artery.

Prognosis

Comparable with transposed basilic vein.

3.3.7 Aneurysms in the Cubital Fossa After AV Anastomoses

Sometimes in giant and odd aneurysms with high flows and numerous collaterals, neither their

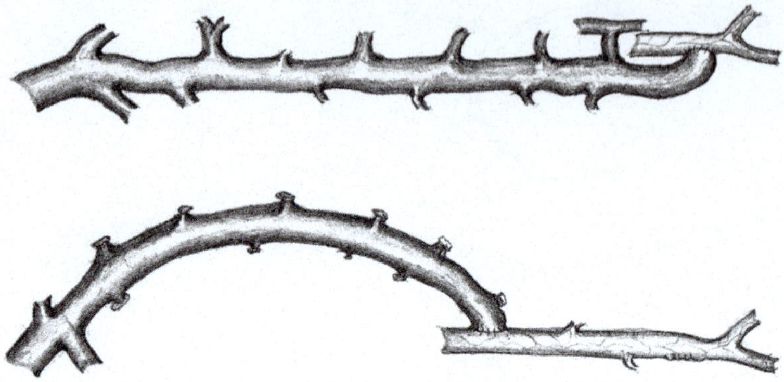

Fig. 3.103 Superficialization of the arterialized deep brachial vein

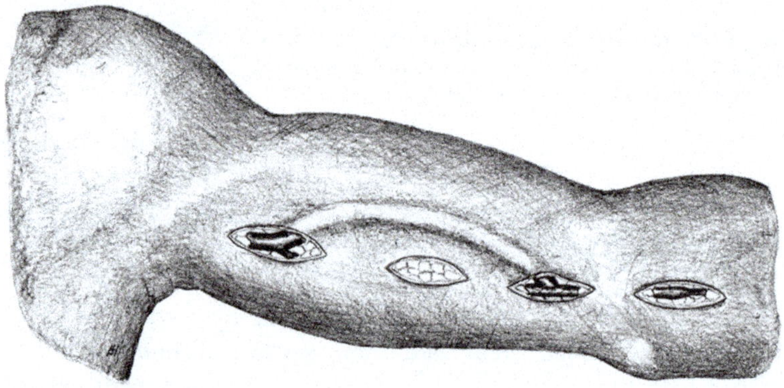

Fig. 3.104 Arterialized and superficialized deep vein in the upper arm

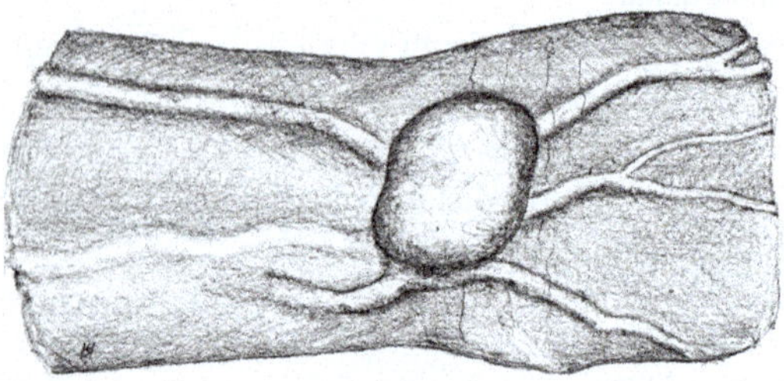

Fig. 3.105 Large aneurysm of an elbow fistula in the cubital fossa

clinical examination, nor sonography, nor phlebography yield satisfactory results as to which vessel they originate from (Fig. 3.105). We recommend an elliptical skin excision over the aneurysm and subtle isolation of every involved vessel (Fig. 3.106). Often there will be a laterolateral anastomosis with retrograde perfusion of the forearm. The reconstruction has two aims:

- Correction of the aneurysm.
- Directing the flow exclusively into the vessel designated for puncture.

Figure 3.107 shows an example of how to proceed.

3.3.8 Great Saphenous Vein as AV Access

If there are no feasible options for AV fistulas of the upper extremities, there are two ways to use the great saphenous vein:

- Femoral loop
- Autologous graft for the upper extremity

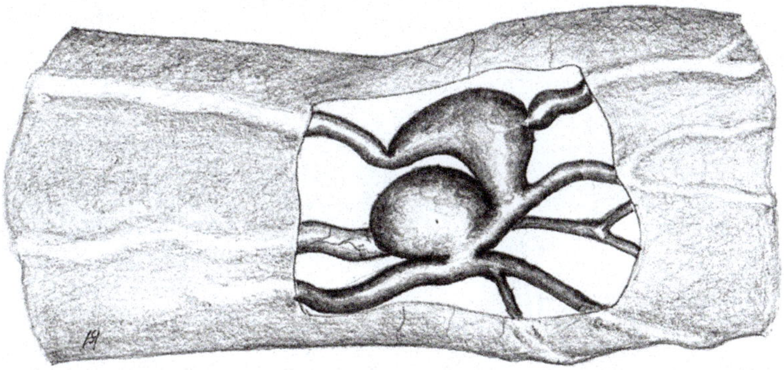

Fig. 3.106 Surgical site after exposure of the vessels (cf. Figs. 3.107 and 3.108)

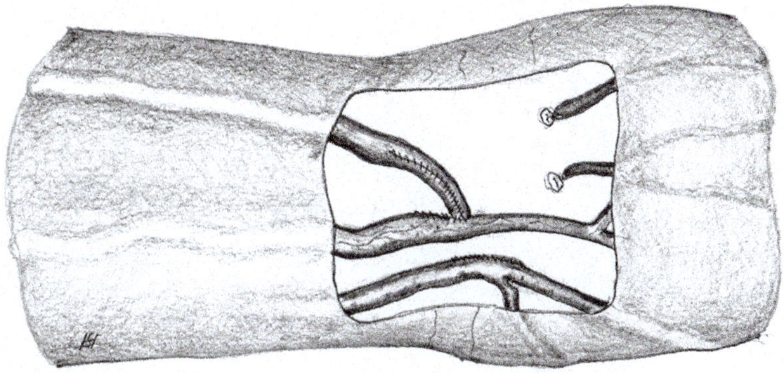

Fig. 3.107 Reconstruction

Despite anecdotal reports of forearm saphenous loops serving for up to 10 years, we see the following limitations and do not use this option:

- Due to its wall structure the dilation of the great saphenous vein may be limited and is not predictable.
- A great saphenous vein that is anastomosed in the cubital fossa requires a good quality basilic or brachial vein. If these vessels can be found, different less demanding surgical options can be realized.
- Depending on pre-existing comorbidities, the great saphenous vein might be needed for potential future coronary bypass surgery.

The arterialization of a great saphenous vein left in situ (if superficially located) is also not a good choice, as from our observation its maturation frequently is insufficient.

Great Saphenous Vein Loop to Femoral Artery

Indication/prerequisites

- AV fistula of upper extremities not feasible.
- Implantation of prosthetic grafts contraindicated because of chronic septic foci (e.g., active osteomyelitis).

Approach

- Exposure of the great saphenous vein via longitudinal incisions from the saphenofemoral junction to just above the knee.
- Creation of a U-shaped subcutaneous tunnel.
- Distal transection of the great saphenous vein, pull out distal end of the vein through the inguinal incision, place vein in U-shaped tunnel.
- Create terminolateral anastomosis to common femoral artery (Fig. 3.108).

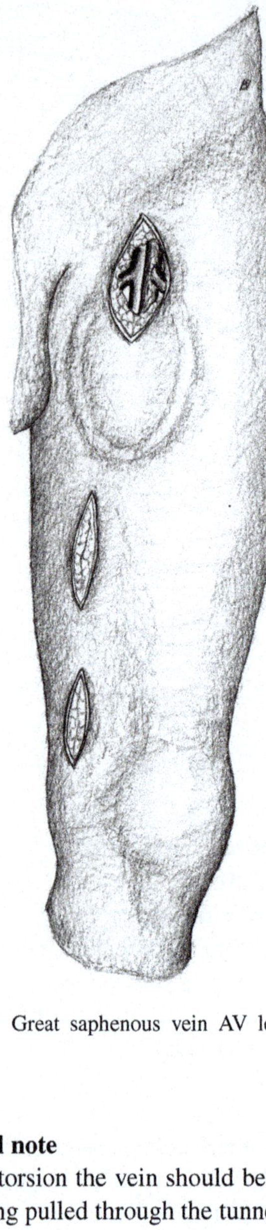

Fig. 3.108 Great saphenous vein AV loop to femoral artery

Technical note

To avoid torsion the vein should be tightly filled when being pulled through the tunnel.

Prognosis

Uncommon vascular access with good results.

Literature

Antoniou GA, Lazarides MK, Georgiadis GS, Sfyroeras GS, Nikolopoulos ES, Giannoukas AD (2009) Lower-extremity arteriovenous access for haemodialysis: a systematic review. Eur J Vasc Endovasc Surg 38: 365–372

Brescia MJ, Cimino JE, Appell K, Hurwich BJ, Scribner BH (1966) Chronic hemodialysis using venipuncture and a surgically created arteriovenous fistula. N Engl J Med 275:1089–1092

Dix FP, Khan Y, Al-Khaffaf H (2006) The brachial artery-basilic vein arterio-venous fistula in vascular access for haemodialysis – a review paper. Eur J Vasc Endovasc Surg 31:70–79

Dixon BS, Novak L, Fangman J (2002) Hemodialysis vascular access survival: upper-arm native arteriovenous fistula. Am J Kidney Dis 39:92–101

Dukkipati R, de Virgilio C, Reynolds T, Dhamija R (2011) Outcomes of brachial artery-basilic vein fistula. Semin Dial 24:220–230

Fitzgerald JT, Schanzer A, Chin AI, McVicar JP, Perez RV, Troppmann C (2004) Outcomes of upper arm arteriovenous fistulas for maintenance hemodialysis access. Arch Surg 139:201–208

Francis DM, Lu Y, Robertson AJ, Millar RJ, Amy J (2007) Two-stage brachio-basilic arteriovenous fistula for chronic haemodialysis access. ANZ J Surg 77: 150–155

Glass C, Porter J, Singh M, Gillespie D, Young K, Illig K (2010) A large-scale study of the upper arm basilic transposition for hemodialysis. Ann Vasc Surg 24: 85–91

Hossny A (2003) Brachiobasilic arteriovenous fistula: different surgical techniques and their effects on fistula patency and diaysis-related complications. J Vasc Surg 37:821–826

Huijbregts HJ, Bots ML, Wittens CH, Schrama YC, Moll FL, Blankestijn PJ, CIMINO study group (2008) Hemodialysis arteriovenous fistula patency revisited: results of aprospective, multicentre intiative. Clin J Am Soc Nephrol 3:714–19

Iyem H (2011) Early follow-up results of arteriovenous fistulae created for hemodialysis. Vasc Health Risk Manag 7:321–325

Jennings WC, Kindred MG, Broughan TA (2009) Creating radicephalic arteriovenous fistulas: technical and functional success. J Am Coll Surg 208:419–425

Kakkos SK, Andrzejewski T, Haddad JA, Haddad GK, Reddy DJ, Nypaver TJ, Scully MM, Schmid DL (2008) Equivalent secondary patency rates of upper extremity Vectra vascular access grafts and transposed brachial-basilic fistulas with aggressive access surveillance and endovascular treatment. J Vasc Surg 47: 407–414

Kakkos SK, Haddad GK, Weaver MR, Haddad RK, Scully MM (2010) Basilic vein transposition: what is the optimal technique? Eur J Vasc Endovasc Surg 39: 612–619

Kakkos SK, Haddad GK, Stephanou A, Haddad JA, Shepard AS (2011) Routine preoperative venous and arterial mapping increases both, construction and maturation rate of upper arm autogenous arteriovenous fistulae. Vasc Endovascular Surg 45:135–141

Koksoy C, Demirci RK, Balci D, Solak T, Köse SK (2009) Brachiobasilic versus brachiocephalic arteriovenous fistula: a prospective randomized study. J Vasc Surg 49:171–177

Korkut AK, Kosem M (2010) Superficialization of the basilic vein technique in brachiobasilic arteriovenous fistula: surgical experience of 350 cases during 4 years period. Ann Vasc Surg 24:762–767

Moossavi S, Tuttle AB, Vachharajani TJ, Plonk G, Bettmann MA, Majekodunmi O, Russell GB, Regan JD, Freedman BI (2008) Long-term outcomes of transposed basilic vein arteriovenous fistulae. Hemodial Int 12:80–84

Paulson KA, Gordon V, Flynn L, Lorelli D (2011) Modified two-stage basilic vein transposition for hemodialysis access. Am J Surg 202:184–187

Petzold M (2012) Die Tabatière-Fistel – av-Gefäßzugang der Wahl. Gefäßchirurgie 17:766–773

Pflederer TA, Kwok S, Ketel BL, Pilgram T (2008) A comparison of transposed brachiobasilic fistualae with nontransposed fistulae and grafts in the Fistula First era. Semin Dial 21:357–363

Rajan DK, Bunston S, Misra S, Pinto R, Lok CE (2004) Dysfunctional autogenous hemodialysis fistulas: outcomes after angioplasty-are there clinical predictors of patency? Radiology 232:508–515

Rao RK, Azin GD, Hood DB, Rowe VL, Kohl RD, Katz SG, Weaver FA (2004) Basilic vein transpostion fistula: a good option for maintaining hemodialysis access site options? J Vasc Surg 39:1043–1047

Rooijens PP, Tordoir JH, Stijnen T, Burgmans JP, de Smet AA, Yo TI (2004) Radiocephalic wrist arteriovenous fistula for hemodialysis: metaanalysis indicates a high primary failure rate. Eur J Vasc Endovasc Surg 28: 583–589

Rooijens PP et al (2005) Autogenous radial-cephalic or prosthetic brachial-antecubital forearm loop AVF in patients with compromised vessels? A randomized, multicenter study of the patency of primary hemodialysis access. J Vasc Surg 42:481–486

Scholz H, Bürger K, Precht K, Matthes G (1990) Subclavio-jugularer av-Shunt (Colliershunt) für die Hämodialyse. Angio 12:151–154

Segal JH, Kayler LK, Henke P, Merion RM, Leavey S, Campbell DA Jr (2003) Vascular access outcomes using the transposed basilic vein arteriovenous fistula. Am J Kidney Dis 42:151–157

Sekar N (1993) Snuff-Box arteriovenous fistulas. Int Surg 78:250–251

Son HJ, Min SK, Min SI, Park YJ, Ha J, Kim SJ (2010) Evaluation of the efficacy of the forearm basilic vein transposition arteriovenous fistula. J Vasc Surg 51: 667–672

Srivastava A, Sharma S (2011) Hemodialysis vascular access options after a failed Brescia-Cimino arteriovenous fistula. Indian J Urol 2:163–168

Taghizadeh A, Dasgupta P, Khan MS, Taylor J, Koffman G (2003) Long-term outcomes of brachiobasilic transpositioin fistula for hemodialysis. Eur J Vasc Endovasc Surg 26:670–672

Weale AR, Bevis P, Neary WD, Lear PA, Mitchell DC (2007) A comparison between transposed brachiobasilic arteriovenous fistulas and prosthetic brachioaxillary access grafts for vascular access for hemodialysis. J Vasc Surg 46:997–1004

Weale AR, Bevis P, Neary WD, Boyes S, Morgan JD, Lear PA, Mitchell DC (2008) Radiocephalic and brachiocephalic arteriovenous fistula outcomes in the elderly. J Vasc Surg 47:144–150

Weiswasser JM, Kellicut D, Arora S, Sidawy AN (2004) Strategies of arteriovenous dialysis access. Semin Vasc Surg 17:10–18

Woo K, Farber A, Doros G, Killeen K, Kohanzadeh S (2007) Evaluation of the efficacy of the transposed upper arm arteriovenous fistula: a single institutional review of 190 basilic and cephalic vein transposition procedures. J Vasc Surg 46:94–99

Yilmaz M, Senkaya I, Saba D, Bicer M (2007) Long-term outcomes of basilic vein transposition fistula for hemodialysis. Vasa 36:29–32

AV Shunts

4

The use of prosthetic material for an AV access is indicated, if:

1. There are no suitable veins for an AV fistula.
2. The expected period of time required before the AV fistula is ready for puncture exceeds 6–8 weeks or is not predictable with the patient already needing hemodialysis.
3. The comparatively more complex surgery using native vessels (e.g., transposition of the arterialized basilic vein of the upper arm) might not be worthwhile if the patient's life expectancy is limited.

The certain availability and the defined dimensions are definite advantages of prosthetic grafts. The disadvantages of all prosthetic materials, however, are their higher thrombogenicity and their susceptibility to infection. The shunt experience presented in this book exclusively concerns vascular ePTFE prostheses produced by the Impra/Bard company.

4.1 Pathophysiology

From a functional point of view, AV shunts have three segments:

- Arterial anastomosis
- Puncturable segment
- Venous anastomosis

4.1.1 Arterial Anastomosis

As with AV fistulas, the proximal part of the artery dilates depending on flow, duration of use, and other individual factors. In contrast to veins, the resistance of prostheses is determined by their metrics, and does not change over the course of time. The dilation of an afferent artery feeding an AV shunt prosthesis is usually less pronounced than that of an artery feeding a native AV fistula. There is however an increase in shunt flow as well because of a diminishing inflow resistance. A lateroterminal anastomosis between a small diameter artery (e.g., 3–4 mm) and large diameter prosthesis (e.g., 7–8 mm) will result in an effective stenosis in 5–35 % (Fig. 4.1a, Asif et al. 2005; Bozof et al. 2008; Choudhury et al. 1995).

If a narrow (4-mm) graft segment is used at the anastomosis, we have not seen a stenosis in more than 4,000 AV shunts over the last 30 years. In the inflow region of the prosthesis a thrill originates, which is caused by low frequency pressure changes (20–50 Hz) and which can also be palpated. This thrill can be noted over the whole length of the prosthesis up to the venous anastomosis and sometimes even beyond; sometimes it is also found in the proximal and distal segments of the artery.

4.1.2 Puncturable Segment

Depending on the time that has passed since implantation and additional individual factors, there is a varied migration of fibroblasts from outside the wall of the ePTFE prosthesis into its lumen. Each puncture destroys the local structure of the prosthesis. At the puncture sites, connective

H. Scholz, *Arteriovenous Access Surgery*,
DOI 10.1007/978-3-642-41139-7_4, © Springer-Verlag Berlin Heidelberg New York 2015

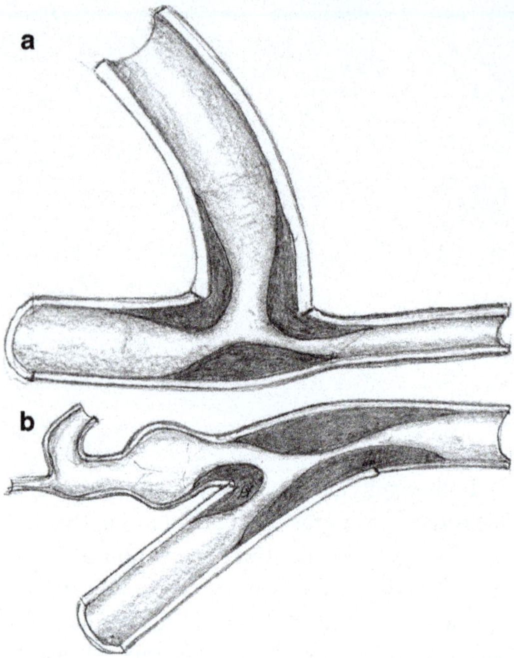

Fig. 4.1 Stenosis at the (**a**) arterial and (**b**) venous anastomosis

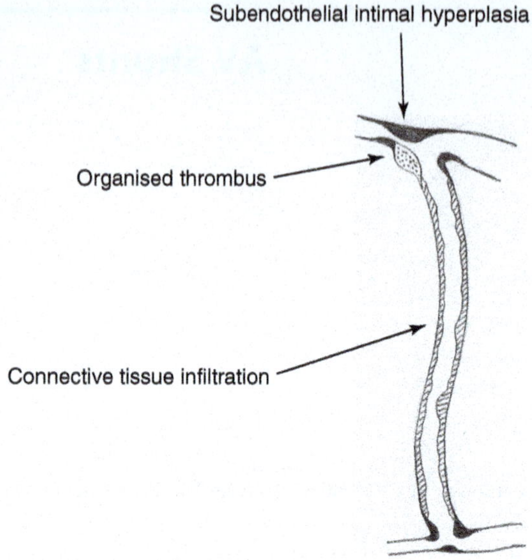

Fig. 4.2 Predilection sites for intravasal tissue proliferation

tissue (sometimes with capillaries) sprouts into the lumen. With multiple punctures close to each other, the whole wall structure of the affected area will be destroyed, leaving mainly scar tissue behind. It is in such areas that aneurysms with wall-adherent thrombi will develop.

4.1.3 Venous Anastomosis

Thrombosis is the most frequent complication of AV grafts. Most frequently it is due to a stenosis of the venous anastomosis caused by hard connective tissue proliferation (Fig. 4.1b).

4.1.4 Tissue Proliferation Inside the AV Shunt

When performing redo surgery, tissue proliferation concerning both anastomoses and the inside of the prosthetic graft can be observed. Irrespective of its location it almost always looks the same. It is a hard, partially callous, grayish-white tissue. In the literature it is frequently referred to as intimal hyperplasia or pseudointima. From a pathogenetic perspective there are three distinct forms as discussed below (Fig. 4.2).

Anastomotic Region of Artery and Vein

Tissue proliferation in this area is likely to be caused by hemodynamic irritation. Intimal hyperplasia is not a suitable term, as this implies hyperplasia of the whole intima consisting of both endothelium and basement membrane. Histology, however, shows a proliferation between endothelium and basement membrane. Therefore we prefer to call this phenomenon subendothelial fibrosis or *subendothelial intimal hyperplasia* (*SIH*). That is what it will subsequently be referred to.

Dead Water Zones Around the Anastomosis

Dead water zones of the vessel are areas which are hardly perfused. Due to the slow or stagnating flow, coagulation is activated locally. These zones are most frequently observed with ill-dimensioned anastomoses in the prosthetic part of the venous anastomosis. Thrombotic material will be transformed into connective tissue, which macroscopically resembles the material described above. The term "pseudointima" is misleading, as it is *organized thrombotic material*.

Prosthesis

After varying periods of time following implantation, frequently circular wall adhesions of hard, grayish-white matter can be observed within ePTFE prostheses. Histologically it is connective tissue. This material, which is also difficult or impossible to remove, can be found everywhere in the prosthesis, even in areas which have not been punctured. The pore size of a prosthesis offers no barrier against the cellular migration from outside. This phenomenon may preferably be characterized as *connective tissue infiltration*.

4.2 Hemodynamics of Arteriovenous Grafts

The following morphologic and functional differences exist between a prosthetic AV graft and an AV fistula:

- The metrics of the anastomotic aperture are defined with prosthetic grafts. (A venous anastomosis tends to dilate in the course of time.)
- The flow resistance of a prosthesis is determined by its metrics. Conversely the flow resistance of a vein decreases following its dilation.
- When using prosthetic grafts, there is an additional terminolateral anastomosis between prosthesis and vein.
- Mostly there is a primarily higher flow in a prosthetic AV shunt than in an AV fistula.

This leads to even more unphysiological flow conditions with grafts at both the arterial and the venous anastomoses. According to the literature (Fillinger et al. 1990; Fung and Liu 1993; Hofstra et al. 1995; Lemson et al. 2000; Liepsch 1989, 1998; Longest and Kleinstreuer 2000; Ojha et al. 1995; Shu and Hwang 1991; Sivanesan et al. 1999; Sottiurai 1990; Tordoir 1999; Zarins et al. 1996) the following hemodynamic conditions favor tissue proliferation in the anastomotic region:

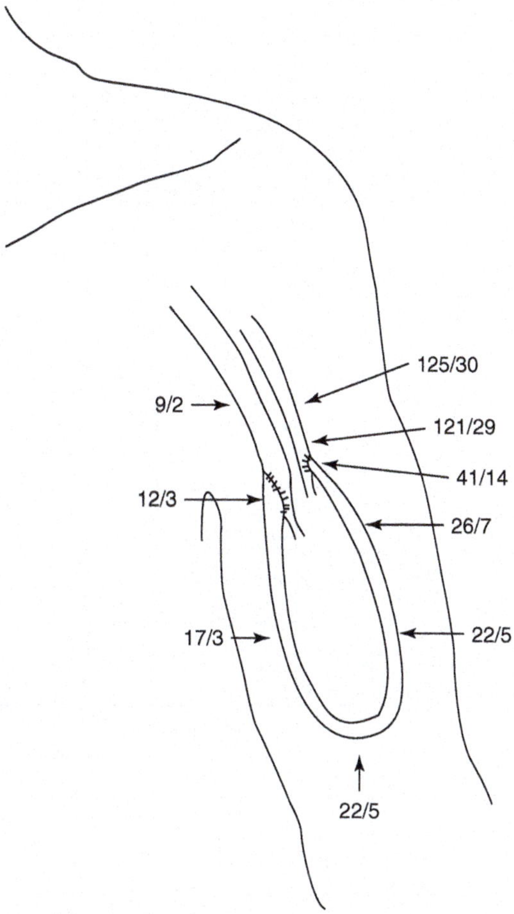

Fig. 4.3 Pressure gradient inside a loop graft (mmHg)

- Elevated and permanently changing shear of the vascular wall
- Oscillations of the flow (pulse synchronous change of flow direction with new orientation of the endothelium)
- Changing pressure load of the venous wall,
- Secondary flow
- Dead water zones at the venous anastomosis

The extent of this unphysiological flow depends on the flow rate. Animal experiments have shown that the degree of a stenosis increases with increasing flow rates (Fillinger et al. 1990). In the region of a sudden pressure drop (Figs. 4.3 and 4.4a), flow disturbances arise which lead to vibrations that are transmitted perivascularly (Fillinger et al. 1990). Palpation of this thrill is

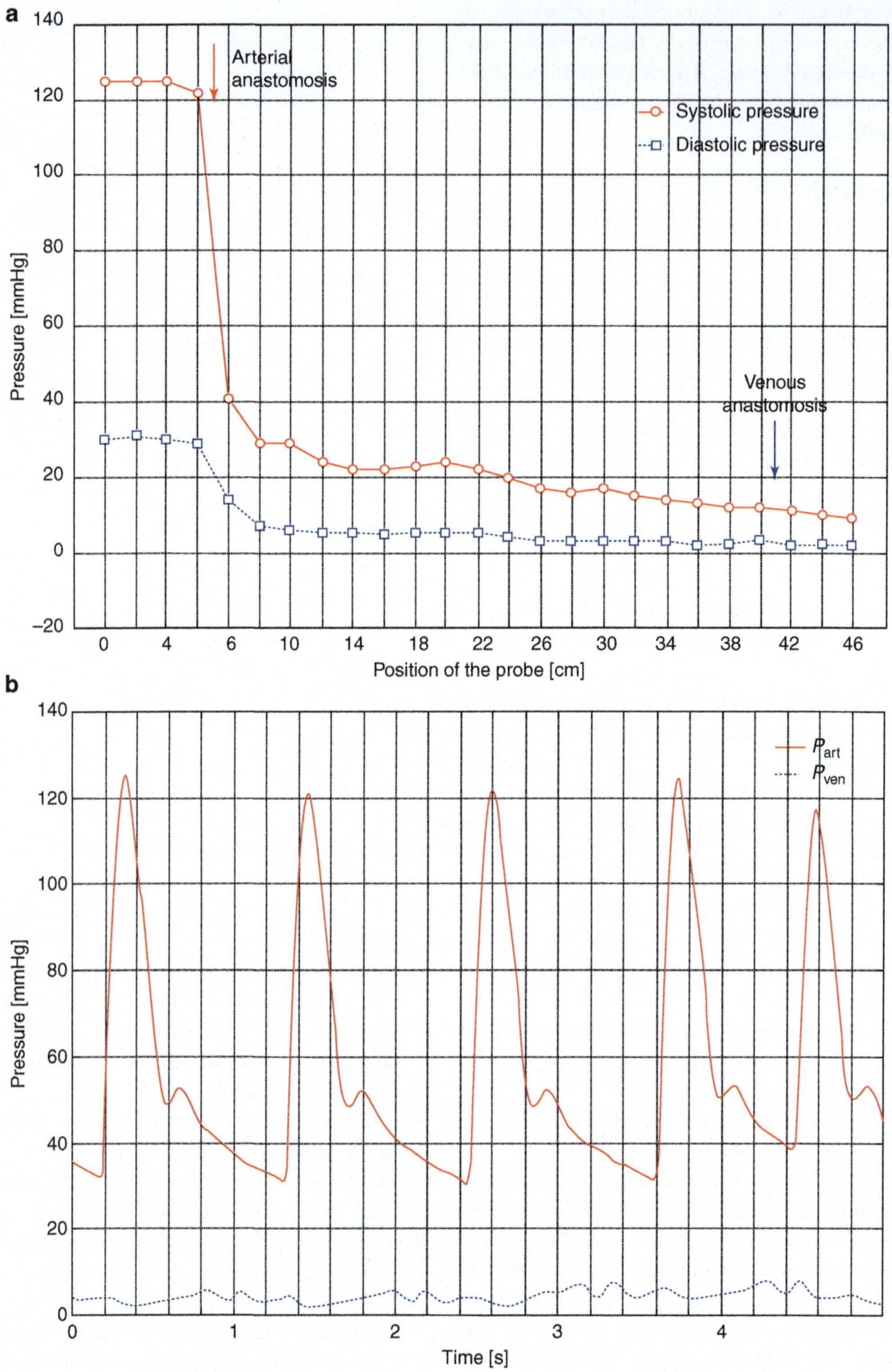

Fig. 4.4 (**a**) Pressure gradient inside a loop graft: pressure dependent on the position of the probe. It is introduced at the apex of the loop and then advanced up to the arterial lumen. Then the venous side of the loop is examined in the same way. For the sketch we assumed a continuous process (i.e., probe-carrying catheter starts in the artery and ends in the vein). (**b**) Pressure inside the artery and 5 cm downstream from the venous anastomosis (same patient as in **a**). In the vein there is a slight pulsation, too

recommended to verify the proper functioning of an AV access for hemodialysis (Richman and Wilson 1991).

In the following, the results of flow dynamic measurements and numerical simulations from the arterial to the venous anastomoses of AV interposition grafts are presented.

4.2.1 Pressure Curves Within an AV Interposition Graft

The aorta and the large arteries determine around 19 % of the resistance of the entire vascular system whilst terminal arteries, arterioles, and capillaries define 75 % (Affeld and Kertscher 2011; Schmidt and Thews 2000). This entails a pressure drop in the venous system to less than 10 mmHg.

The presence of an AV access almost excludes the pressure-lowering part of the vascular system. The high energy of the arterial system directly reaches the venous low pressure system. Figure 4.3 shows the pressure readings within a loop-shaped AV shunt of the upper arm depending on the position of the pressure probe. There is a rapid decrease in pressure within the graft. Already 1 cm downstream from the arterial anastomosis, the systolic pressure drops to a third of its initial value. Figure 4.4 shows the corresponding pressure curves. Pulsation of the venous pressure can still be observed several centimeters downstream from the venous anastomosis.

4.2.2 Influence of the Sudden Change of Diameter Between a Narrow Artery and a 7-mm Prosthesis on Blood Flow

In the literature, the incidence of stenoses of the arterial anastomoses ranges from 5 to 35 % (Asif et al. 2005; Bozof et al. 2008; Choudhury et al. 1995). These stenoses are mainly caused by SIH. We investigated the influence of a sudden change of diameter between an artery and a prosthesis following the clinical observation of a stenosis in the transition zone between a 3-mm artery and a 7-mm prosthesis (Huhle et al. 2002; Krueger et al. 2004).

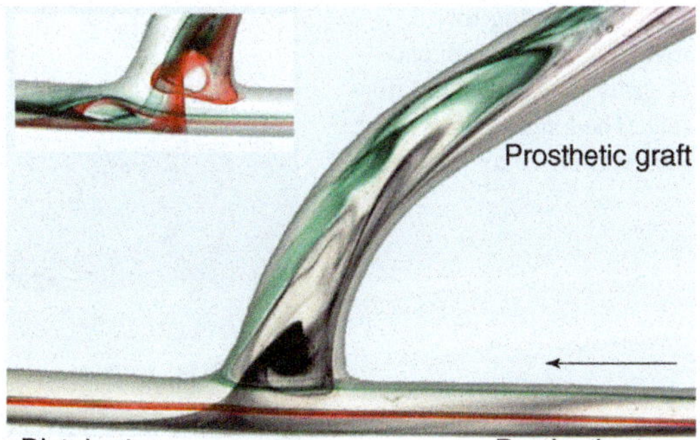

Fig. 4.5 Flow visualization with direct anastomosis of a small caliber artery and a large caliber prosthesis. The *arrow* marks the direction of the inflow

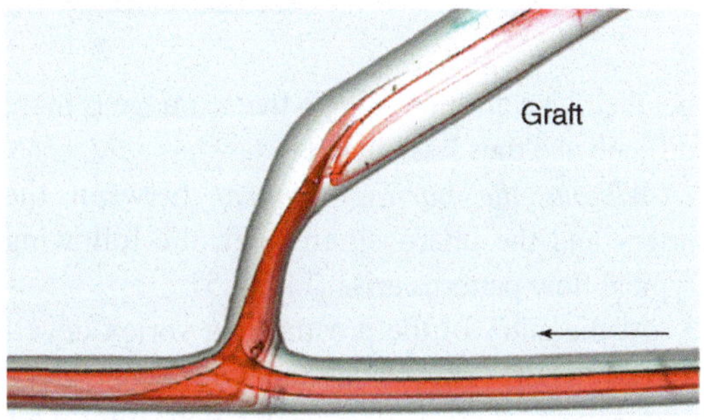

Fig. 4.6 Flow visualization with interposition of a narrow segment (length 10 mm) between a small lumen artery and a large lumen graft

The typical flow patterns between a 4-mm artery and a 7-mm prosthesis are depicted in Fig. 4.5. Figure 4.6 shows the same situation with an additional narrow intercalated 4-mm segment upstream from the 7-mm prosthesis.

The experiments were conducted using a pulsatile flow system as described in the literature (Petzold 2001; Huhle 2002; see Chap. 21). The metrics of the models corresponded to those of straight interposition grafts of the upper arm. The diameters of artery and vein varied over a wide range. For the figures we present here, we selected a 7-mm prosthesis and a 4-mm artery. The narrow segment started with a diameter of 4 mm which conically merged into the prosthesis. Dye injection helped visualize flow patterns. For better illustration an (atypical) flow rate of 100 mL/min was chosen. Higher flow rates do not change the flow patterns,

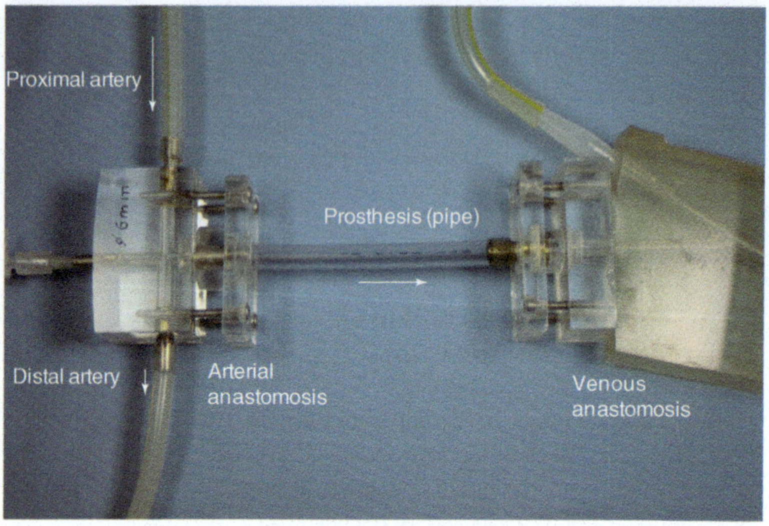

Fig. 4.7 Setting for investigating the influence of graft length on shunt flow rate. The length of the pipe varied from 10 to 50 cm

but their visualization using a freeze image is more difficult and thus less obvious.

Without the narrow segment between the artery and the interposition graft, the following typical flow patterns arise (Fig. 4.5):

- At the entry of the prosthesis a vortex develops whose expansion and rotational speed increases with an increasing flow rate. This vortex's rotation slows down as it drifts towards the proximal anastomotic angle during diastole (lower part of Fig. 4.5, slightly altered position of the injection needle).
- Maximum flow velocity is prevalent in the central stream which runs from the proximal to the distal artery. Only a few millimeters downstream from the distal anastomotic margin, a partial backflow develops during systole (as can be seen on the arterial floor). This backflow induces a deflection of the central stream towards the anastomotic aperture at the distal anastomotic angle.
- The lateral stream on the arterial floor runs into the distal artery. During systole its collision with the backflow fraction of the central stream leads to its perpendicular deflection from the arterial floor to the entry of the prosthesis. The point of impact of this lateral stream shifts distally during diastole. It also shows pronounced pulse-synchronous oscillations.
- Both phenomena increase as the difference in diameter between the artery and the interposition graft increases.

If a narrow segment (length 4 mm, diameter 10 mm) is inserted between artery and graft, the following changes of flow phenomena occur (Fig. 4.6):

- The vortex at the entry into the prosthesis near the anastomotic aperture vanishes.
- In the region of the conical widening of the prosthesis, a stationary vortex develops due to the flow detachment from the prosthetic wall.
- The oscillating changes in flow direction on the arterial floor diminish considerably. (The reasons are the altered metrics of the anastomosis.)

Lengthening of the narrow segment does not entail a different quality of the flow patterns (Krueger et al. 2001).

The narrow segment reduces unphysiological flow in the anastomosis. The flow oscillations on the arterial floor diminish while the vortex at the entry vanishes. Both phenomena reduce the strain on the arterial endothelial cells.

4.2.3 Influence of the Design and Length of a Graft on Flow Rate

The knowledge of the influence of the prosthesis length on shunt flow is clinically important. For our experiments on the influence of the design and length of a graft prosthesis we used a model pulsatile flow system as shown in Fig. 4.7. For these experiments, the arterial anastomosis did not have a narrow segment. Straight pipes with diameters of

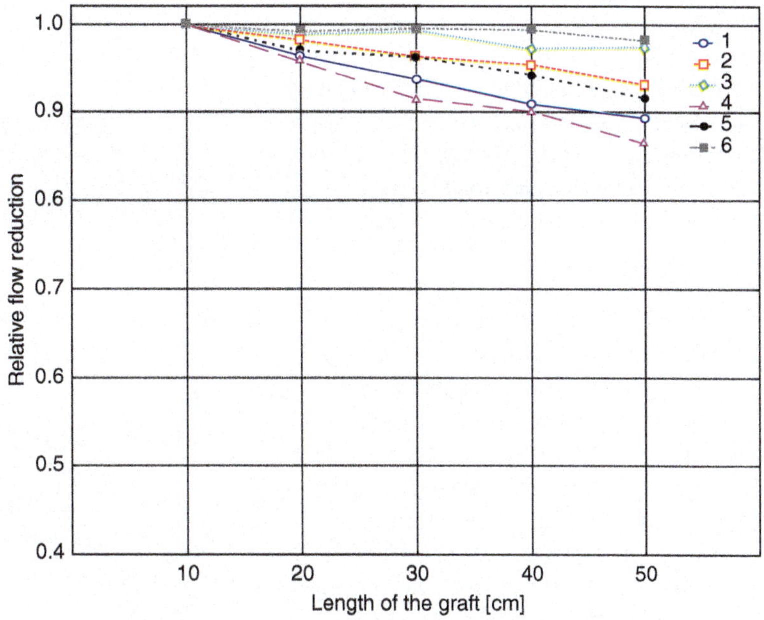

Fig. 4.8 Relative flow reduction dependent on the length of a straight AV graft. For curves 1–3 the arterial diameter was 4 mm, but 7 mm for curves 4–6. Graft diameters were 5 mm (curves 1 and 4), 6 mm (curves 2 and 5), and 7 mm (curves 3 and 6)

5, 6, and 7 mm connected the arterial to the venous model anastomosis. The pipes'lengths varied from 10 to 50 cm. To simulate loop grafts we placed the pipes in bent mountings with radii of curvature of 30, 45, or 60 mm. We used two different models with arterial diameters of either 4 or 7 mm.

Figure 4.8 shows a summary of the readings at a mean pressure of 100 mmHg. The readings of respective combinations of arterial diameters and interposition grafts were related to a standardized pipe length of 10 cm. The curve in Fig. 4.8 illustrates that the length of an interposed graft hardly influences the shunt flow. With 7-mm prosthetic grafts the maximum mean flow hardly changes for increasing lengths of the grafts (curves 3 and 6). A prosthetic diameter of 5 mm influenced length-dependent shunt flow more than other diameters (curves 1 and 4). Still the impact remains small, showing a decrease in flow of only 13 % as the respective lengths change from 10 cm to 50 cm. In a clinical situation a 5-mm prosthesis to a 7-mm artery would be highly unlikely. With the most frequently used 7-mm prostheses, the influence of their lengths on flow rates in the interposition graft may be neglected.

In comparison with a straight graft, a loop does not change the flow rate. Even a decrease of the radius of curvature from 60 to 30 mm changes the flow by less than 1 % (mean of all readings under three different arterial pressures, and combinations of diameters as described above). Therefore we do not show these results. The influence of the length of a prosthesis on flow characteristics that might favor thrombosis was not examined.

4.2.4 Venous Anastomosis

Progressive stenoses of the venous anastomosis are the most frequent causes of prosthetic access failure. We have examined the flow in the venous anastomosis for different constellations:

1. Comparison between a conventional terminolateral anastomosis and a prosthetic anastomosis whose venous side shows a bulb-shaped patch design (patch prosthesis/patch anastomosis; Fig. 4.32).
2. Finding the adequate patch size for different venous diameters.
3. Not or incorrectly trimmed patch prosthesis.
4. Influence of a venous side branch near the anastomosis (ligation recommended?)
5. Influence of the angle between prosthesis and vein.
6. Influence of inflow radius with loop grafts.
7. High grade stenosis on the venous floor of a conventional terminolateral anastomosis

(starting point for further stenoses of the venous runoff path?)

For these examinations we used both transparent silicone casts in the pulsatile flow system and numerical simulations (Chap. 21). There were identical boundary conditions:

- Duration of the pulsatile cycle: 1 s (corresponds to a pulse rate of 60 min^{-1}).
- Prosthesis entry: systolic flow rate 1,500 mL/min with Reynolds number *Re* 1,389, and mean flow 700 mL/min with *Re* 648.
- The distally-directed venous outflow is one-third of the inflow into the prosthesis. Two-thirds remain for the centrally-directed venous outflow. This flow distribution mirrors a frequent situation found in vivo. It is caused by increasingly insufficient distal venous valves with ensuing venous dilatation (Gordon 1996).
- Fluid characteristics: density $\rho = 1.1$ g/cm^3, dynamic viscosity $\eta = 3.6$ mPa·s.

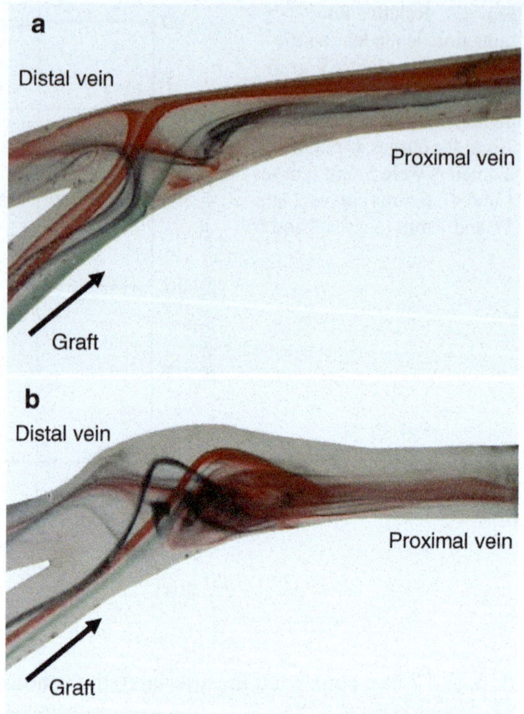

Fig. 4.9 (**a**) Flow visualization in a conventional terminolateral anastomosis. (**b**) Flow visualization in a patch anastomosis

Comparison Between a Conventional Terminolateral Anastomosis and a Patch Anastomosis

Since 1998 an ePTFE prosthesis (Bard, Inc) with a patch area for the venous anastomosis that we developed has been available. Hereafter we refer to it as patch prosthesis.

Visualization of the Flow in a Pulsatile Flow System

The observed flow patterns are highly complex. Figures 4.9 and 4.10 summarize their main characteristics. After entry into the recipient vein, the flow is diverted to the venous outer wall in both models (conventional and patch anastomosis). In the conventional anastomosis a stagnation point occurs (Fig. 4.9a).

There the flow is divided according to the configuration (one-third distally, two-thirds proximally). The location of the stagnation point is time-dependent. During the acceleration phase it moves upstream towards the distal vein. During diastole it moves downstream to the proximal vein. In the patch anastomosis, the flow is also divided, but there is no stagnation point (Fig. 4.9). Its main characteristic is the

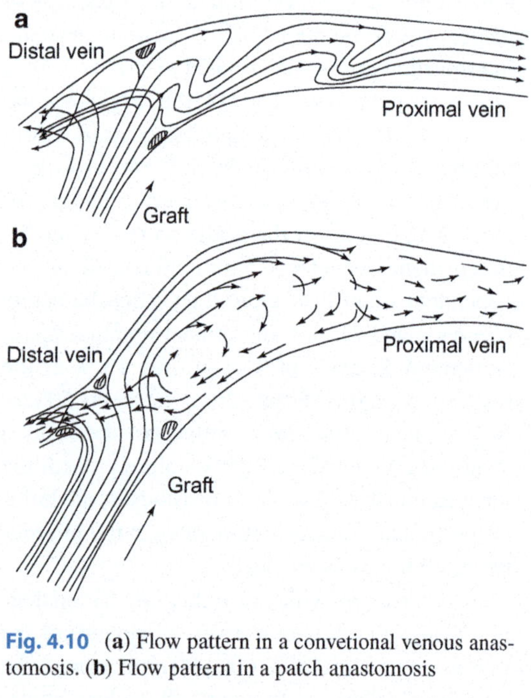

Fig. 4.10 (**a**) Flow pattern in a convetional venous anastomosis. (**b**) Flow pattern in a patch anastomosis

flow detachment from the venous wall and the development of a large vortex whose rotational speed is slow. This vortex keeps its sense of rotation during the entire simulated cycle without oscillations of the flow. The mixing of the dyes indicates a better wash out effect, which leads to a calmed down outflow in the proximal vein. Size and location of the vortex depend on the flow rate. As a result a significant reduction or disappearance of the thrill may also be observed clinically with patients (Petzold 2001).

Numerical Simulation

The numerical simulations were carried out with a non-Newtonian fluid (Cross 1965). The viscosity at zero shear rate was defined as 120 mPa·s, and the infinite shear rate viscosity at 3.6 mPa·s. Furthermore, the vessel walls were defined by their no slip condition: zero velocity at the walls (see Chap. 20).

Compared to the other pictures of the venous anatomosis, the results of the numerical simulation are shown vertically mirrored. The lowest readings are shown in dark blue, and the highest in red. If not stated otherwise, the flow is shown at the systolic maximum, as then the differences between the anastomotic configurations are most pronounced. The side of the prosthesis which faces the vein is called the inner side. The floor of the vein lies opposite to the entry into the prosthesis.

Distribution of Velocity in the Symmetry Plane

With both anastomotic configurations the main flow is deflected to the proximal vein according to the flow distribution. As the visualization is restricted to the symmetry plane, Fig. 4.11a renders only a limited impression of the complexity of the flow. The symmetry plane is the plane that yields two mirrored halves of the model. Once again a stagnation point can be seen directly on the floor of the vein, where the flow is divided into a proximal and distal portion. The highest velocities are at the venous floor. The stagnation point migrates during the simulated heart cycle. During the acceleration phase it moves downstream, and in diastole distally. By contrast, the distribution of velocities in the patch anastomosis is much more harmonious on the floor of the recipient vein (Fig. 4.11). Between the floor of the venous wall and the jet stream marked in yellow there is a narrow band of low velocities. This indicates a distinctively lower shear at the venous wall. There is no stagnation of the flow (dark blue). After entry into the anastomosis the flow is detached from the venous wall while forming a vortex. This vortex persists during the entire simulated heart cycle (Fig. 4.12) without further flow oscillations and leads to an improved wash out effect.

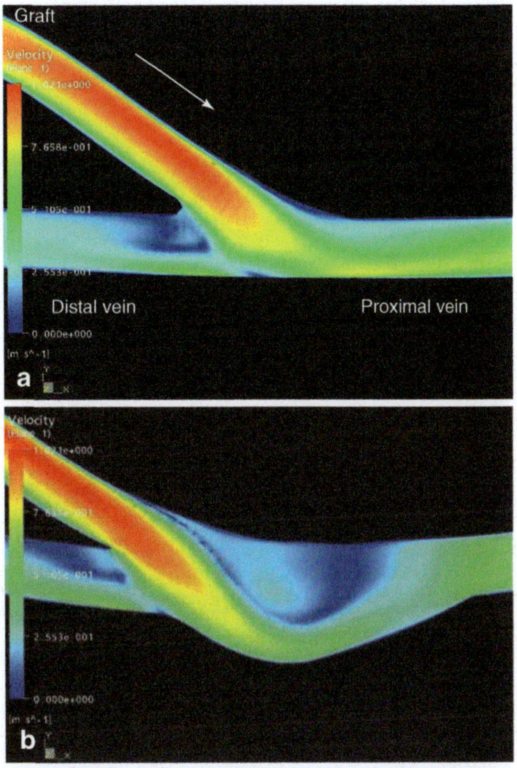

Fig. 4.11 (**a**) Velocity distribution in a conventional terminolateral anastomosis. The *arrow* marks the direction of the inflow (valid for all figures in Sect. 4.2.4, and for all vessel denominations unless stated otherwise). (**b**) Velocity distribution in a patch anastomosis

Velocity Vectors

A cross section area perpendicular to the venous floor is the origin of these vectors in the middle of the conventional anastomosis in Fig. 4.12a. The vectors demonstrate the formation of a secondary flow (Chap. 20) perpendicular to the main

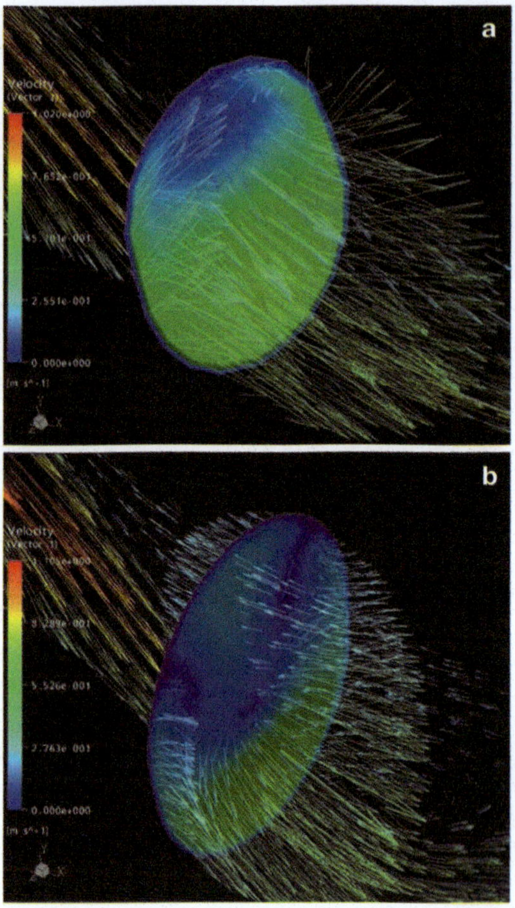

Fig. 4.12 (**a**) Velocity vectors in a conventional anastomosis. These vectors originate from a cross section area perpendicular to the venous floor in the middle region of the anastomosis. (**b**) Velocity vectors originating from the cross section area in a patch anastomosis

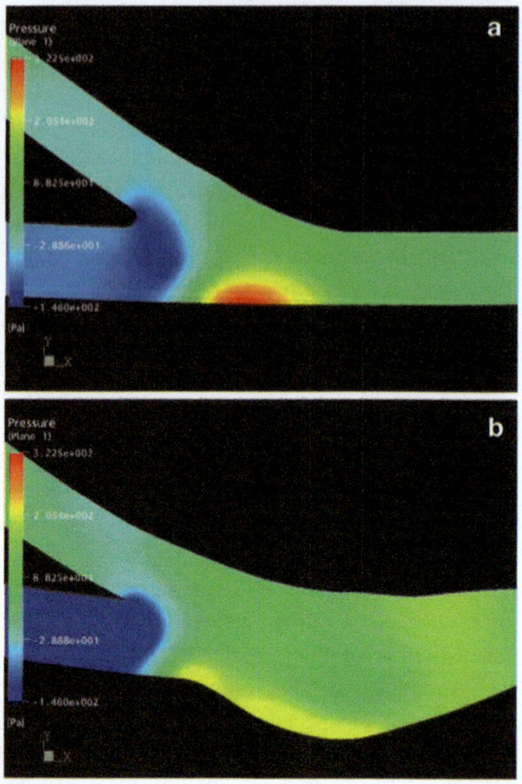

Fig. 4.13 Pressure distribution (**a**) in a conventional anastomosis and (**b**) in a patch anastomosis

flow. The direction of the vectors changes with the ongoing cycle. Thus an additional stimulus would be exerted on the venous endothelium (change of flow direction) in vivo. In the patch anastomosis, the 3D shape of the said vortex is depicted in Fig. 4.12b.

Static Pressure in the Symmetry Plane

The figures show the distribution of the relative static pressure in the anastomotic regions. The normalized static pressure is set to that of the proximal exit for comparison. Thus only the increase in pressure caused by the flow deceleration is depicted. In the conventional anastomosis, there is a local pressure maximum on the venous floor (Fig. 4.13a). Also taking into account the velocity distribution (Fig. 4.11a), it becomes clear that here a flow stagnation occurs. The kinetic energy of the flow is transformed into local pressure strain on the venous wall (for estimates of the absolute values see Chap. 20). In the patch anastomosis, the increase in pressure is much less pronounced. The enlarged anastomotic space can accommodate the high energy flow and conduct it to the vortex described above (Fig. 4.13b).

Wall Shear Stress

Figure 4.14 shows the distribution of the wall shear stress. This stress is distinctly lower in the patch anastomosis (Krueger et al. 2002). The highest readings may be found in the conventional anastomosis on the floor of the recipient vein. They correspond to the high velocities of the proximal outflow (Fig. 4.11a).

Results of the Experiments Comparing a Conventional Terminolateral Anastomosis to a Patch Anatomosis

The bulb-shaped design of a patch anastomosis offers the following advantages over a conventional anastomosis:

- Better wash out effect of the anastomotic space.
- Calmed down outflow into the proximal vein.
- Less pressure strain on the venous wall in the anastomotic space.
- Lower shear stress.
- No flow oscillations (flow reversal) at the wall.

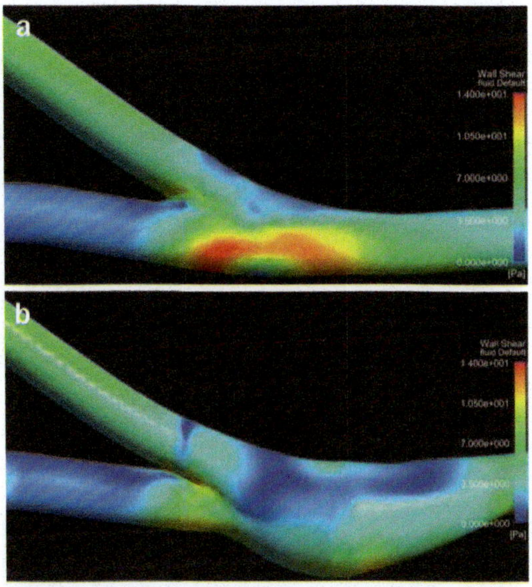

Fig. 4.14 Distribution of the wall shear stress (**a**) in a conventional anastomosis and (**b**) in a patch anastomosis

Investigations Concerning the Adaptation of the Patch Size to the Venous Diameter

In the pulsatile flow system we examined several constellations with different patch sizes and venous diameters between 3 and 9 mm so as to prove the advantages mentioned above as criteria for the correct anastomotic design. The findings show that only a patch whose dimensions are adapted to the respective venous diameter yields optimum hemodynamic results (no extra diagram). The lines printed on the commercially available ready-to-use patch graft exploit the results of these experiments to make the ideal trimming possible (Fig. 4.40).

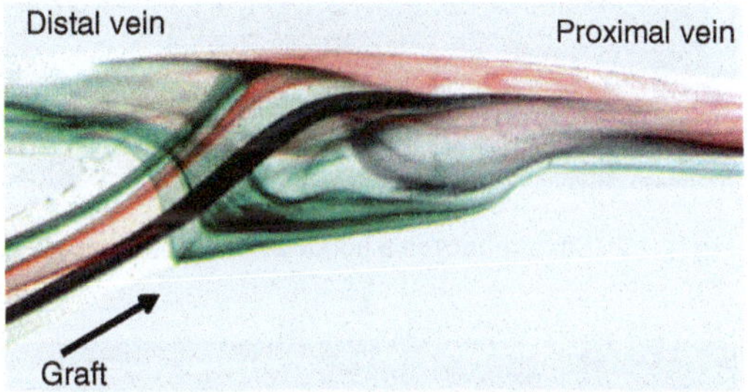

Fig. 4.15 Flow visualization in a hooded patch anastomosis

Investigations Concerning Anastomoses with Not or Incorrectly-Trimmed Patches

The desired effects of a patch anastomosis are closely linked to the correct design (size) of the patch which determines its hemodynamic characteristics. It is almost always necessary to trim the patch prosthesis. The diameter of the vein when it is dilated to the max determines the cut. A mismatched patch or a patch whose trim is too blunt cannot adopt the desired bulb-shaped, harmoniously tapering configuration, but results in an undesirably hooded anastomosis between the prosthetic patch and the vein (Figs. 4.14, 4.15, 4.16, 4.17, and 4.18).

Visualization of the Flow in a Pulsatile Flow System

We recreated an untrimmed model patch prosthesis. As with the conventional terminolateral anastomosis, there is a stagnation point (Fig. 4.15). The vortex detected in this kind of patch anastomosis is reduced. In the hooded region, the dye remains for a long time (dead

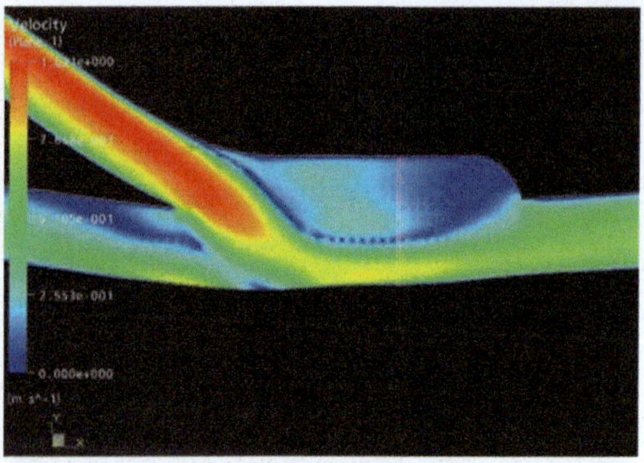

Fig. 4.16 Velocity distribution in a hooded patch anastomosis

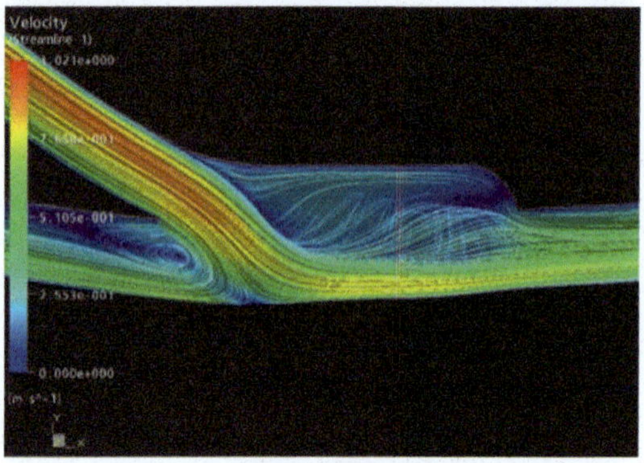

Fig. 4.17 Stream lines in a hooded patch anastomosis

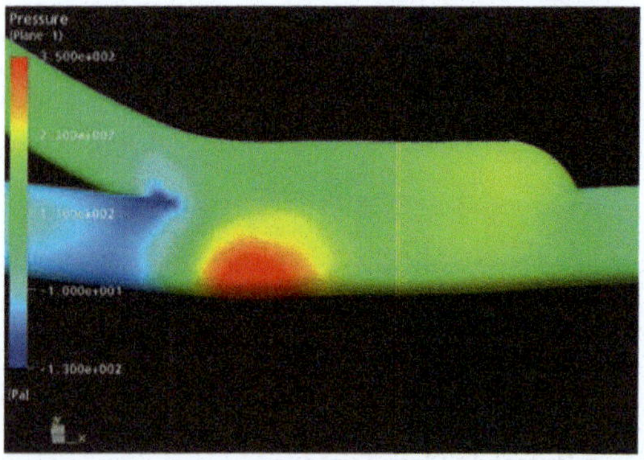

Fig. 4.18 Pressure distribution in a hooded patch anastomosis

water zone; Chap. 20). Dead water zones are known to be regions where thrombi preferentially form. The impact of the blood flow on the exterior venous wall is comparable to that in

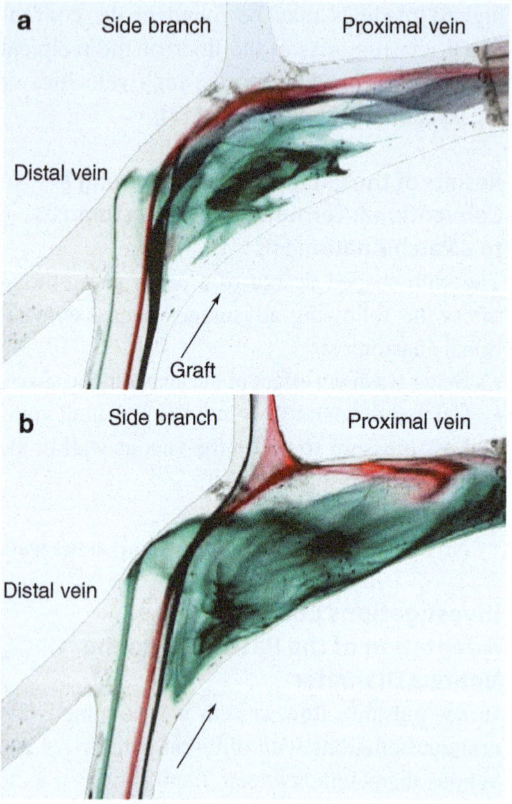

Fig. 4.19 Flow visualization in a patch anastomosis (**a**) with a closed side branch and (**b**) with an open side branch

a conventional anastomosis. The stress on the venous wall is not reduced.

Numerical Simulation

In a hooded patch anastomosis, velocities at the venous floor are higher than in a correctly-trimmed anastomosis (Fig. 4.16). In the hood the flow becomes separated from the outer wall. The resulting vortex is smaller than in correctly-trimmed patch prostheses. It only persists during systole. During the entire heart cycle, velocities are rather low (dead water zone). The stream lines (Fig. 4.17) show that there is only sparse movement. At the outer wall of the hood the fluid comes to a standstill. Figure 4.18 shows the pressure distribution at the anastomotic wall. The local pressure maximum on the venous floor corresponds to that of a conventional anastomosis. It results from the strong impact of the flow

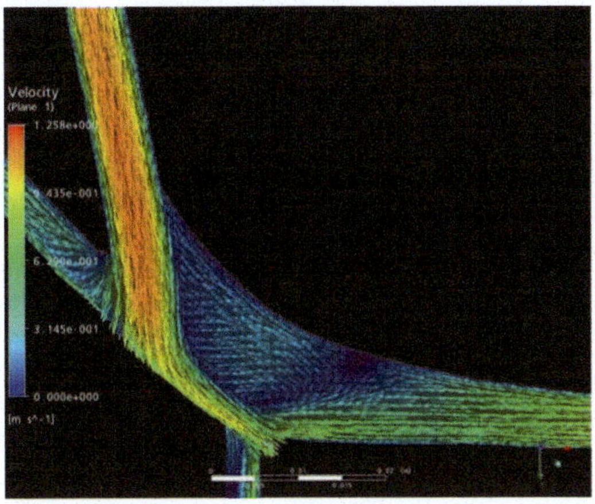

Fig. 4.20 Velocity vectors in a patch anastomosis with an open side branch

on the venous wall. The desired calming down of the flow does not occur.

> The precise harmonious trimming of the prosthetic patch is essential in order to obtain the desired hemodynamic advantages.

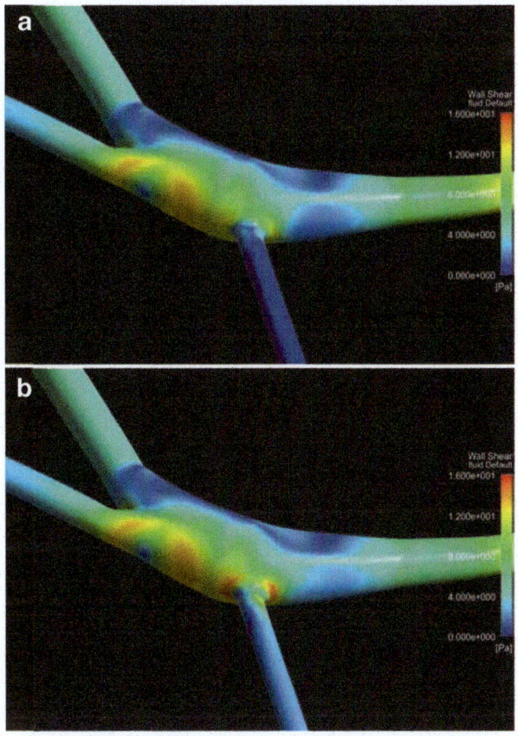

Fig. 4.21 Distribution of the wall shear stress in a patch anastomosis (**a**) with closed side branch and (**b**) with open side branch

Influence of a Venous Side Branch Close to the Anastomosis

The clinical observation that leaving a venous side branch may cause a high-grade stenosis near the venous anastomosis prompted our investigations of this situation in the model pulsatile flow system (Fig. 4.19). The results of the numerical simulations confirmed the results obtained in the circular flow system (Figs. 4.20 and 4.21). Both methods recorded hemodynamics in the anastomosis when the side branch was either open or closed. While the flow with a closed side branch (Figs. 4.19a and 4.21a) corresponds to the flow in an undisturbed patch anastomosis, (cf. Figs. 4.9b, 4.11b, and 4.14b), a totally different hemodynamic situation arises with an open venous side branch near the anastomosis (Figs. 4.19, 4.20, and 4.21b). It is characterized by:

- Disappearance of the bulb function.
- Lack of a calmed down flow.
- Occurrence of dead water zones.
- Impact of the main flow on the venous wall flow at the ostium of the side branch.
- Increased wall shear stress exerted on the venous wall at the ostium of the side branch.

These mechanical irritations favor subendothelial intimal hyperplasia.

Venous sidebranches near the anastomosis should be ligated.

Investigations on the Angle Between Prosthesis and Vein

With terminolateral anastomoses, the anastomotic angle influences hemodynamics (Staalsen et al. 1995). For investigations on the influence of the inflow angle between prosthesis and vein, we produced a model with an acute angle between the patch anastomosis and the vein (Fig. 4.22a).

An acute angle leads to the harmonization of the flow in the anastomosis. Again a large vortex

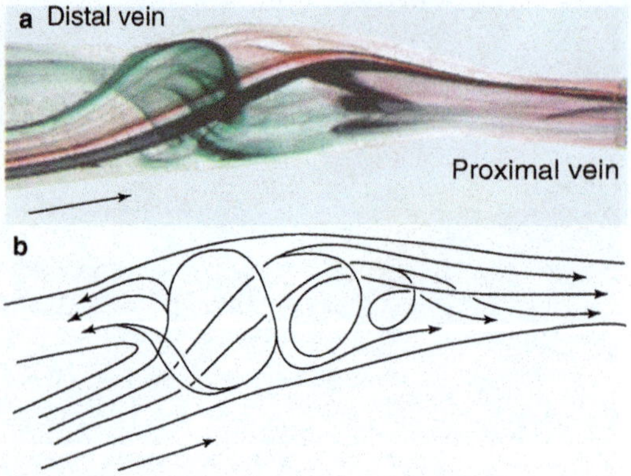

Fig. 4.22 (**a**) Flow visualization and (**b**) flow patterns in a patch anastomosis with an acute angle between graft and vein

becomes visible that persists over the entire simulated cardiac cycle and does not change its rotation. Small portions of the lateral flow (green) hit the venous wall during systole, divide, and flow both distally and laterally. The velocities of the flow portions close to the wall are considerably smaller than those of the central stream. That is why their impact is not critical. Over the course of the heart cycle all flow portions are deflected in a proximal direction and either directly follow the venous outflow or feed the large vortex from which the distal outflow originates during diastole (Fig. 4.22).

An acuter anastomotic angle leads to more physiologic flow changes.

Investigation of the Inflow Radius in Loop Grafts

The flow takes a different course when it is submitted to a radial acceleration in a curve (Munson et al. 1994). Inertia and centrifugal forces deflect the central flow to the outside, whereas at the inner side of the curve the central flow becomes detached. Furthermore there are secondary flows which are superimposed on the longitudinal flow. A picturesque description of this phenomenon can be found with aerial views or maps of meandering rivers like the Moselle (Chap. 20). These flow phenomena also occur in AV loops.

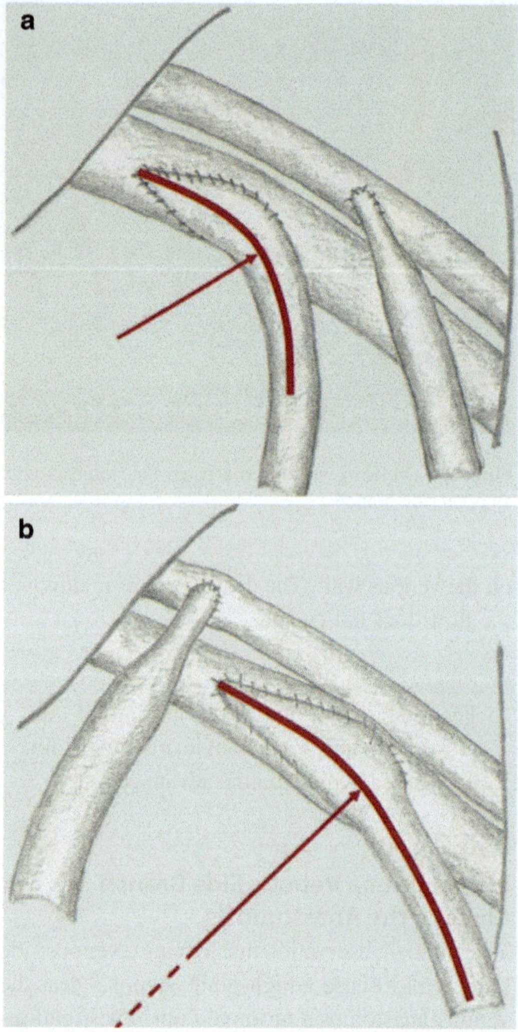

Fig. 4.23 Definition of the term "inflow radius". (**a**) Subclavian loop with a narrow inflow radius of the graft into the vein. (**b**) Wide inflow radius

The inflow radius of the graft as related to the vein influences the flow in the anastomosis. Figure 4.23 illustrates the term *inflow radius*. Figure 4.23a depicts a prosthesis with a small radius joined to the vein. The most expressed curvature is close to the anastomosis, whereas in Fig. 4.23b there is an expressed curvature directly downstream from the arterial anastomosis, but close to the vein the prosthesis shows a large radius. The angle between the vein and the

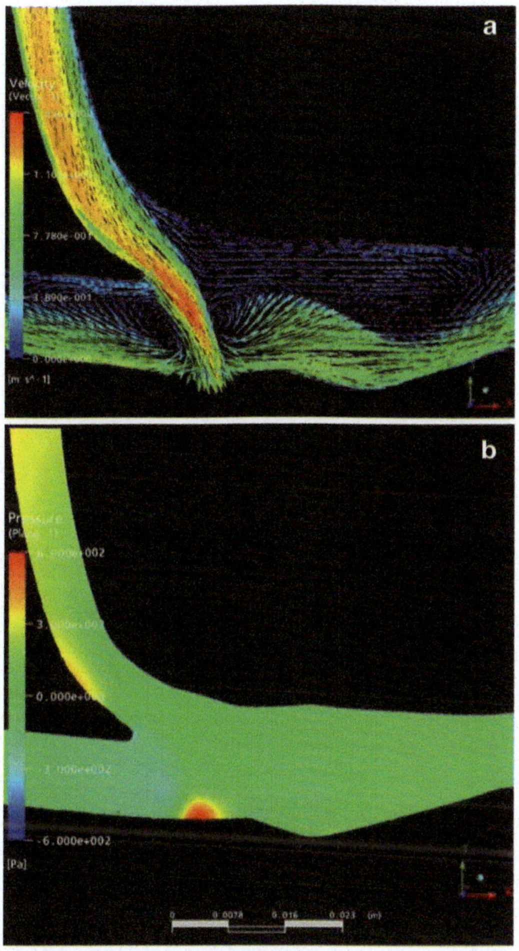

Fig. 4.24 (**a**) Velocity distribution within a narrow inflow radius anastomosis. The impact of the main flow on the venous floor is well visible. (**b**) Pressure load in a narrow influx. The site of maximum pressure corresponds to the impact site of the main flow.

venous end of the prosthesis (anastomotic angle) was the same in both situations for numerical simulations.

Velocity Vectors in the Symmetry Plane

In a small inflow radius prosthesis, a strong impact of the main flow on the venous floor can be observed at the systolic maximum. According to the preset flow division, the flow is directed mainly proximally. When entering the anastomosis there is a flow separation from the anastomosis, which persists during the whole cycle. Where the flow separation occurs there is also a retrograde flow. There are noteworthy flow portions directed to the inside of the anastomosis which originate from the impact area of the main flow on the venous floor. In contrast, in a large inflow radius prosthesis, a gentle deflection of the main flow into the anastomotic space and further into the proximal vein can be seen (comparable to Figs. 4.11a and 4.12b).

Pressure Load in the Symmetry Plane

Figure 4.24b shows the relative pressure distribution with regard to the proximal outlet of the anastomotic wall. Again a high strain at the systolic maximum can be seen. This maximum corresponds to the point of impact of the main flow. It shows a stagnation point.

Wall Shear Stress

In the small radius anastomosis, the wall shear stress is elevated over a larger area and a longer period of time especially at the sharp curvature and on the floor of the distal outflow path (Krüger and Scholz 2008).

The inflow radius of loop grafts should be as large as possible. A small inflow radius counteracts the advantages of a patch anastomosis.

Influence of a Pre-existing Stenosis in a Terminolateral Anastomosis on the Outflow Path

The mechanisms why multiple stenoses develop in the venous outflow path are not totally clear (Fig. 4.25). In the pulsatile flow system with a stenosis near the venous anastomosis of the silicone models, considerably altered flow patterns could be seen. In order to investigate the influence of these flow patterns on the formation of further stenoses, two configurations were numerically simulated:

- A conventional terminolateral anastomosis (reference).
- The same anastomosis with an additional 77 % stenosis at the venous floor.

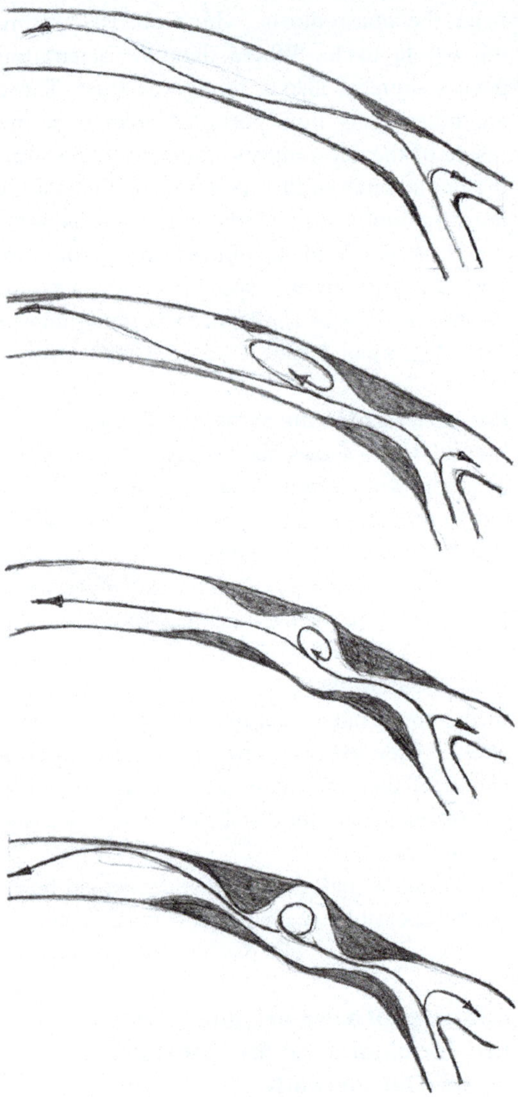

Fig. 4.25 Development of a second stenosis downstream from a pre-existing high-grade stenosis in the proximal venous outflow path

We compared the flow downstream from the venous anastomosis. Therefore we changed the boundary condition at the inlet to facilitate the recognition of clear differences.

The systolic flow was set to 2,200 mL/min ($Re = 2{,}037$) and the mean flow to 1,000 mL/min ($Re = 926$). Based on these Reynolds numbers the flow was still laminar (cf. Chap. 20).

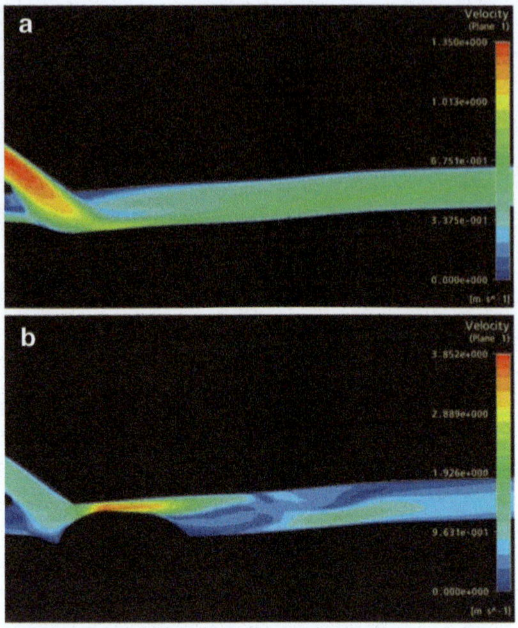

Fig. 4.26 (**a**) Velocity distribution in a conventional anastomosis and the proximal vein. (**b**) Velocity distribution in a conventional highly stenotic anastomosis and the procimal vein (different scale than **a**)

The velocity distribution at the systolic maximum in the conventional anastomosis and in the proximal vein are shown in Fig. 4.26a (symmetry plane). A jet stream hits the venous floor and divides into two portions (cf. Fig. 4.11a). The main flow leaves via the proximal vein (two-thirds of the total flow; see boundary conditions in the introduction to Sect. 4.2.2). The angle between the inner wall of the vein and the prosthesis is too large to prevent the flow detachment from the inner wall. Consequently a backflow zone appears. Apart from these unphysiological characteristics near the anastomosis, no other disturbances can be found in the course of the venous efflux. The farther the distance from the anastomosis becomes, the calmer the flow pattern seems.

Conversely, a pre-existing stenosis on the venous floor changes the flow within the vein decisively (Fig. 4.26b). Within the stenosis the maximum velocity is three times as high as the maximum velocity in an anastomosis without a

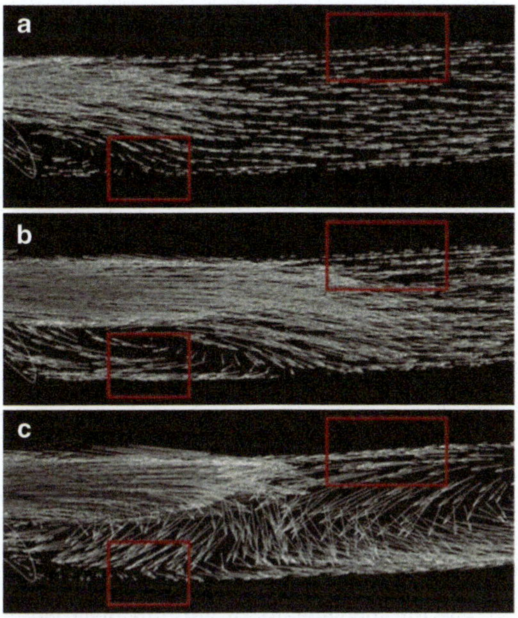

Fig. 4.27 Velocity vectors downstream from a stenosis. The stenosis reaches the left margin of the image. (**a**) Start of systole. (**b, c**) Velocity vectors downstream from the stenosis: (**b**) 40 ms after start of systole, (**c**) 200 ms after start of systole

stenosis. (Note the different scales in Fig. 4.26a, b). Here the poststenotic velocity distribution is highly disturbed. In several regions flow separation occurs. Oscillating backflows and vortices consequently develop. Figure 4.27 shows the velocity vectors in the symmetry plane downstream from the stenosis at different points in time (a: start of systole, b: 40 ms later, c: 200 ms later). The poststenotic vortex on the venous floor can be seen in Fig. 4.27b. The vectors mark the retrograde flow. The change of the flow direction at the inner wall of the vein can be seen in Fig. 4.27c. Whereas there is an early orthograde flow (Fig. 4.27a, b) in this region, it later turns back and shows no further changes till the end of diastole.

A pre-existing stenosis in the venous anastomotic region considerably changes flow patterns in the poststenotic area. The alterations of the flow direction during a heart cycle as well as the regions with high oscillating wall shear stress (not shown) can cause further poststenotic lesions of the venous wall (Krueger et al. 2009).

4.2.5 Evaluation of the Results

The results prove the significant influence of geometry on the hemodynamics of anastomoses. Several authors report on the formation of SIH in the venous anastomosis (Fillinger et al. 1990; Lemson et al. 2000; Shu and Hwang 1991; Heise et al. 2011). In these studies, maximum SIH always occurred on the venous floor opposite the entry into the prosthesis. Various in vitro studies and numerical simulations showed a high velocity stream portion (jet stream) that hit the venous floor (Longest and Kleinstreuer 2000; Shu and Hwang 1991). The enlargement of the anastomotic space can decrease the strain on the venous floor and in particular the wall shear strain (Figs. 4.14 and 4.12). This approach led to the development of a patch prosthesis (Scholz et al. 1999a, b). The advantages of a patch prosthesis over a prosthesis with a standard venous anastomosis have been confirmed several times (Berard et al. 2003; Escobar et al. 1999; Lau et al. 2007; Liu et al. 2006; Nyberg et al. 2001; Sorom et al. 2002; Tsoulfas et al. 2008; Ko et al. 2009; Kan et al. 2009).

There are conflicting views concerning wall shear stress and its influence on SIH formation Some authors emphasize the correlation between low shear stress and SIH in arteries (e.g., Bassiouny et al. 1992; Lemson et al. 2000; Salam et al. 1996; Staalsen et al. 1995; Zarins et al. 1996). They consider this kind of hyperplasia an "adaptive response" of the arteries to the low shear rates which normalizes the shear near the wall (Zarins et al. 1996). The effective wall shear rates were around 0.5 Pa (Salam et al. 1996). Other authors, however, are convinced that high shear rates cause SIH (Sottiurai 1990; Hofstra et al. 1996; Haruguchi and Teraoka 2003; Kleinstreuer 2006), especially in AV interposition grafts (Fillinger et al. 1990) and veins used as arterial bypass grafts (e.g., Heethaar 1993; Lemson et al. 2000; Thubrikar 2007). There wall shear stress values were around 10 Pa (calculated from the presented hemodynamic data with blood viscosity of 3.6 mPa·s; Fillinger et al. 1990). The respective wall shear rates for SIH formation in arteries and veins thus show more than a tenfold difference.

This discussion is probably due to diverging views concerning the histomorphologic manifestation of the so-called *intimal hyperplasia*.

Correlation between wall shear stress and SIH

- *High shear rates* and alternating pressure load (at the stagnation point) can lead to *SIH* in both vein and artery (e.g., femoro-crural bypass anastomoses) by mechanical irritation.
- *Low shear rates* can lead to local thrombus formation in both arteries and veins. After some time these thrombi are transformed into connective tissue (*organized thrombi, also* called *pseudo intima*). The resulting tissue macroscopically resembles SIH. From a hemodynamic perspective, unnecessary spaces are thus "corrected" by the interaction of coagulation and connective tissue activities.

The longitudinal axes of endothelial cells are usually oriented parallel to the blood flow. Cell shapes are also dependant on flow. If the flow increases as in a stenosed lumen, the cells will take a longish form and lie closer to each other (Matsuda et al. 2003; Thubrikar 2007). In poststenotic areas, cells are rounder and shorter. The intercellular gaps become larger. Oscillating flows constitute a strong mechanical irritation. They cause cycle-dependent changes of shapes and orientations in endothelial cells (Matsuda et al. 2003; Sottiurai 1990). Under extreme flow conditions cells can become partially detached and form tower-like structures, which protrude into the lumen. Towards the subendothelium, large gaps open. The migration of cells as well as the opening of these gaps entail increased contacts between blood and subendothelium, where SIH starts.

4.2.6 Hemodynamics and Shunt Thrombosis

The thrombosis of a shunt prosthesis results from an imbalance of three factors (Virchow's triad):

- Thrombogenicity of the vascular wall
- Coagulation
- Hemodynamics

The thrombogenicity of all graft materials is significantly higher than that of native vessels. Therefore prosthetic grafts require higher flow velocities near the wall than native vessels in order to avoid thrombosis. The flow velocity is determined by:

- Diameter of a vessel
- Flow rate
- Flow characteristics

A prosthetic shunt should offer a large enough surface for puncturing in a clinical setting. Therefore its predetermined *diameter* should be at least around 7 mm.

The *flow rate* is determined by:

- Inflow resistance of the artery
- Blood pressure
- Flow resistance of the prosthesis
- Resistance of the venous outflow path
- Blood viscosity

With common prosthesis dimensions, the impact of its *flow resistance* may well be neglected. The same is true for the resistance of the venous outflow path unless there is a venous stenosis. The *arterial inflow resistance*, however, can be influenced by the position of the arterial anastomosis (see Chap. 11).

The influence of the *flow characteristics* on thrombosis becomes clear when comparing the infrarenal aorta to the vena cava. Whereas a thrombosis is a rare event in a prosthesis after aortic replacement, the risk of thrombosis is much higher in a caval prosthesis despite similar flow rates. Flow characteristics are quite different, though. In the aorta, prevailing characteristics are:

- Pulsatility
- Plenty of turbulence

In the vena cava, there is/are:

- No pulsatility
- Hardly any turbulence
- Predominantly smooth laminar flow

This predominantly constant, laminar flow in the vena cava leads to a lower flow velocity near the wall when compared to the aorta, which explains the higher risk of thrombosis in the vena cava.

The less pulsatile the flow, the higher the risk of thrombosis in a prosthetic graft.

In an AV shunt there is a laminar, slightly pulsatile flow with turbulence. With a growing distance from the arterial anastomosis, there is less turbulence, the flow calms down, and the flow velocity near the vessel wall decreases. Therefore the risk of thrombosis may rise with an increasing length of the prosthetic graft even if the flow rate stays the same. A significant change of flow characteristics also occurs with curved vessels (shunt loop). At the inside there is recirculation downstream from the curve which also contributes to the decrease in flow velocity near the vessel wall (see Chap. 20). This recirculation is more pronounced with a smaller radius.

According to the Hagen–Poiseuille law, the flow rate is inversely proportional to the viscosity. The viscosity at a hematocrit (HCT) of 40 % is twice as high as at 25 % (Opitz and Pfeiffer 1984), and thus exerts a definite influence on the flow rate. Experience shows, however, that the patency of an AV shunt is only threatened when raising the HCT to physiological levels if the initial flow rate has already been marginal. To decrease the risk of thrombosis, the following conclusions may be drawn for surgery:

1. The flow rate in a prosthetic alloplastic AV shunt needs to be considerably higher than in a native AV fistula.
2. A higher risk of thrombosis requires a higher flow rate, which can be influenced by the choice of the position for the arterial anastomosis. Thrombogenicity can also be lowered by additional anticoagulants.
3. The radius of a looped interposition graft should not be too small so as to avoid unfavorable flow characteristics.
4. Prosthetic shunt grafts should not be longer than necessary.

Figure 4.28 lists the influencing factors. Based on the hemodynamics presented here, the practical considerations mentioned below should be followed when creating AV accesses with prosthetic grafts:

1. A *narrow segment* (e.g., 4 mm diameter) for the arterial anastomosis eliminates the vortex there and reduces the oscillation on the arterial floor. Undesirable flow patterns are reduced. It hardly influences the flow rate at all.
2. The *length of an interposition graft* hardly influences the flow rate. These grafts should not be longer than necessary to minimize the risk of thrombosis.
3. The flow rate in a *looped shunt* is basically the same as in a straight graft. The radius should be as large as possible.
4. The bulb shape of a *venous patch anastomosis* calms down the high energy arterial inflow. The large vortex in this kind of anastomosis leads to an improved wash out effect. The comparably low pressure and the decreased shear put less stress on the venous wall.
5. Trimming the patch so that it is *matched to the venous diameter* is necessary to obtain the advantages of a patch anastomosis. Thus an overly hooded configuration of an oversized patch can be avoided.
6. A patent *venous side branch* near the venous anastomotic space should be transected.

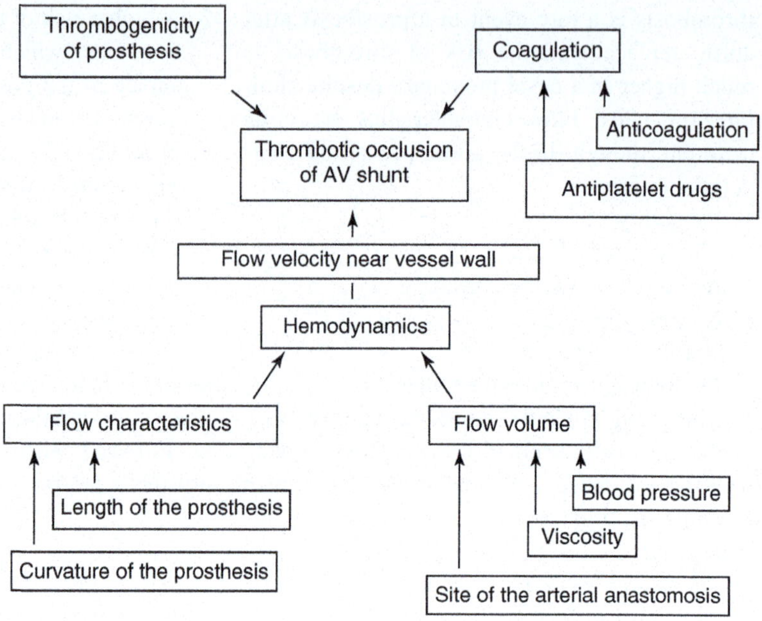

Fig. 4.28 Influence of graft, coagulation, and hemodynamics on shunt thrombosis

7. The *angle between the graft and the vein* should be as acute as possible in order to harmonize the intraanastomotic flow. An almost perpendicular blunt angle should be avoided. Then the impact of the flow on the venous wall would be much stronger.
8. The *inflow radius* of a looped graft should be as large as possible.

4.3 Principles for the Implantation of Prosthetic Shunt Grafts

Observing the following principle has proved to be worthwhile in our clinical practice.

4.3.1 Preoperative Vascular Diagnostics

Before the implantation of a vascular prosthesis we conduct duplex ultrasound examinations of the feeding artery and the draining vein. If we still have doubts we add contrast medium studies to the diagnostics. Should it be possible to create an AV fistula using the patient's native vessels only, we always prefer this option.

4.3.2 Anesthesia

With cooperative patients, most shunt procedures of the upper extremities may be carried out under infiltration anesthesia. Frequently patients complain of lower back pain during surgery. We recommend administering an appropriate pre-medication. We prefer infiltration anesthesia, while others prefer plexus anesthesia. For central AV shunts, we almost always use general anesthesia.

4.3.3 Prevention of Infections

The implantation of an AV shunt prosthesis entails a high risk of infections in the frequently immunocompromised patients.

Therefore we strictly adhere to the following rules:

- Thorough shave of the whole field.
- Incise film for the whole operative field.
- Intraoperative administration of antibiotics.

- Covering of the prosthetic graft by subcutaneous adipose tissue at the incision sites.
- Meticulous hemostasis.
- Layered technique for wound closure.

4.3.4 Isolation of the Vessels

If artery and vein are to be isolated separately (straight interposition grafts), we will always start with the vein. Only the intraoperative findings show whether a successful venous anastomosis is likely. The suitability of the artery can mostly be judged by the preoperative findings.

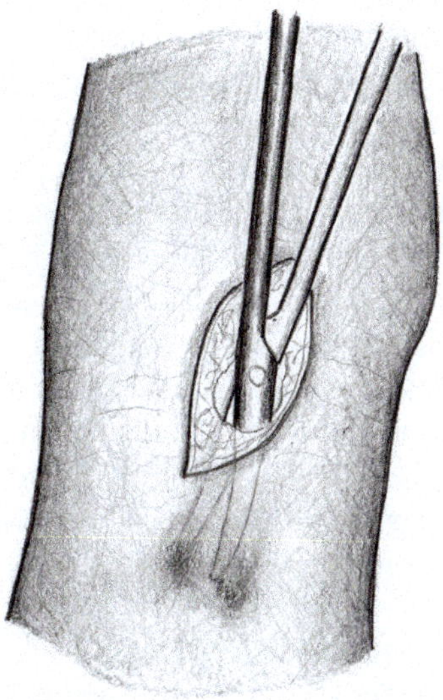

Fig. 4.29 Creating a subcutaneous tunnel with a pair of scissors

4.3.5 Tunnel for the Prosthetic Graft

To create an area for puncturing which is as large as possible, with normal skin conditions the prosthesis should be placed subcutaneously as close to the surface as possible. For this purpose the concave side of the curved scissors is directed towards the skin surface (Fig. 4.29).

The size of the puncturable area of a prosthesis depending on its distance from the surface is shown in Fig. 4.30. In order to prevent impaired wound healing, we take care that the prosthesis is sufficiently covered by subcutaneous tissue (Fig. 4.31).

4.3.6 Fibrin Sealing of ePTFE Graft (cf. Chap. 10)

In up to a third of our hemodialysis patients, fluid leakage (filtration) of ePTFE grafts by different manufacturers led to perigraft seromas. In patients without renal insufficiency – who do not need hemodialysis – we observed this filtration in only around 1 %. Postoperatively the filtration of a prosthetic graft causes subcutaneous edemas, a delayed healing process, and thus a longer period of time till the graft may be punctured for the

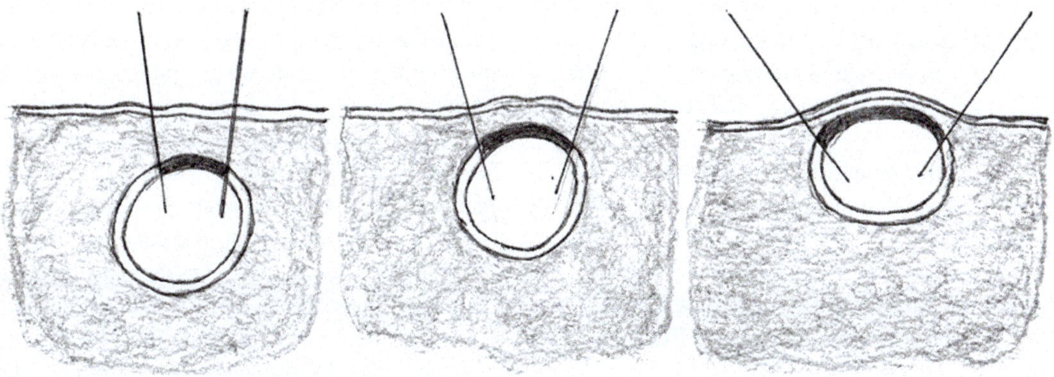

Fig. 4.30 Surface area which can be used for puncture dependent on the distance of the prosthesis from the surface. With a deep prosthesis position, the needle may have to be inserted perpendicularly

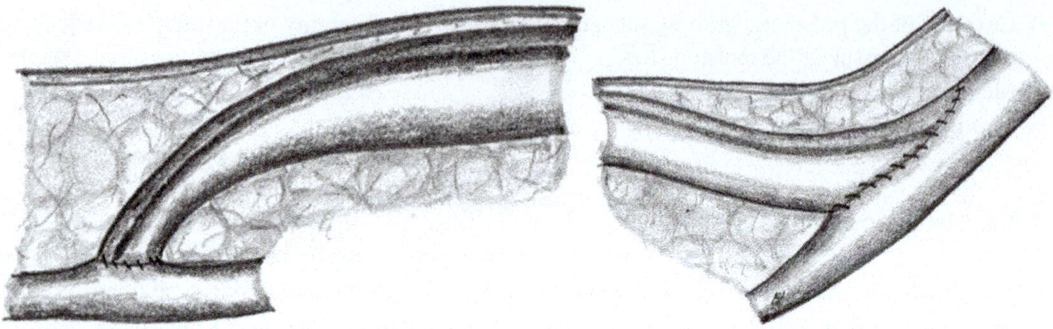

Fig. 4.31 Subcutaneous cover of the anastomotic region

first time. Depending on the extent and time of filtration, as well on the absorptive capacity of the surrounding subcutaneous tissue, perigraft seroma may develop. Resulting fistulas may lead to graft infections.

This filtration is caused by molecules which transform the hydrophobic surface of ePTFE into a hydrophilic one. We examined the sealing of the graft wall by sequential fibrin application to the outer surface. In ePTFE prostheses without exterior wrap-around layers this proved feasible and effective. With exterior wrap-around layers, the small pore size prevents the fibrin from penetrating these outer layers. Thus fibrin can easily be removed like a film. Since 1992 we have been using fibrin sealant with all AV graft prostheses. Since then with more than 2,500 AV grafts we have observed filtration worth mentioning in seven grafts: Twice this was due to pathologically increased fibrinolysis and five times due to faulty techniques.

Techniques for Fibrin Sealing

1. Apply fibrinogen to the graft's entire surface.
2. Rub it in while extending and compressing the graft.
3. Apply thrombin in the same way.
   Attention: clamping destroys the fibrin seal.

4.3.7 Placing the Prosthetic Graft in the Subcutaneous Tunnel

Before we create the anastomoses we always place the prosthetic graft in its subcutaneous tunnel. Only when the prosthesis has been placed in its final position can the optimal configuration of the anastomoses be found from a hemodynamic point of view. As we exclusively use reduced caliber patch grafts (4/7-mm), we describe the choice of the correct prosthetic length and the pull through technique for this type of prostheses. Caliber-reduced patch prostheses are available in lengths of 20–45 cm with 5 cm intervals. The length includes the 7-cm narrow segment (4 mm diameter) (Fig. 4.32). Not more than 1–2 cm of the narrow segment should be used. Thus a 30-cm prosthetic graft will be shortened to 24–25 cm. The positioning of straight grafts and looped ones is different and will therefore be dealt with separately.

Straight Interposition Grafts

The correct length of the prosthesis is determined by the distance between the vein and the artery which have to be connected. The graft should be pulled through the tunnel beginning at the incision over the vein towards the artery in order not to damage the patch for the venous anastomosis. The arterial end, where we grasp the graft will be shortened anyway. We insert an aortic clamp at the arterial skin incision and grasp the long end of the narrow segment of the prosthesis (Fig. 4.33). Then the graft is placed in the best position for the patch anastomosis with the vein. If the graft is too long, a 7 mm diameter segment close to the arterial anastomosis will be excised and the continuity then re-established (Fig. 4.34). The flow rate is hardly influenced by shortening the 7-cm narrow segment, so its total length of either 1 or 2 cm hardly makes a difference. A longer

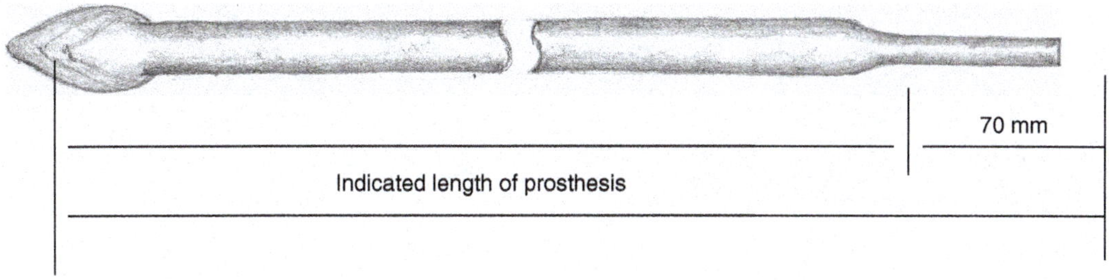

Fig. 4.32 Length of the patch prosthesis

Fig. 4.33 Aortic clamp in place before pulling through the prosthesis

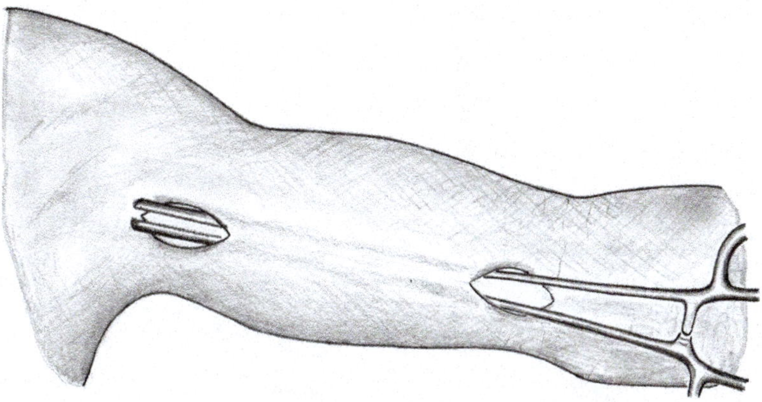

Fig. 4.34 Shortening and re-establishment of the continuity of a prosthesis that is too long

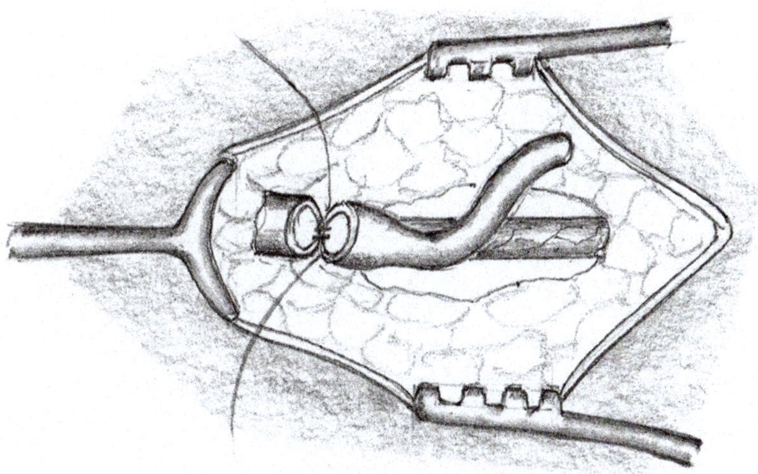

narrow (not suited for puncture) segment, however, means that there is less area for dialysis needle placement.

Looped Interposition Grafts

Finding the correct length for a looped graft is much easier than for a straight graft. After isolating the vessels we choose a 35–45-cm prosthesis depending on the available space and the distance between the vessels and the skin surface. We place the graft on the surface and draw its path on the incision film, taking care to sketch a larger radius (Fig. 4.35).

The U-shaped subcutaneous tunnel begins at a transverse skin incision 2.5–3 cm distal to the previously marked turning point without removing

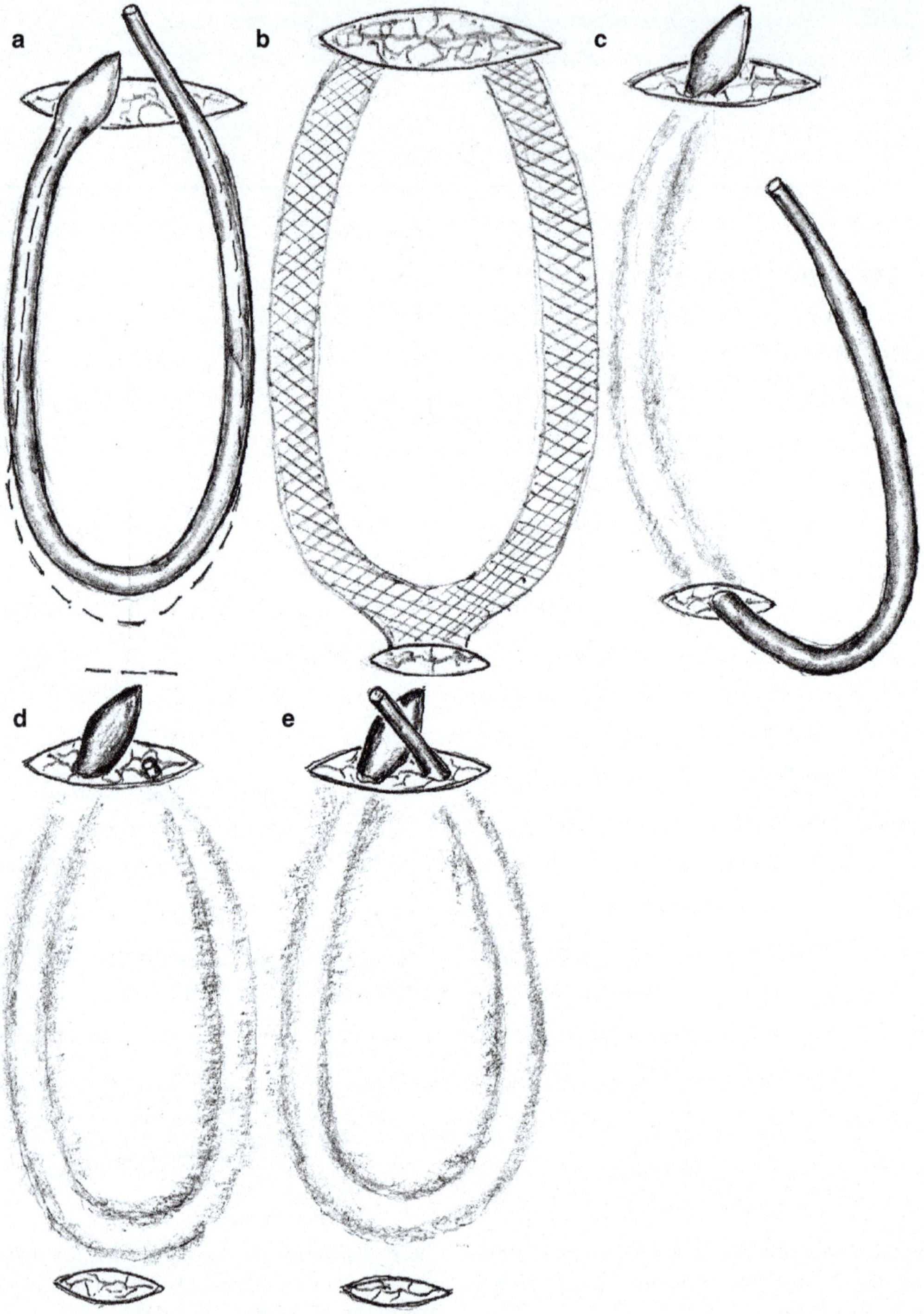

Fig. 4.35 Subcutaneous positioning of a loop prosthesis. (**a**) Mark the path on the skin. (**b**) Subcutaneous tunnel. (**c**) Pulling through of the venous graft segment. (**d**) Pulling through of the arterial segmenent. (**e**) Correction of the position

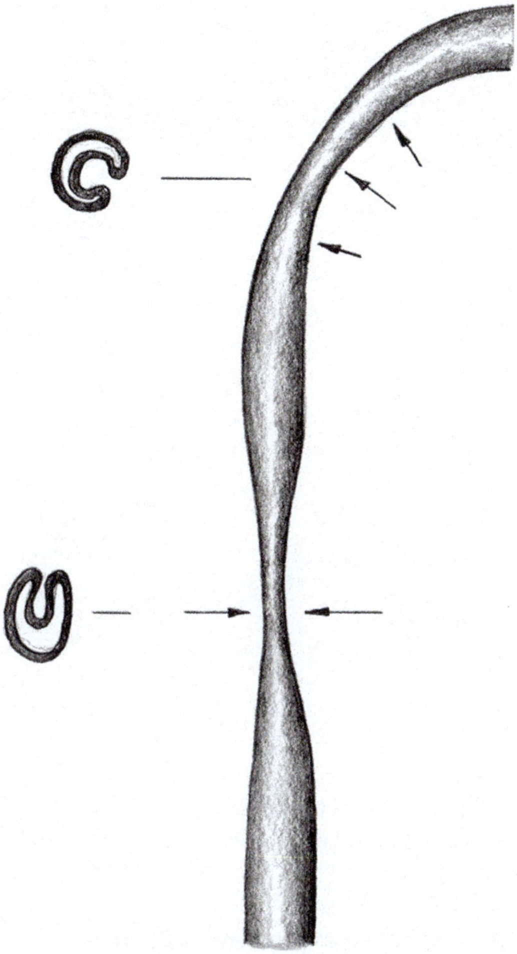

Fig. 4.36 Stenosis caused by U-shaped deformation of the graft caused by a tunnel that is too narrow or a radius that is too small

any subcutaneous tissue. Just as with a straight graft, the arterial end is pulled through by grasping the narrow segment. The prosthetic patch is placed in the best positions for the venous anastomosis (Fig. 4.35c) Then we place the arterial end (Fig. 4.35d). If the prosthesis is too short, the radius of the tunnel will be decreased by incising the subcutaneous tissue at the turning point (Fig. 4.35e). Once the narrow arterial segment (desired length 1–2 cm) is in the right position, we use a lid retractor to visualize the path of the prosthesis near its apex. We correct it if necessary. With strong tensile forces or a tunnel that is too narrow, the graft may show a U-shaped deformation (Fig. 4.36). We flush the graft from its narrow end to exclude stenoses which might be hidden in the tunnel.

4.3.8 Position of the Venous Anastomosis

For the placement of the venous anastomosis, joints have to be avoided. If placed too close to a joint (elbow, axilla, groin), the anastomosis might be submitted to compression (Fig. 4.37).

4.3.9 Creating an Anastomosis

The design of the anastomoses is essential for the long term functioning of a graft. For two reasons,

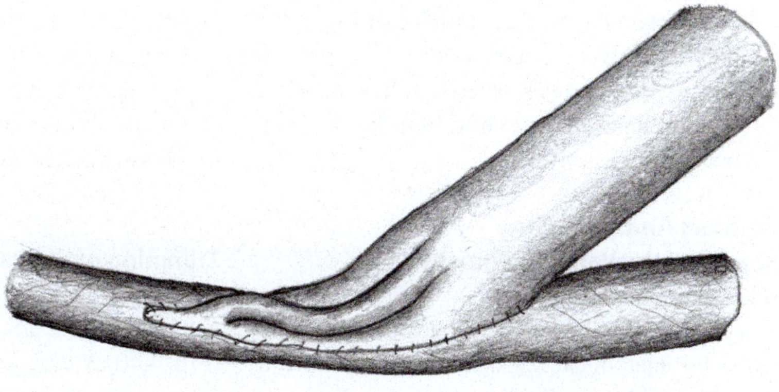

Fig. 4.37 Stenosis of a venous anastomosis caused by compression (e.g., near a joint)

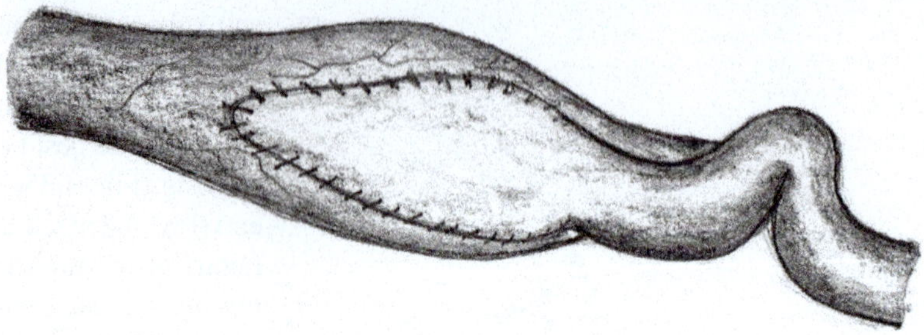

Fig. 4.38 Bending of a prosthesis that is too long

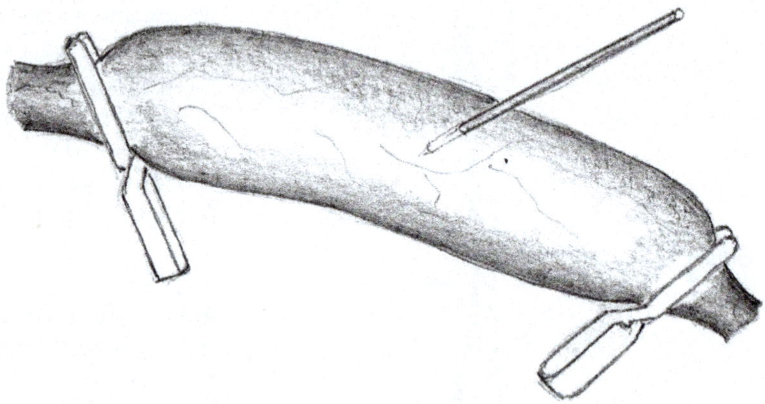

Fig. 4.39 Dilation of the vein by injecting heparin solution so as to figure out the diameter

the venous anastomosis should be completed first:

- Should the prosthetic graft prove too long after the completion of the anastomosis, kinking can be avoided simply by pulling towards the planned arterial anastomosis (Fig. 4.38).
- After the completion of the venous anastomosis, we clamp the graft near the patch and declamp the patient's native vein so that blood flow within the native vessel returns. Clamping of the graft wall locally destroys the fibrin layer. As the pressure close to the venous anastomosis is lower than near the arterial anastomosis, filtration hardly ever occurs.

Venous Anastomosis

Choice of the Venous Segment

The anastomosis should not be too close to venous valves. Should such a position be inevitable for anatomical reasons, the valves have to be excised. Venous side branches near the anastomosis should be ligated and transected as their influence on hemodynamics could favor the proliferation of connective tissue and the formation of stenoses.

Determination of the Venous Diameter

The patch size of a prosthesis has to be adapted to the venous diameter to achieve the best hemodynamic results. We determine the venous diameter as follows:

- Distal and proximal clamping of the vein (Schwartz clamps).
- Puncturing of the clamped venous segment using a thin cannula, with tight filling of the clamped venous segment with Heparin solution to achieve maximum dilation (Fig. 4.39).
- Measurement of the venous diameter.
  The venous diameter should be at least 3 mm.

Trimming of the Patch

For hemodynamic reasons, the trimming of the patch should be adjusted to the venous diameter (Fig. 4.40). Cutting along the printed lines which also signal the corresponding venous diameter facilitates this step. A hooded anastomosis caused by wrong trimming should be avoided (Fig. 4.41).

Suture Technique

We prefer the following technique for creating the anastomosis:

- Bilateral clamping of the vein.
- Longitudinal venotomy and flushing of both sides with heparin solution.
- Start of the anastomosis with a U shaped suture (6-0) at the distal patch (Fig. 4.42).
- Continue with running suture to the tip of the anastomosis, extending venotomy if necessary (Fig. 4.43).
- Continue suturing to the other side and dilate anastomosis using a dissector (Fig. 4.44).
- Complete sutureline starting with the other side of the U-shaped suture.
- Clamping of the graft close to the patch and declamping of the vein for free blood flow (Fig. 4.45).

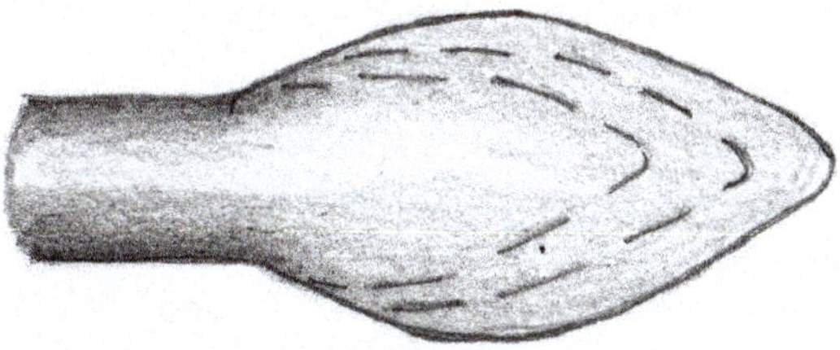

Fig. 4.40 Printed lines to trim the patch for different venous diameters

Arterial Anastomosis

After completing the venous anastomosis it is necessary to check and possibly correct the length of the graft.

- Shortening of the narrow segment to 1–2 cm. Should the graft be too long, a 7 mm wide segment is excised near the exposed artery and the continuity re-established (cf. Fig. 4.34).
- Bilateral clamping of the artery, longitudinal arteriotomy, running suture (6-0) for a lateroterminal anastomosis of artery and graft (Fig. 4.45).
- The angle of the prosthetic take-off should always be acute so as to allow the passage of a thrombectomy catheter into the artery (Fig. 4.46) in case of thrombosis (Fig. 4.47).

4.4 AV Grafts in the Forearm

There are two possible variants in the forearm.

4.4.1 Straight Graft

Indication/prerequisites

Very rare indication:

1. Usually only possible if a preexisting AV fistula has led to the dilation of the feeding artery. With arteries that have kept their

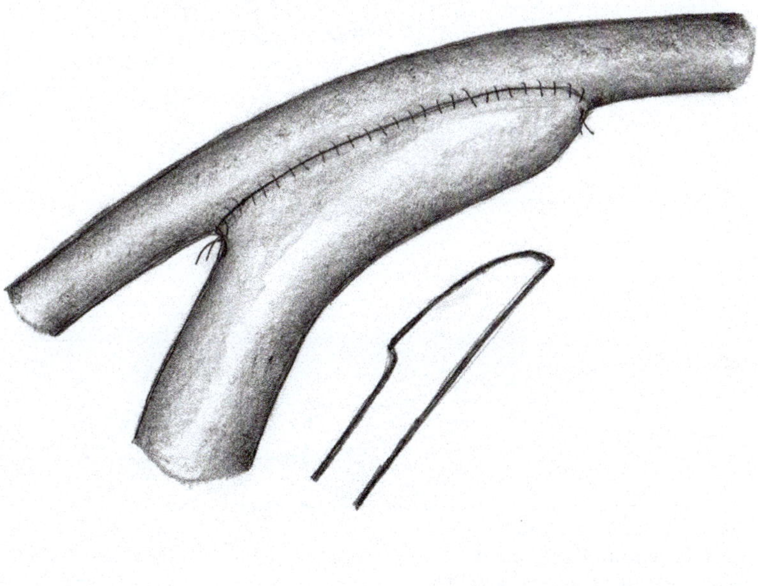

Fig. 4.41 Wrongly-trimmed patch prosthesis

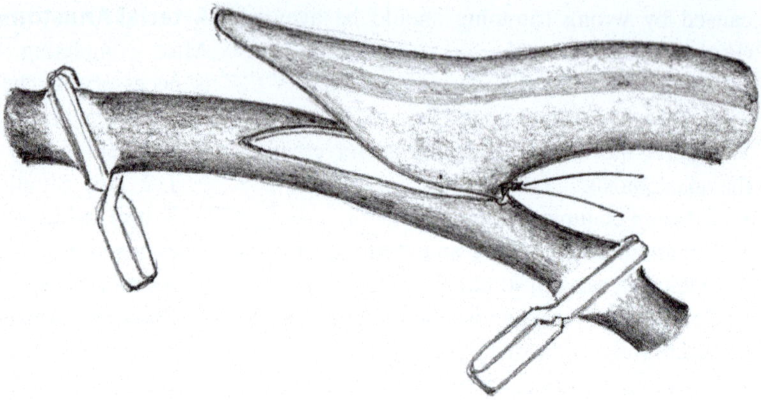

Fig. 4.42 Start suturing at the distal end of the patch (heel)

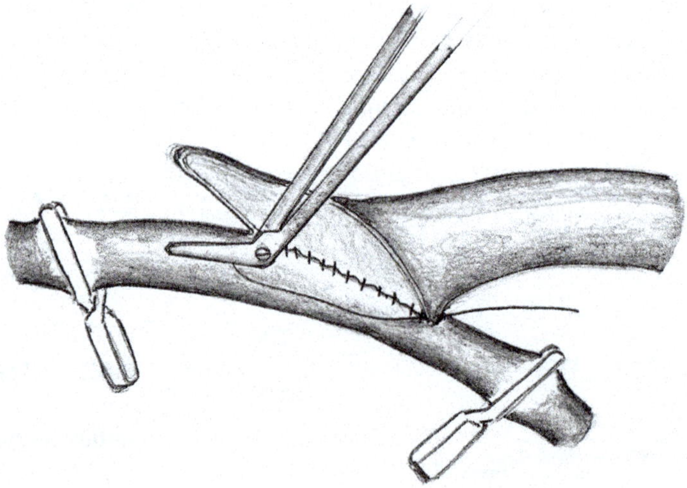

Fig. 4.43 Correct lengthening of the venotomy after unilateral fixation of the suture

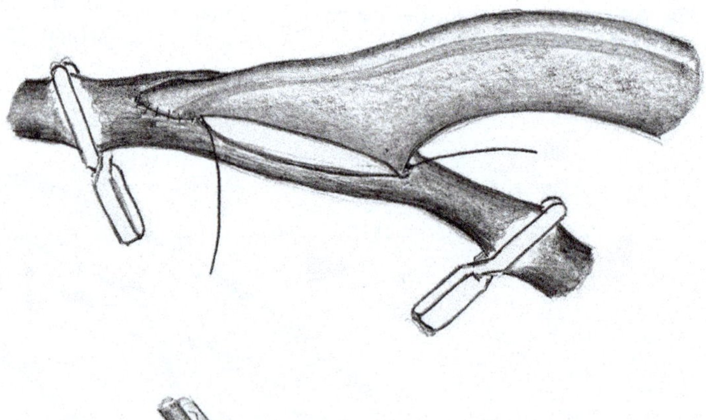

Fig. 4.44 Continue suturing on the other side of the anastomosis

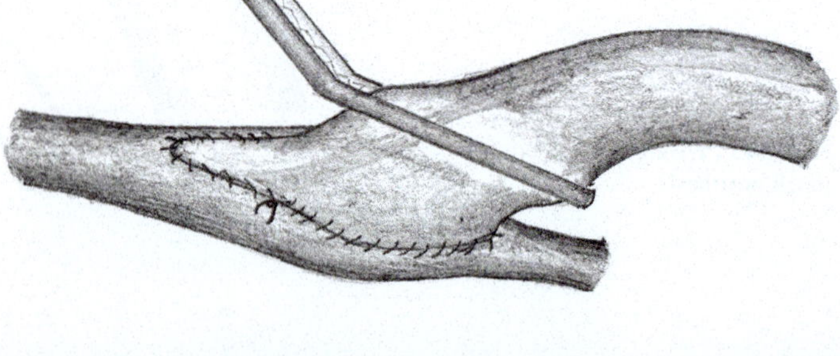

Fig. 4.45 After completion of the suture, clamp prosthesis near the anastomosis and release venous flow

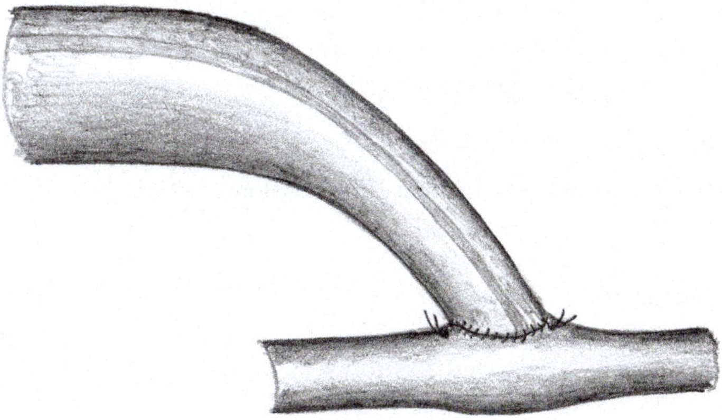

Fig. 4.46 Acute angle of the arterial anastomosis

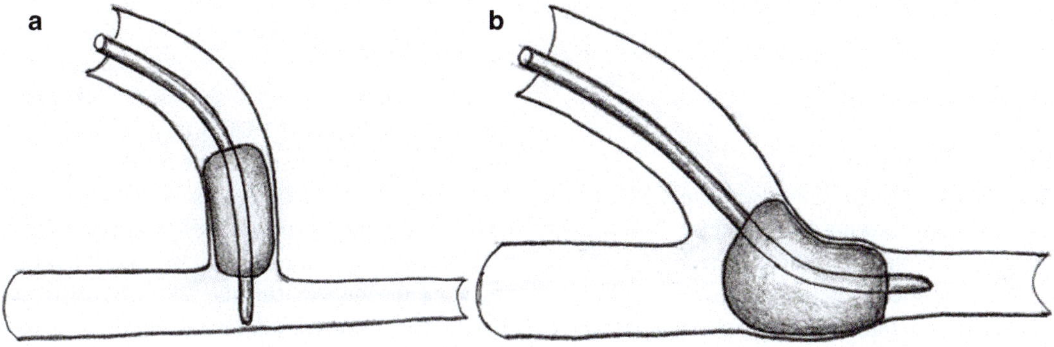

Fig. 4.47 Possible courses of a Fogarty catheter depending on the angle of the arterial anastomosis

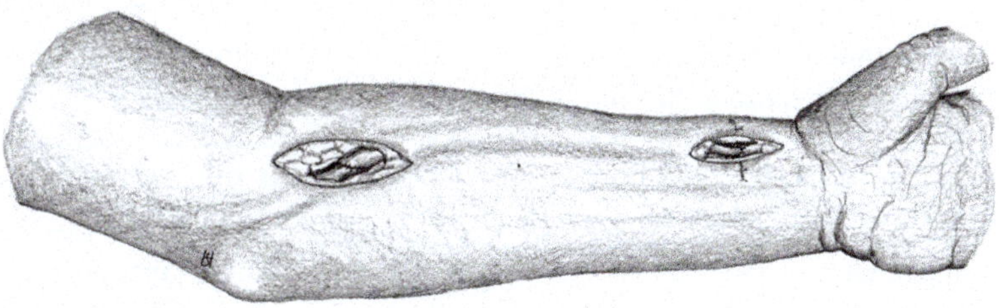

Fig. 4.48 Straight AV shunt in the forearm

normal diameters of 2–3 mm there will only be a low flow rate of around 300 mL/min. This will be insufficient to prevent thrombosis.

2. There should also be a suitable vein with a diameter of at least 3 mm. The anastomosis should be at a venous segment without side branches if possible. The elbow joint should be avoided as otherwise there might be kinking. Should a suitable vein exist, the alternative option for a native AV fistula should be verified.

Contraindication

Vein close to the elbow that seems to be suitable for creating a (native) AV fistula that may also be ready for early puncturing.

Approach

Exposure of the vessels via longitudinal incisions. Check first whether the vein is suitable. If so also expose the artery and create a subcutaneous tunnel as far lateral/radial as possible to allow for easy and less painful punctures (Fig. 4.48). Should the venous anastomosis be situated proximal to the elbow, the prosthesis passes through the (lateral) turning point at the elbow to avoid kinking when flexing the elbow.

Prognosis
Dependent on the maturation of the anastomosed vein.

Evaluation
Aspects:

1. Always verify whether AV fistula in the elbow region is possible alternatively.
2. Veins in the elbow regions may mature for potential future AV fistulas.

4.4.2 Loop Graft

Indication/prerequisites
Rare indication. We only use them in extremely adipose patients whose veins lie far from the surface. A suitable vein should be ready for anastomosis near the elbow. Alternatively a distal AV fistula in the forearm with superficialization of the vein should be considered. The decisive criterion is the length of time till a puncturable vascular access is needed.

Contraindication
Suitable vein close to the elbow that will mature for puncturing in the foreseeable future if an AV fistula is created.

Approach
Exposure of vein and artery via a longitudinal incision close and distal to the elbow. Additional incision in the forearm, creation of a U-shaped tunnel, passage of the prosthesis and anastomosis (Fig. 4.49).

Prognosis
Depends on the maturation of the anastomosed vein.

Evaluation

- Alternative to the superficialization of a distal AV fistula.
- Alternative to an elbow fistula which is superficialized in the upper arm.
- Conditioning of upper arm veins.

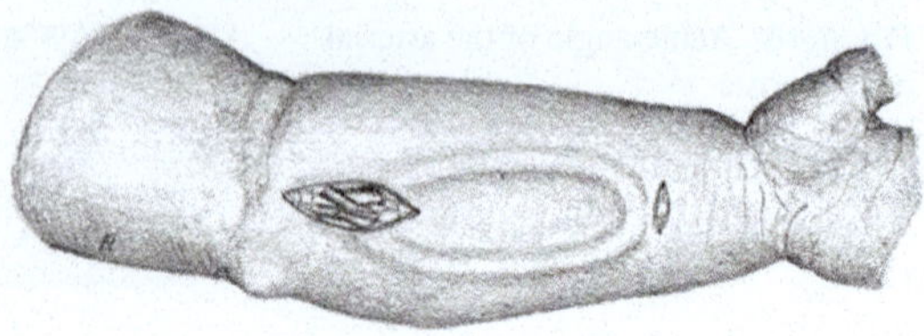

Fig. 4.49 Looped AV shunt in the forearm

4.4.3 Repair of Forearm Interposition Grafts

A venous stenosis at or proximal to the anastomosis is the most frequent complication. PTA should be the first treatment option. We disapprove of stents in the elbow region because of their high risk of thromboses. If PTA is unsuccessful or an early restenosis occurs, we opt for surgery. With short stenoses, patch plasties should be tried. With long stenoses, or occlusions of the veins in the elbow region combined with large diameter veins in the upper arm, the venous runoff can be improved by prosthetic interposition grafts. Principally the cephalic vein (Fig. 4.50), the basilic vein, and the brachial vein (Fig. 4.51a, b) may be worth considering. Care should be taken to guide the interposition graft laterally to the joint to avoid kinking with flexion.

4.5 AV Grafts in the Upper Arm

An AV interposition graft in the upper arm may be either straight or looped. For both choices the venous anastomosis should be placed in an infraaxillary position.

4.5.1 Anatomy of the Infraaxillary Veins

To start with, a suitable vein should be exposed via an infraaxillary longitudinal incision. Due to anatomical variations, several veins may serve this purpose. The pertinent literature does not give precise names to the infraaxillary veins. The two narrow lumen concomitant veins of the brachial artery in the distal and middle upper arm

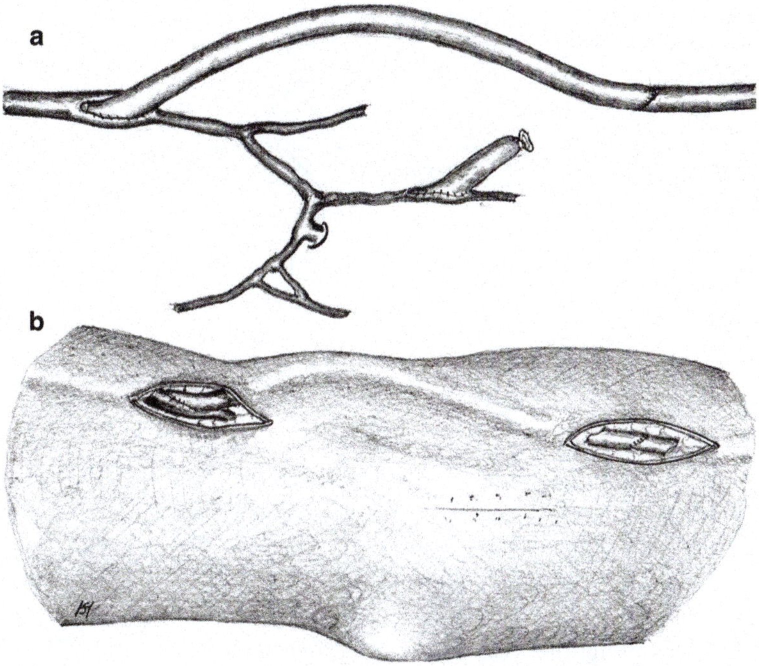

Fig. 4.50 (**a**) Long stenosis of the draining vein of an AV shunt in the forearm. (**b**) Reconstruction using an interposition graft to the cephalic vein in the forearm

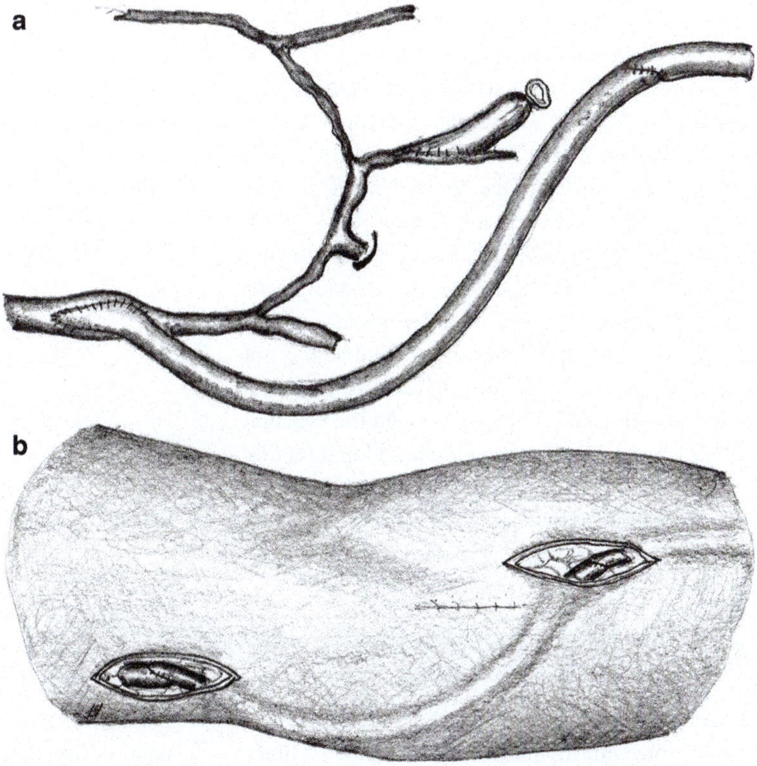

Fig. 4.51 (**a**) Long stenosis of an efferent vein of a forearm AV shunt.
(**b**) Reconstruction using an interposition graft to the basilic vein in the forearm

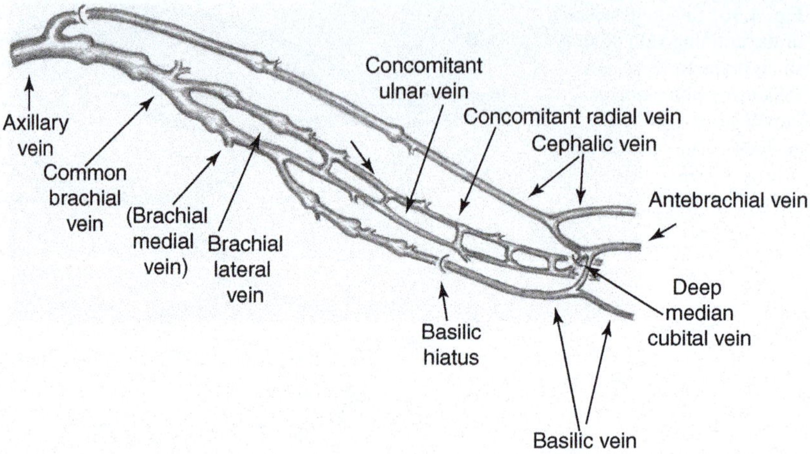

Fig. 4.52 Diagram of the veins of the upper extremity

are called radial and ulnar concomitant veins. In the infraaxillary region, both veins show a wide lumen and run more or less independent of the artery. We use the following terms: medial brachial vein for the wide vein which originates from the ulnar concomitant vein and drains into the basilic vein, and lateral brachial vein for the vein that originates from the radial concomitant vein. After the medial and lateral brachial veins merge, we call the resulting proximal vessel the common brachial vein.

Figure 4.52 shows a sketch of the veins in the upper arm. The site where the medial and lateral brachial veins merge to form the brachial vein varies widely just like the site where the basilic vein joins the medial brachial vein. Most often the medial brachial vein is suited. It is situated directly beneath the neurovascular sheath (neurovascular tunic) accompanied by nerves on both sides (Fig. 4.53). If the medial brachial vein is not suited, the lateral brachial vein has to be exposed. It is situated dorsal to the nerves and the brachial artery (Fig. 4.54). As the vein is hidden laterally, we recommend an approach between the brachial artery and the median nerve. Extra care should be taken in order to avoid nerve damage.

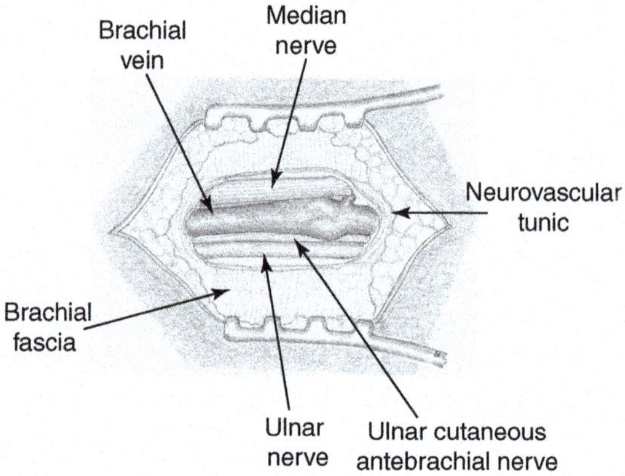

Fig. 4.53 Infraaxillary field after isolation of the median brachial vein

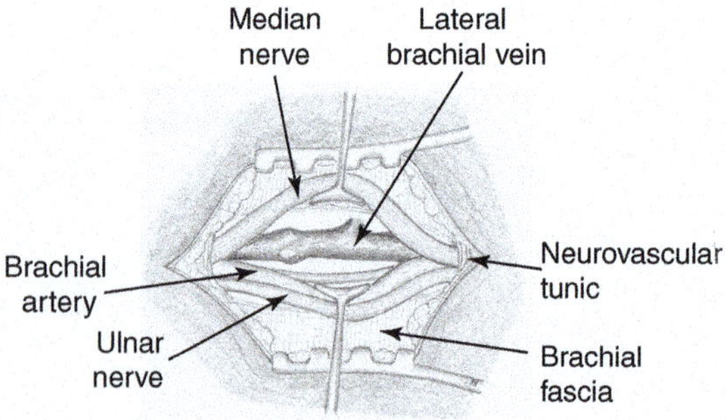

Fig. 4.54 Infraaxillary field after isolation of the brachial vein

4.5.2 Straight Graft

Interposition graft between the brachial artery directly proximal to the elbow and an infraaxillary vein.

Indication

- AV fistula or AV shunt in the forearm not possible.
- Arterial hypertension, for thus relatively low shunt flow (as an alternative to a looped

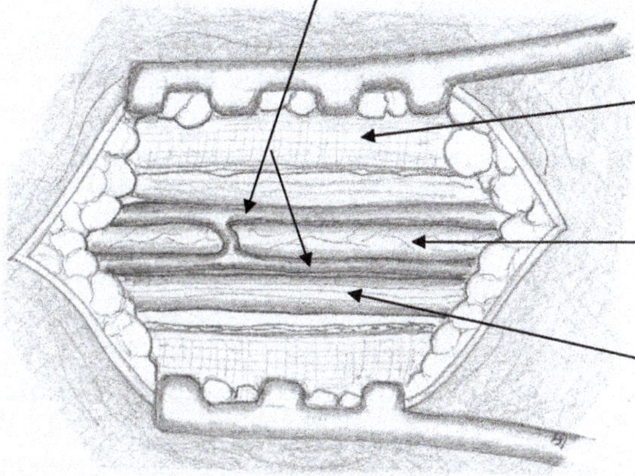

Fig. 4.55 Surgical field after exposure of the brachial artery just promixal to the elbow

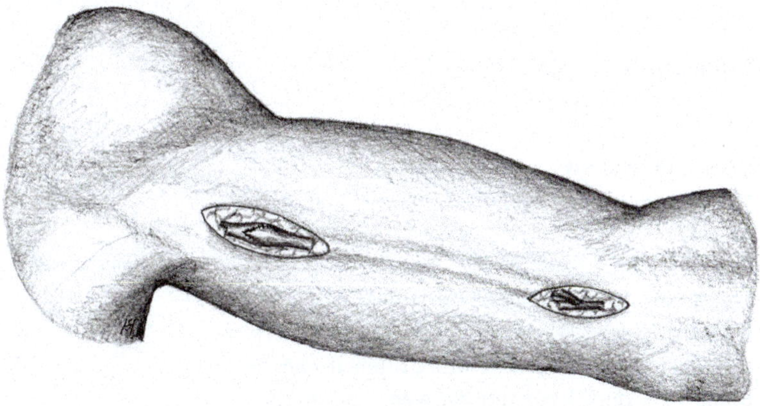

Fig. 4.56 Straight AV shunt in the upper arm

interposition graft in the upper arm which is anastomosed to the infraaxillary brachial artery).

Prerequisites

- Systolic pressure constantly above 100 mmHg.
- Suitable artery and vein.

Contraindication

- Preoperatively insufficient perfusion of the forearm.

Access

The exposure of a suitable vein has been described (Figs. 4.53 and 4.54). The exposure of the brachial artery begins with a longitudinal incision directly proximal to the elbow. After the longitudinal opening of the fascia and the vasoneuronal sheath, a wound retractor between the medial fascial margin and the biceps brachii muscle helps maintain a better view. The brachial artery with its two concomitant veins may be found lateral/radial to the median nerve (Fig. 4.55). There are diverging views as to whether a straight (Fig. 4.56) or a slightly curved path of the prosthesis is better.

Prognosis

Good long term prognosis dependent on possible venous stenoses and puncture-associated lesions.

Evaluation
Frequent interposition graft with our patients.

4.5.3 Loop Graft

Looped interposition grafts between the brachial artery and the axillary vein.

Indications
- AV fistula or AV shunt of forearm not possible.
- Brachial vein in cubital fossa not suited.
- Systolic blood pressure too low (below 100 mmHg).
- Insufficient perfusion of forearm already before surgery.
- Normotensive patients with hypercagulopathy and contraindications to anticoagulants.

Prerequisite
- Suitable infraaxillary vessels.

Contraindication
- No particular contraindication.

Access
The access to the vein has already been shown (Figs. 4.53 and 4.54). The same approach is used to isolate the artery. Most often it can be found in a dorsal position between the median nerve and the medial brachial vein. It may help to keep the nerve to one side using a lid retractor (Fig. 4.55). For the U-shaped tunnel one small transverse extra incision proximal to the cubital fossa should be sufficient (Figs. 4.57 and 4.58).

Prognosis
Good long term prognosis dependent on possible venous stenosis and puncture-associated lesions.

Evaluation
- Frequent interposition graft with our patients.
- Long segment which may be used for puncturing.

4.5.4 Repair of Upper Arm Grafts

In our patients the most frequent complications comprise stenoses and occlusions of the draining veins at or central to the anastomosis, aneurysmatic alterations of the prosthesis at frequent puncture

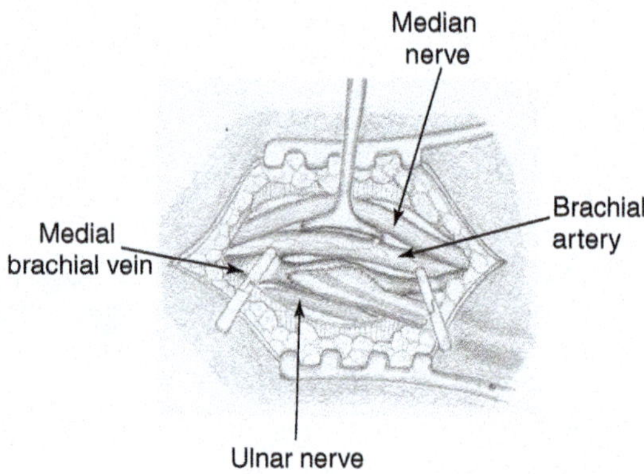

Fig. 4.57 Infraaxillary field after completion of the venous anastmosis, and with the exposed brachial artery

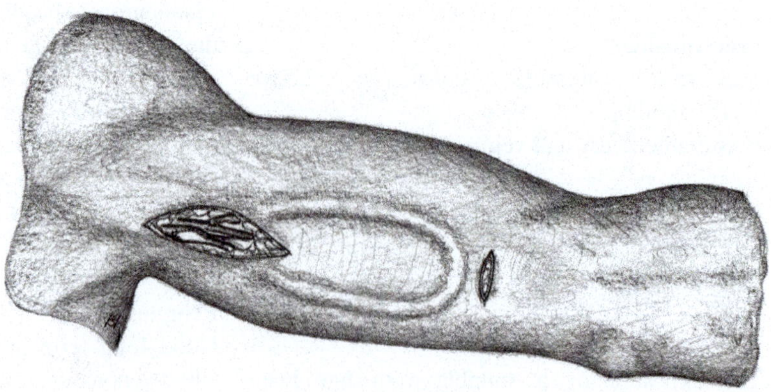

Fig. 4.58 Looped upper arm AV shunt

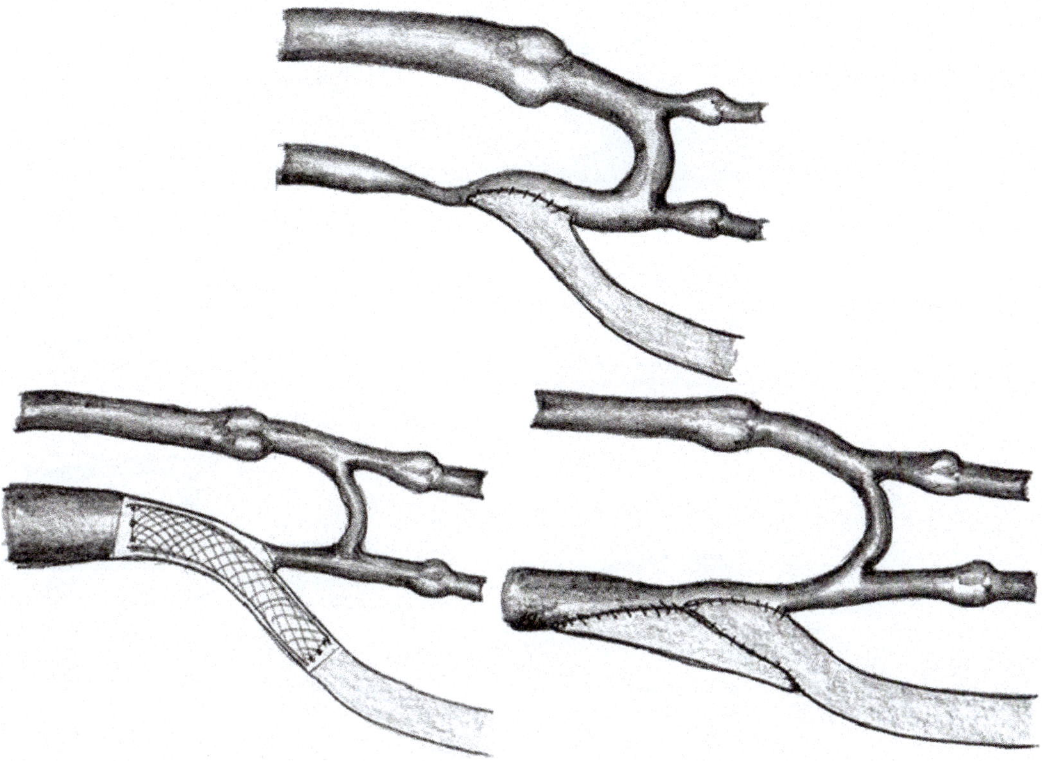

Fig. 4.59 Therapy for a short venous stenosis close to the anastomosis by stent or patch plasty

sites (less frequently), and rarely infections. The arterial anastomosis has not been involved.

Repair of Stenoses and Occlusions of the Veins

In addition to duplex sonography we also rely on preoperative angiograms.

Short Stenoses at the Venous Anastomosis

There are two treatment options. Based on the high rate of restenosis and thrombosis of endovascular stent placement, we usually prefer open surgery with patch plasty (Fig. 4.59) for its better long-term results, especially in younger patients whose AV-interposition grafts are worth preserving.

Short Stenoses Proximal to the Anastomosis

Stenoses proximal to the anastomosis are situated in the highly mobile axillary region. In this position we always use prosthetic interposition grafts. According to the findings, these grafts are either sutured to the vein proximal to the stenosis (Fig. 4.60) or to the lateral brachial vein (Fig. 4.61) if possible.

Long Stenosis or Occlusions Close to the Axilla

Should the axillary vein be patent close to its entry beneath the clavicula, the interposition of a prosthetic graft seems advisable (Fig. 4.62). For this purpose we expose the vein via an infraaxillary longitudinal incision slightly distal to the anastomosis. The axillary vein is exposed via an infraclavicular transverse incision. We place the prosthetic graft in a curved subcutaneous tunnel which passes the ventral pivot point of the shoulder joint (Fig. 4.63). Thus the motion-dependent compression of the prosthesis can mostly be avoided.

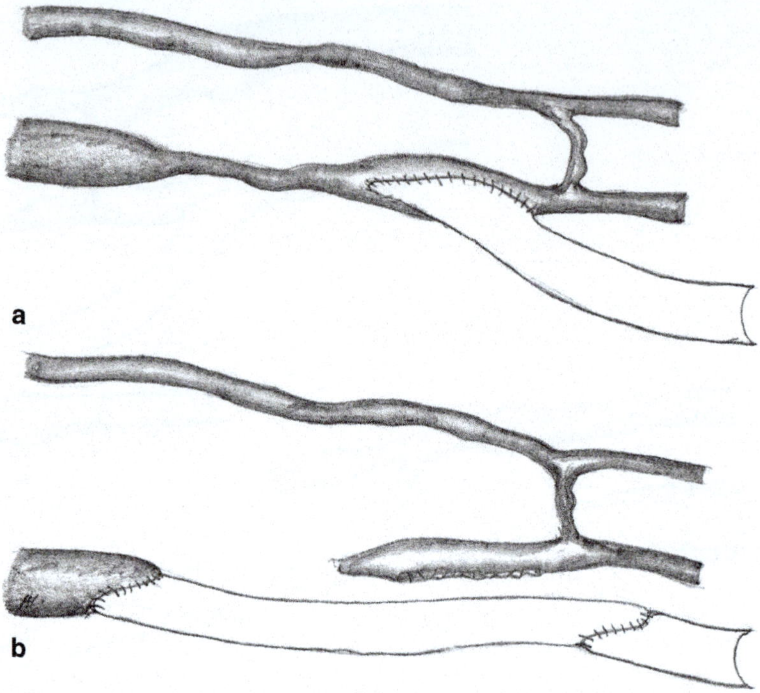

Fig. 4.60 Reconstruction of a long stenosis of the efferent vein (**a**) by inserting a graft (**b**)

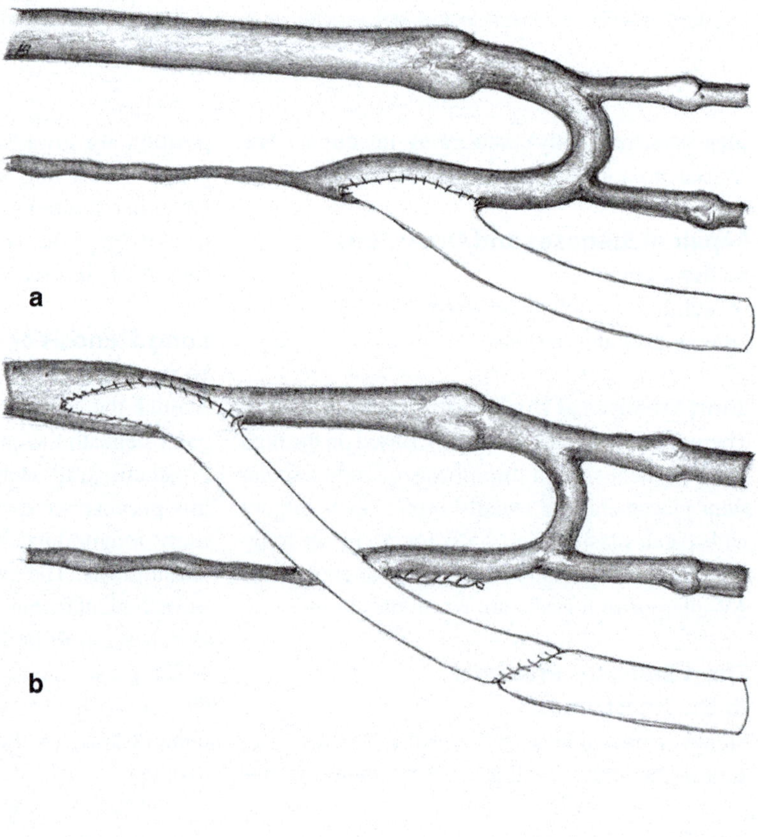

Fig. 4.61 Reconstruction of a long stenosis of the efferent vein (**a**) by transposing and inserting a graft (**b**)

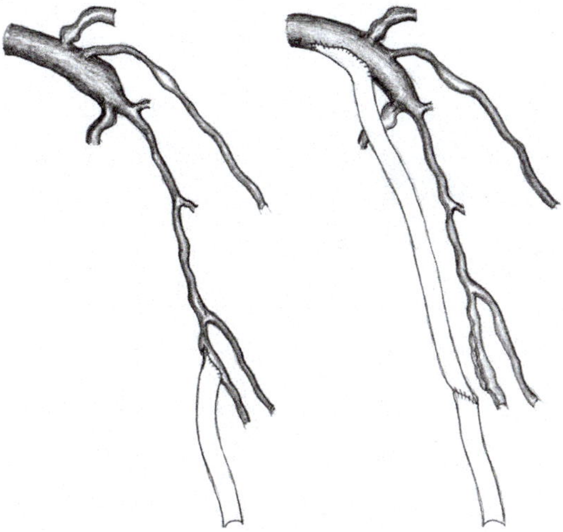

Fig. 4.62 Long axillary occlusion of the vein. Reconstruction using a graft to the infraclavicular axillary vein

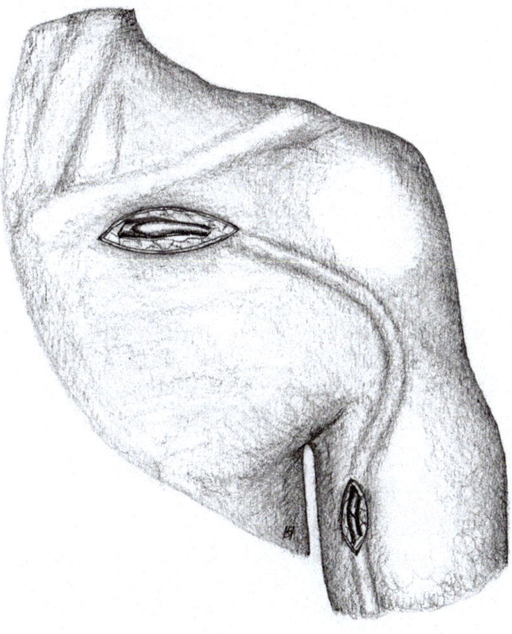

Fig. 4.63 Site of Fig. 4.62

Long Stenoses or Occlusions of the Brachial, Axillary, and Subclavian Veins

With a patent internal jugular vein and patent brachiocephalic vein, it is possible to facilitate drainage by inserting a graft directly to the internal jugular vein in case of stenosed or occluded axillary and subclavian veins (Fig. 4.64).

4.6 Infraclavicular Graft

The placement of a looped infraclavicular interposition graft in the thoracic wall between the axillary artery and vein is one of the most demanding operations of AV access surgery. Therefore it will be presented in detail.

Indication

- Occlusion of the peripheral deep veins of the upper extremities.
- Arterial hypotension (systolic blood pressure below 80 mmHg).
- Hypercoagulability.
- Insufficient peripheral perfusion of an upper extremity.
- Ipsilateral amputation of the arm (so that the sound arm is left intact).
- Ipsilateral spastic paresis of an arm which renders puncturing difficult.
- Preferable to femoral AV shunt loops.

Prerequisite

- Suitable axillary artery and vein.

Contraindication

- Heart failure refractory to therapy because of extra cardiac stress due to high shunt flow.

4.6.1 Access and Technical Advice

Exposure of Axillary Artery and Vein

The exposure of the infraclavicular vessels starts with an infraclavicular transverse incision (Fig. 4.65). The arm should be positioned close to the torso. It might be beneficial to palpate the artery in order to choose the optimum incision. Having passed the subcutaneous adipose tissue, the fascia of the pectoralis major muscle is opened (Fig. 4.66), and the muscle fibers are separated following their orientation (Fig. 4.67). Beneath the pectoralis major muscle, numerous vessels and nerves cross the considerably varying layer of adipose tissue. Here also the palpation of the artery may help find the shortest route. More often than not it is necessary to nick the pectoralis minor muscle that may be found laterally

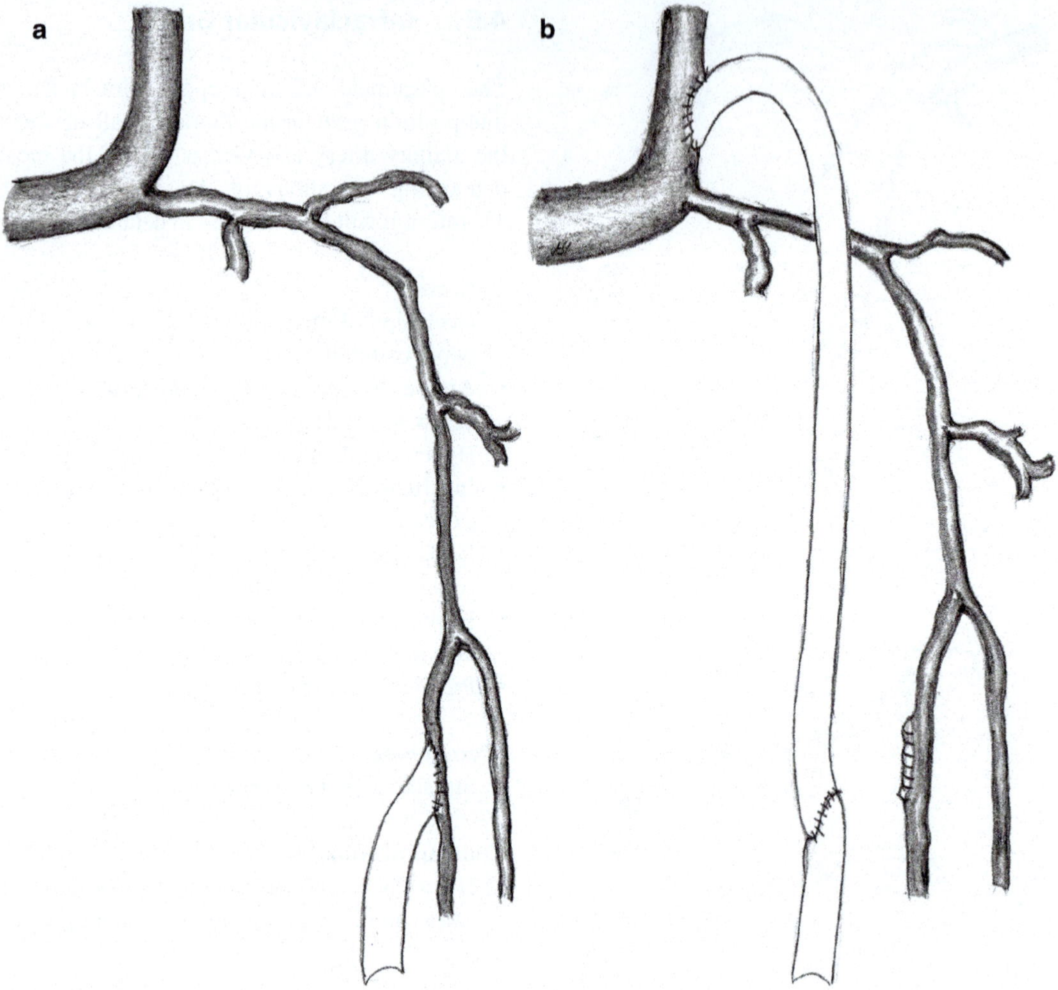

Fig. 4.64 (**a**) Occlusion of the axillary and subclavian veins. (**b**) Reconstruction using a graft to the jugular vein

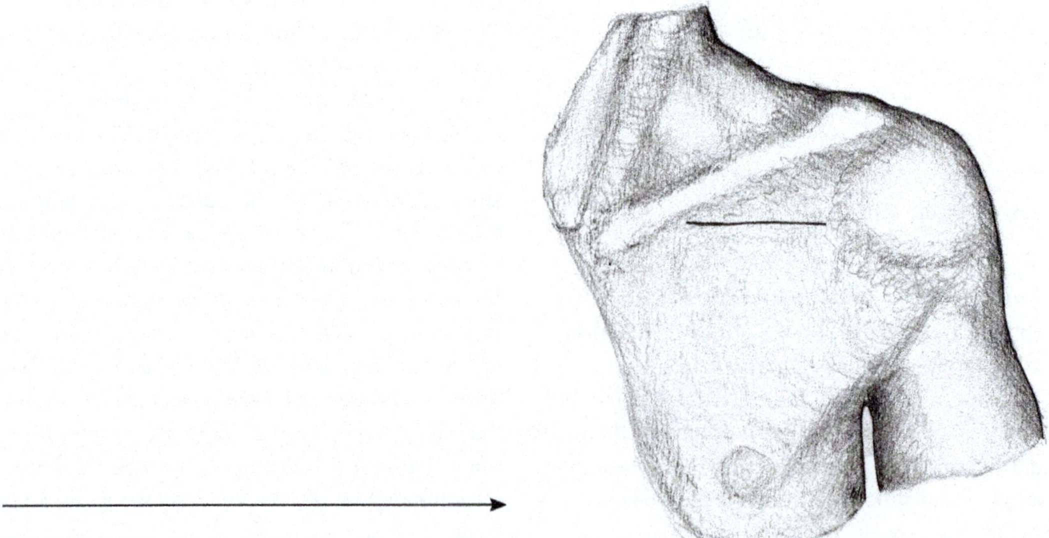

Fig. 4.65 Skin incision to isolate the axillary vessels

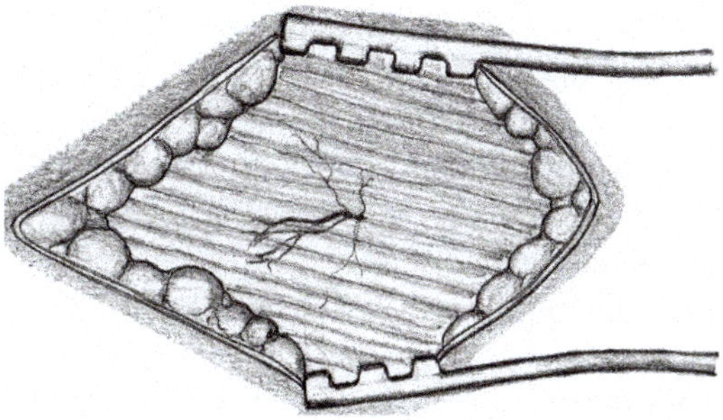

Fig. 4.66 After dissection of the fascia of the major pectoral muscle

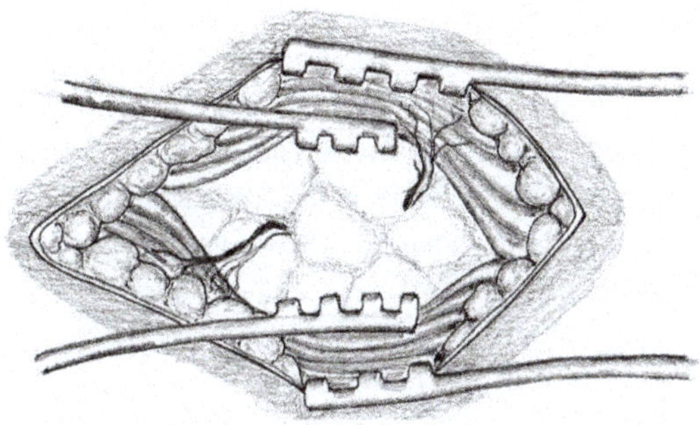

Fig. 4.67 After longitudinally opening the major pectoralis muscle

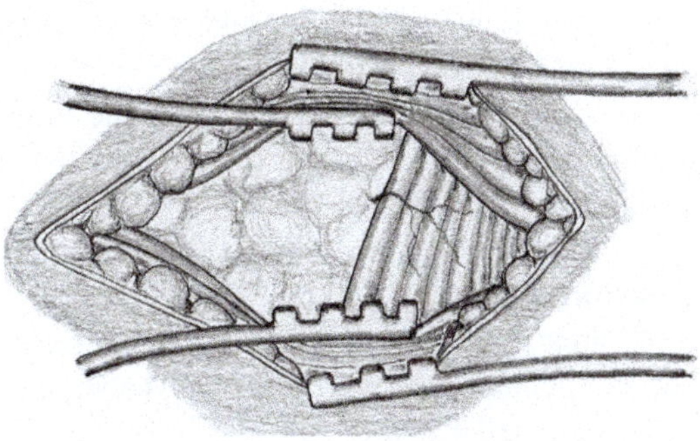

Fig. 4.68 After dissection of the minor pectoral muscle

(Fig. 4.68). Then the axillary vein can typically be seen first (Fig. 4.69). We recommend severing the side branches of the vein (Fig. 4.70) to expose the axillary artery accompanied by nerves (Fig. 4.70).

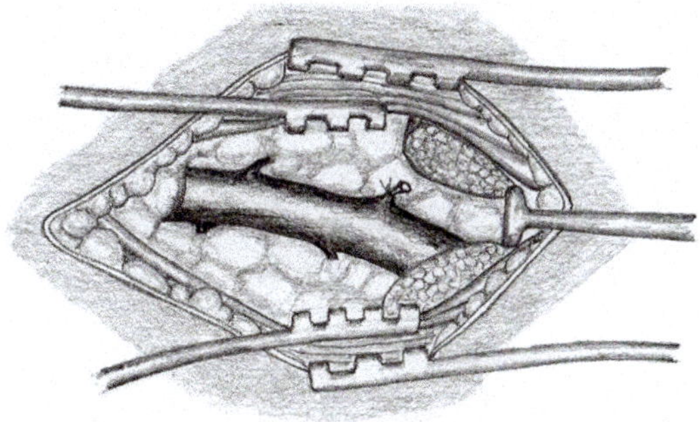

Fig. 4.69 After dissection of the axillary vein

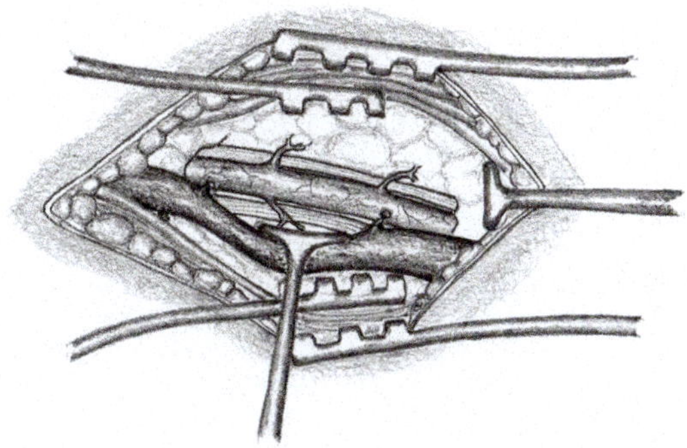

Fig. 4.70 After dissection of the axillary artery

Position of the Anastomosis

Once the axillary artery and vein have been exposed, the position of the anastomosis has to be determined. The anatomical position of the artery and the vein and the maximum reasonable size of the operative site are fixed. For a correct anastomosis there are three requirements:

- The angle of the venous anastomosis should be as acute as possible.
- The inflow radius of the venous anastomosis should be as large as possible.
- The venous anastomosis should not be compressed by the crossing arterial part of the prosthesis.

Different anatomical variations of the infraclavicular axillary vein and artery are depicted in Fig. 4.71.

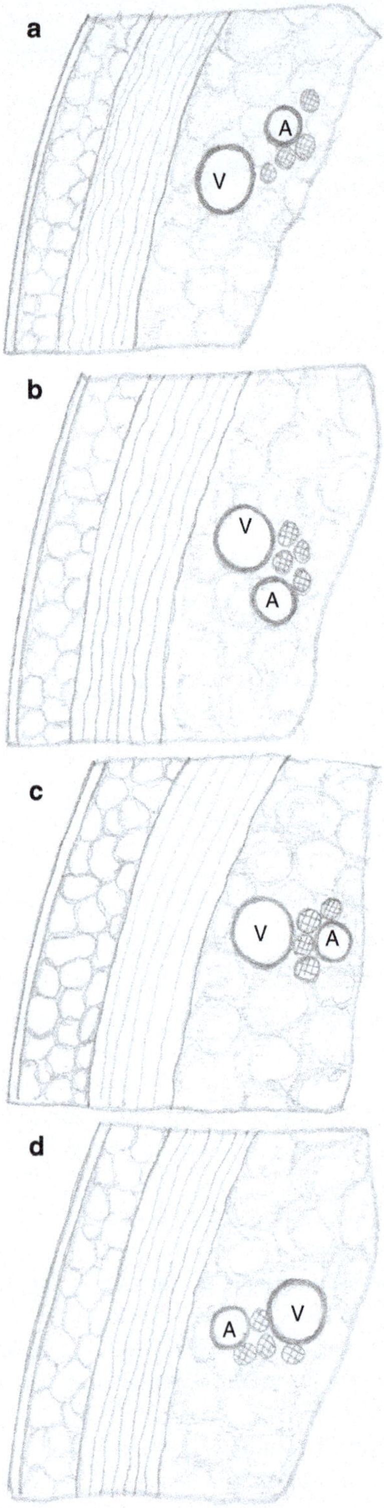

Fig. 4.71 Different anatomical variations of the infraclavicular axillary vein and artery. *A* artery, *V* vein

Most frequently the artery is located dorsal and slightly cranial to the vein (Fig. 4.71a). Several positions for anastomoses are possible (Fig. 4.72a–d). With a wide access to the vessels, option a (Fig. 4.72a) should be chosen as it can accommodate the most acute angle for the anastomosis as well as the largest inflow radius of the prosthesis. Should this prove impossible for topographical reasons, option b offers an alternative, albeit with a considerably smaller inflow radius (Fig. 4.72b). A narrow access leaves space for option c (Fig. 4.72c) with the arterial side of the prosthesis dorsally crossing the venous side. The venous side should only be placed anterior to the arterial side. Otherwise the venous side would almost certainly be compressed (Fig. 4.72d). In rare cases with the artery lying caudad, or caudad and dorsal, to the vein (Fig. 4.71b, c), positions as shown in Fig. 4.72e, f would make sense.

Placement of the Prosthesis

After deciding on the best location for the anastomoses, the prosthesis may be placed in the newly-created subcutaneous tunnel. We recommend marking the path of the loop on the incision film before making an extra incision for the tunnel. As the infraclavicular vessel run relatively far from the surface, both sides of the loop should begin a gentle descent 3–5 cm before entering the surgical field through the subcutaneous adipose tissue and the pectoralis muscle tissue.

Anastomoses

Only after placement in the tunnel do we suture the anastomoses starting with the venous side (Figs. 4.73 and 4.74).

Prognosis/evaluation

Hemodynamically stable AV-access (if indication correct). Of all AV-interposition grafts presented here, most frequently venous stenosis by connective tissue proliferation develops. The infraclavicular axillary vein and subclavian vein seem to react quite strongly to unphysiological flow situations. Therefore great care should be taken to establish an acute angle venous anastomosis with a large inflow radius.

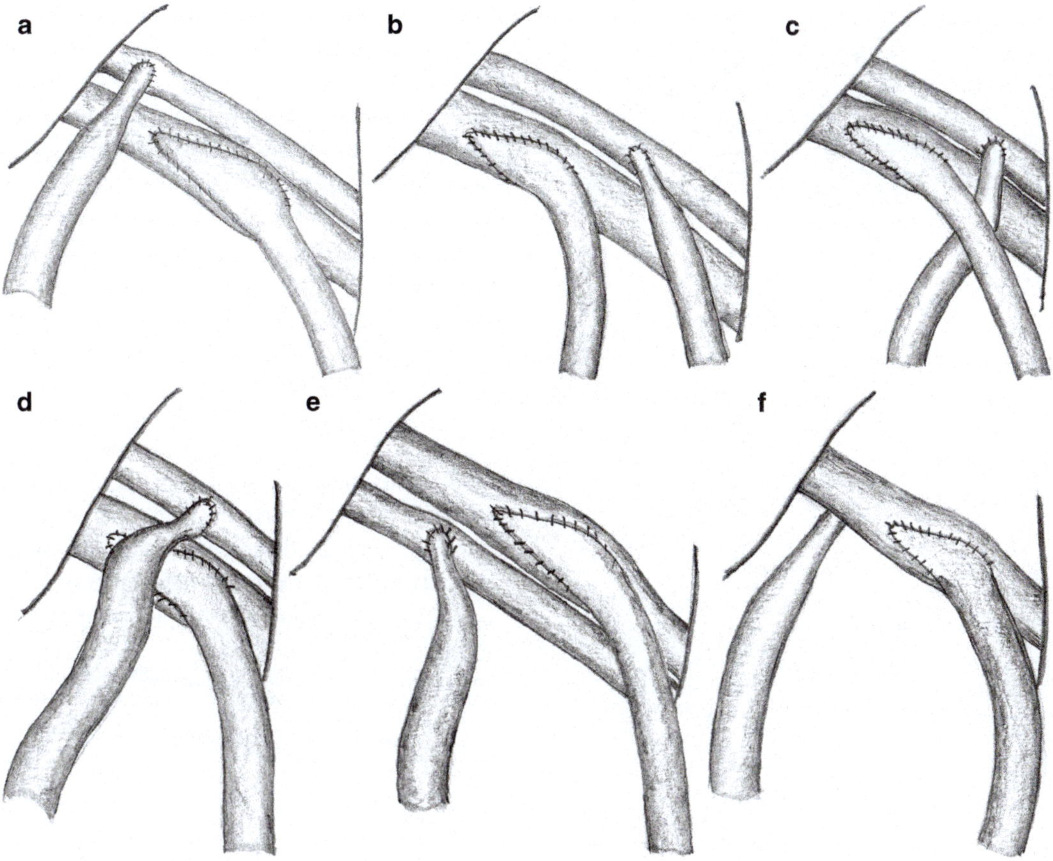

Fig. 4.72 Possible positions for infraclavicular arterious and venous anastomoses (**a–f**)

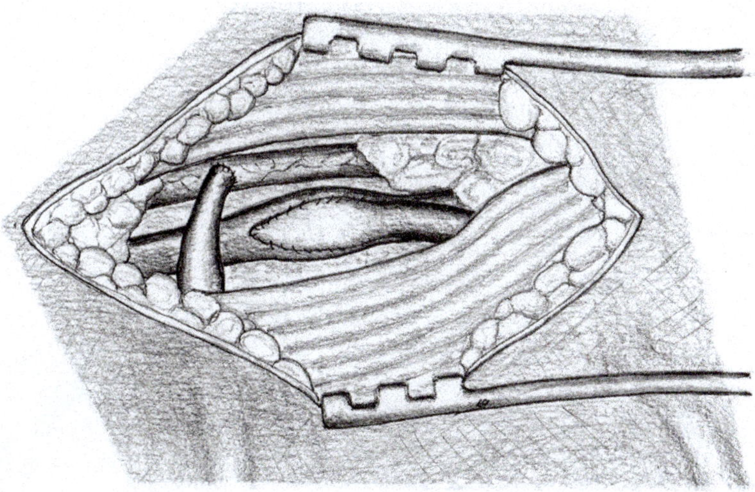

Fig. 4.73 Anastomosis of a subclavian AV loop

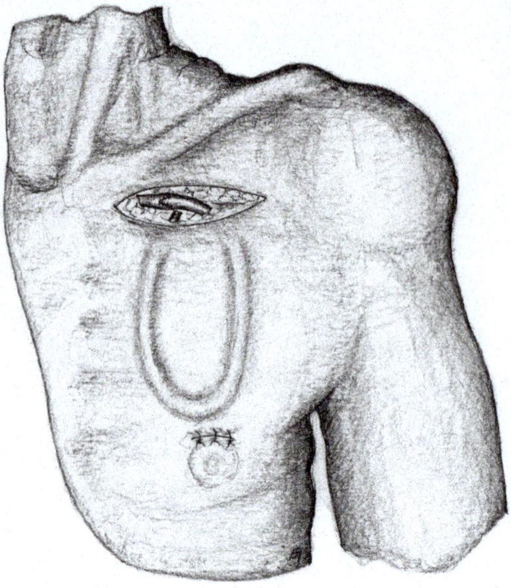

Fig. 4.74 Subclavian AV loop

4.6.2 Repair of Infraclavicular AV Grafts

The most frequent complications comprise stenoses of the venous anastomosis and the subclavian vein, and aneurysm of the prosthetic graft at frequent puncture sites.

Venous stenoses

Treatment depends on the location in relation to the clavicula (Fig. 4.75a, b). We favor pre-treatment phlebography.

- Unless a stenosis reaches the clavicula (Fig. 4.75a), we favor surgical repair (dissection and patch plasty) for better long term results in comparison with endovascular therapy. Frequently marked scarring leads to relatively long times required for surgery. Extra care should be taken to avoid nerve injury.

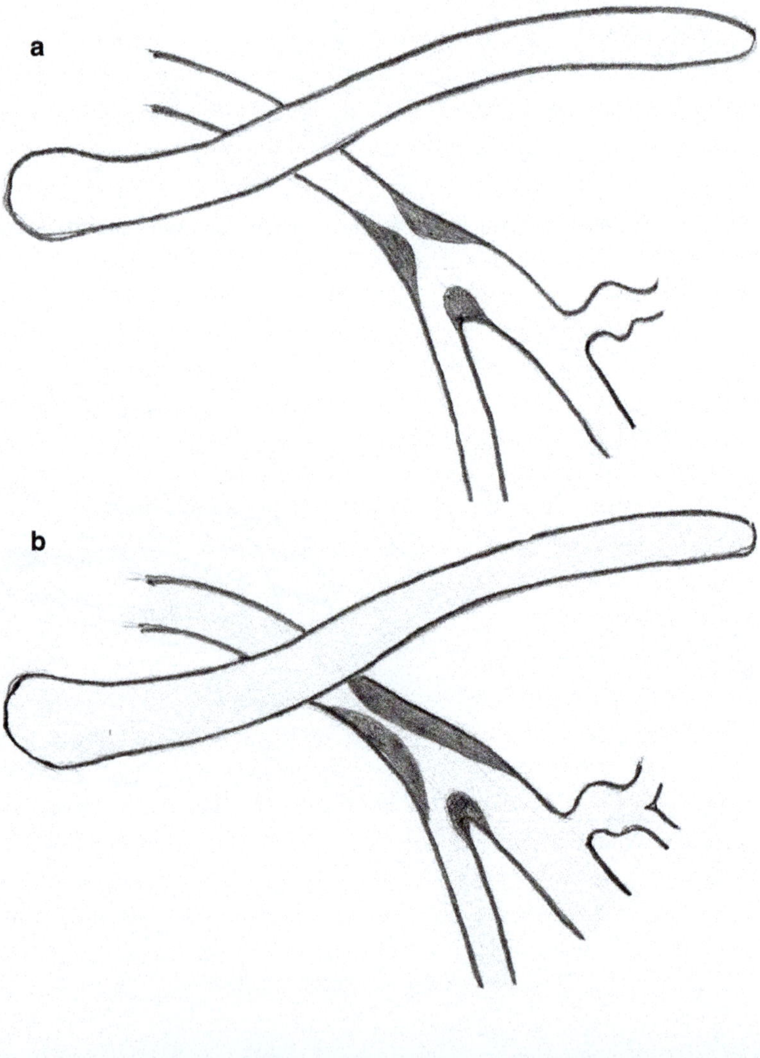

Fig. 4.75 Stenosis of the axillary artery: (**a**) distal to the clavicula and (**b**) reaching the clavicula

- Should a stenosis reach the anterior margin of the clavicula or even farther central regions (Fig. 4.75b), it is not accessible for surgery. Then we see an indication for PTA and stent placement.

Long Stenosis or Occlusion of the Subclavian Vein

In case of a restenosis or occlusion after PTA and stent placement, or with a long occlusion of a graft which is worth preserving, we extend the prosthesis to the internal jugular vein (Fig. 4.76). For this purpose we expose the internal jugular vein via a longitudinal incision and then the venous side of the AV loop graft in order to create a subclavianjugular AV shunt.

4.7 Subclavianjugular AV Grafts

Looped interposition grafts between the axillary artery in the infraclavicular position and the internal jugular vein.

Indications

- Only two of the six large deep veins are patent (jugular, subclavian, and femoral veins). One of these should be preserved as an emergency access.
- Femoral AV loop not feasible or temporarily contraindicated.
- Very rare indication.

Prerequisite

- Definite proof of unimpaired central runoff of the internal jugular vein (respiratory phasicity in color Doppler studies, MR angiography, phlebography via direct venous puncture).

Contraindication

- Just one patent internal jugular vein is the only patent large deep vein (see above). It should be preserved as an emergency access. In this case an arterioarterial interposition graft is indicated.

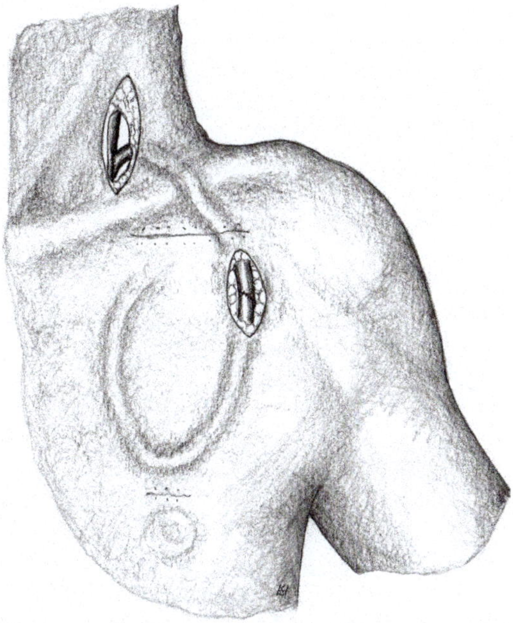

Fig. 4.76 Extension of a subclavian loop to the jugular vein using a graft

Approach to the Internal Jugular Vein and Creation of the Anastomosis

Via a longitudinal incision in the minor supraclavicular fossa (Fig. 4.77), the platysma is dissected and the clavicular head of the sternocleidoid muscle is divided. Then the internal jugular vein is dissected free centrally as far as possible. After the subcutaneous placement of the prosthesis, a terminolateral anastomosis of the prosthesis to the vein is created with the central angle being as acute as possible. For this purpose the graft performs an almost complete U-turn. To prevent kinking or compression of the graft, the radius of this curve should be as large as possible. It may prove useful to nick transversely the longitudinally-divided sternocleidomastoid muscle (Fig. 4.78). The graft pierces this gap. Simple interrupted sutures unite the muscle (Fig. 4.79) without compressing the prosthesis. The access to the infraclavicular axillary artery has been described above.

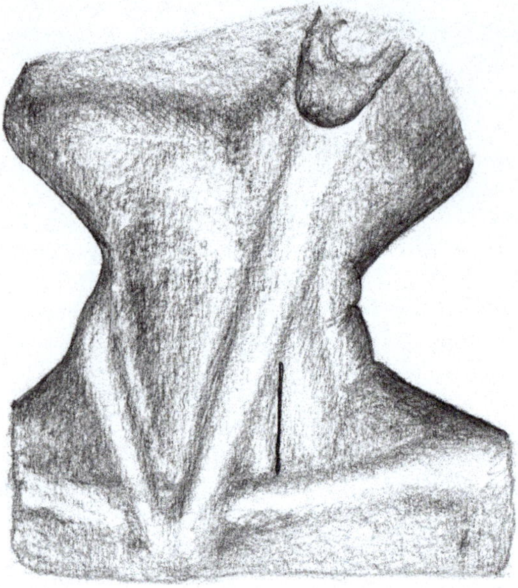

Fig. 4.77 Skin incision for the exposure of the internal jugular vein

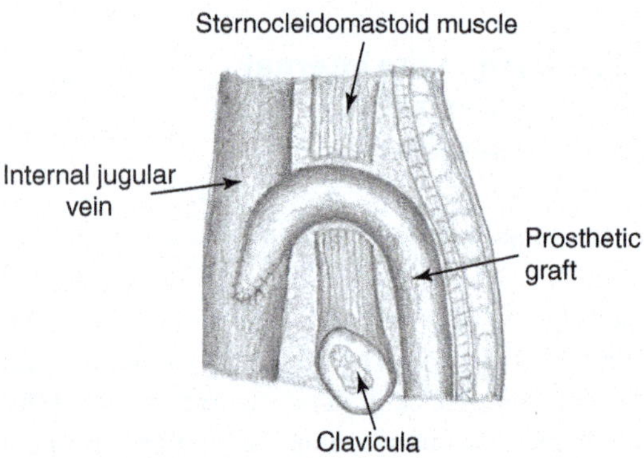

Fig. 4.78 Transverse nicking of the sternocleidomastoid muscle to accommodate the curved path of the graft

Variants

Depending on whether the axiallary artery and internal jugular vein are suitable and on local factors (scars, catheters), there are unilateral or bilateral solutions.

Unilateral Subclavianjugular Shunt (Fig. 4.80)

If possible the unilateral option should be preferred.

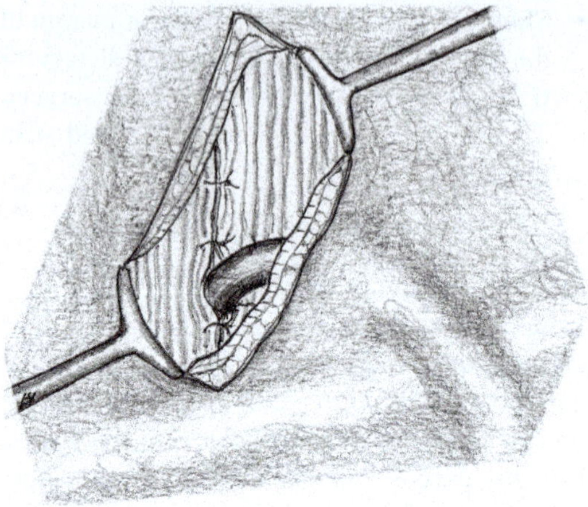

Fig. 4.79 Position of the prosthesis after closing the longitudinally-divided sternocleidomastoid muscle

Bilateral Subclavianjugular Shunt (Necklace Shunt) (Fig. 4.81)

The bilateral option offers a longer graft segment that may be used for puncture. Most often it is not fully used, though, due to painful puncturing.

Prognosis and evaluation

Effective long term vascular access. Most frequent complications include false post puncture aneurysms and stenoses of the jugular anastomoses, which can usually be successfully treated surgically.

4.8 Femoral AV Graft

Looped graft between the femoral artery and vein in the ventral thigh.

Indication

- Only two of the six large deep veins are patent (jugular, subclavian, and femoral veins).
- One of these should be preserved as an emergency access.

Prerequisites

- Femoral vein definitely patent for undisturbed runoff.
- Exclusion of clinically relevant insufficient arterial perfusion of lower extremity.

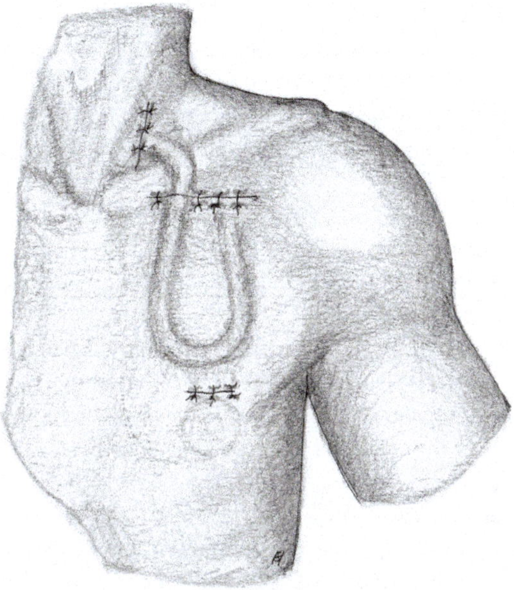

Fig. 4.80 Unilateral subclavianjugular AV shunt

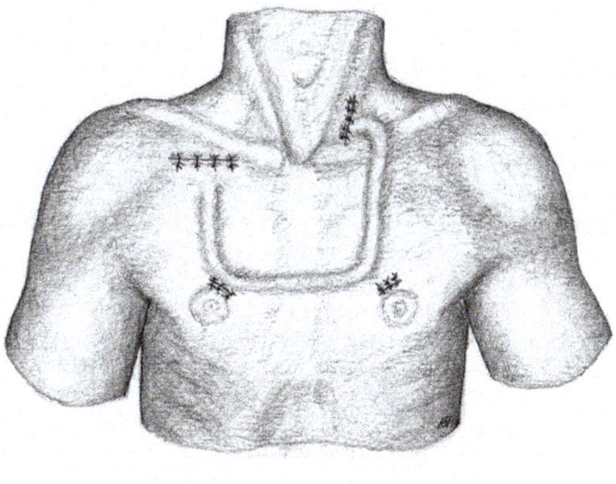

Fig. 4.81 Bilateral subclavianjugular AV shunt

- Exclusion of potential compression of a planned shunt by lower limb prosthesis in above-knee amputees

Contraindication

- Clinically relevant insufficient arterial perfusion of the lower extremity which cannot be improved.

4.8.1 Femoral Loop

Access

The palpable common femoral artery and common femoral vein are exposed via a longitudinal inguinal incision (Fig. 4.82). An additional small transverse incision is made for the U-shaped subcutaneous tunnel. After having pulled the prosthesis through the tunnel, the venous anastomosis is completed (Fig. 4.83). For two reasons it should be situated as far distally as possible (Fig. 4.84):

- Should a stenosis develop near the anastomosis, there is still sufficient space for reconstructions distal to the inguinal ligament.
- The risk of compressing the anastomosis while sitting cross-legged increases the closer the anastomosis is located to the inguinal ligament.

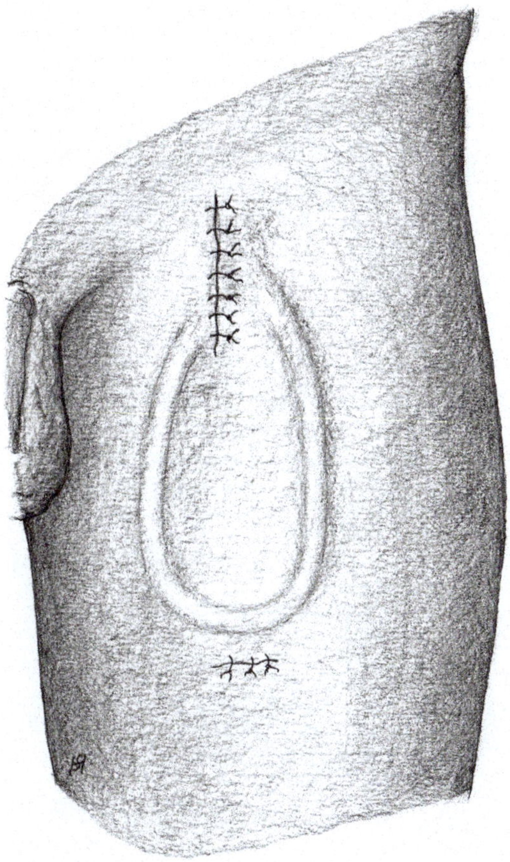

Fig. 4.82 Femoral AV loop

Prognosis and evaluation

Effective long-term vascular access that is not particularly prone to infections. Its most frequent complications are stenoses of the venous anastomoses and false aneurysms at frequent puncture sites.

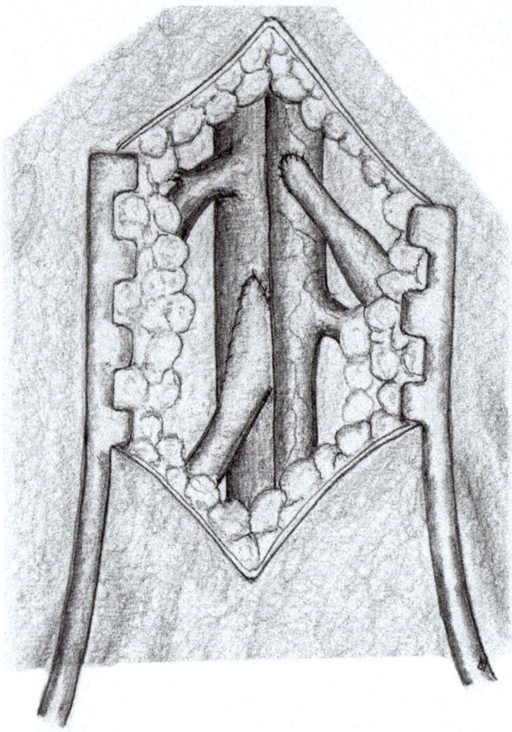

Fig. 4.83 Anastomoses of a femoral loop

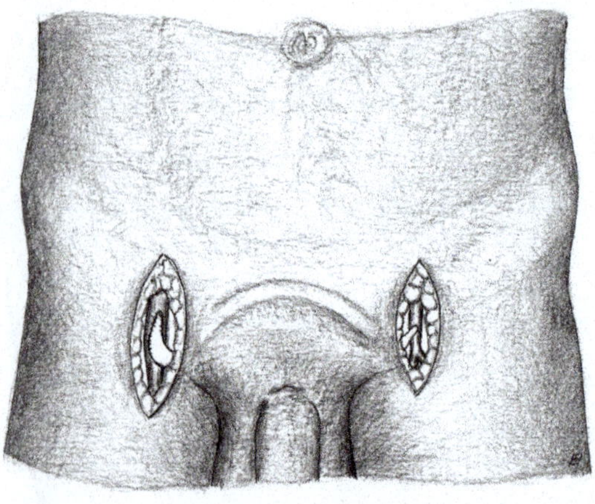

Fig. 4.84 Femorofemoral crossover shunt

4.8.2 Femorofemoral Crossover Shunt

Interposition graft between the femoral artery and contralateral vein crossing suprapubically (Fig. 4.84).

Indications

Only two of the six large deep veins are patent (jugular, subclavian, and femoral veins). One of these is to be preserved as an emergency access.

- The suitable artery and vein are on contralateral sides.

Prerequisites

- Femoral vein definitely patent with uncompromised runoff.
- Exclusion of clinically relevant insufficient arterial perfusion of the lower extremity.
- No compression of the planned shunt by lower limb prosthesis in above knee amputees.

Contraindication

- Clinically relevant insufficient arterial perfusion of the lower extremity which cannot be improved.

Access

See above.

Prognosis

Our own experience is limited as this operation has only been performed twice by us.

Evaluation

In this extremely rare constellation the disadvantageous suprapubic path of the prosthesis causes punctures to be painful. The desired acute angle of the venous anastomosis and its desired distal position might prove hard to realize.

4.8.3 Repair of Femoral Grafts

Stenoses near the venous anastomosis and/or of the femoral vein proximal to the anastomosis constitute the most frequent complications. Distal to the inguinal ligament, effective surgical repair including patch plasty is possible. We think that near or cranial to the inguinal ligament PTA is always indicated although its success may be short-lived. *Therefore the venous anastomosis should be placed as distal as possible.*

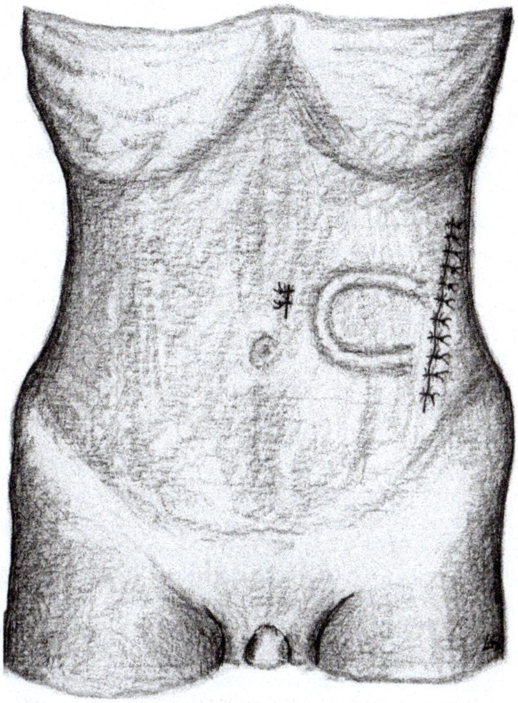

Fig. 4.85 Aortocaval AV shunt

4.9 Other AV Shunts

In the literature a whole variety of other rare AV accesses have been described such as arterialized and superficialized femoral veins or interposition grafts to the superior caval and renal veins. These operations put the patients under a lot of stress. We have never performed them. We have encountered several patients with severe complications after using the common carotid artery as the feeding vessel.

The common carotid artery must never be used as the feeding artery of an AV vascular access. With the armamentarium presented here it has been possible to create *effective* hemodialysis accesses in more than 17,000 operations over a 30-year period. We haven't yet had to establish an aortocaval AV shunt which is reserved for extremely rare circumstances (Fig. 4.85). Then the retroperitoneal exposure of the aorta and vena cava and their connection via a shunt prosthesis passing through the subcutaneous tissue of the ventral abdominal wall would be an option.

4.10 First Puncture of AV Grafts

With an ePTFE prosthesis we wait for 2–3 weeks before the first puncture. Under exceptional circumstances with no other choices, though, we have already started puncturing on the first postoperative day without complications.

References

Affeld K, Kertscher U (2011) Vorlesungsskript "Strömungsmechanik in der Medizin – Biofluidmechanik". www.charite.de/biofluidmechanik/downloads/SkriptBiofluidmechanik1.pdf

Akoh J (2009) Prosthetic arteriovenous grafts for hemodialysis. J Vasc Access 10:137–147

Asif A, Gadalean FN, Merrill D, Cherla G, Cipleu CD, Epstein DL, Roth D (2005) Inflow stenosis in arteriovenous fistulas and grafts: a multicenter, prospective study. Kidney Int 67:1986–1992

Bassiouny HS, White S, Glagov S, Choi E, Giddens DP, Zarins CK (1992) Anastomotic intimal hyperplasia: mechanical injury or flow induced. J Vasc Surg 15:708–717

Beradinelli L (2006) Grafts and graft materials as vascular substitutes for haemodialysis access construction. Eur J Vasc Endovasc Surg 32:203–211

Berard X, Baste JC, Sassoust G, Du Bourguet L, Combe C, De Precigout V, Midy D (2003) Retrospective study of the one-year patency of a cuffed polytetrafluoroethylene Venaflo-type graft placed for venous hemodialysis access. J Mal Vasc 28:73–78

Bittl JA (2010) Catheter interventions for hemodialysis fistulas and grafts. JACC Cardiovasc Interv 3:1–11

Bozof R, Kats M, Barker J, Allon M (2008) Time to symptomatic vascular stenosis at different locations in patients with arteriovenous grafts. Semin Dial 21:285–288

Chang TI, Paik J, Greene T, Desai M, Bech F, Cheung AK, Chertow GM (2011) Intradialytic hypotension and vascular access thrombosis. J Am Soc Nephrol 22:1536–1543

Choudhury D, Lee J, Elivera HS, Ball D, Roberts AB, Ahmed Z (1995) Correlation of venography, venous pressure, and hemoaccess function. Am J Kidney Dis 25:269–275

Cross MM (1965) Rheology of non-Newtonian fluids: a new equation for pseudoplastic systems. J Coll Sci 20:417–437

Cull DL, Carsten CG 3rd, Kalbaugh CA, York JW, Campbell TR, Cass AL, Taylor SM (2008) The reverse J arteriovenous graft configuration for hemodialysis access: rationale, technique, and outcomes. Am Surg 74:620–624

Davies MG, Huynh TT, Hagen PO (2000) Pathophysiology of access failure. In: Colon PJ, Schwab SJ, Nicholson

ML (eds) Hemodialysis vascular access: practice and problems. Oxford University Press, Oxford/New York, pp S 23–S 51

Escobar FS, Schwartz SA, Aboulijoud M, Douzdjian V, Escobar MD, Besarab A, Elliott JP (1999) A preliminary study comparing a new "hooded" vs. conventional ePTFE graft in hemodialysis patients. In: Henry ML (ed) Vascular access for hemodialysis VI. W.L. Gore & Associates, Inc. and Precept Press, Chicago, pp S 205–S 211

Fillinger MF, Reinitz ER, Schwartz RA, Resetarits DE, Paskanik AM, Bruch D, Bredenberg CE (1990) Graft geometry and venous intimal-medial hyperplasia in arteriovenous loop grafts. J Vasc Surg 11:556–566

Flarup S, Haimeri H (2003) Arteriovenous PTFE dialysis access in the lower extremity: a new approach. Ann Vasc Surg 17:581–584

Fung YC, Liu SQ (1993) Elementary mechanics of the endothelium of blood vessels. J Biomech Eng 115:1–12

Geenen IL et al (2010) Prosthetic lower extremity hemodialysis access grafts have satisfactory patency despite a high incidence of infection. J Vasc Surg 52(6):1546–1550

Gordon IL (1996) Physiology of the arteriovenous fistula. In: Wilson SE (ed) Vascular access – principles and practise. Mosby-Year-Book Inc, St. Louis, pp S 335–S 345

Haruguchi H, Teraoka S (2003) Intimal hyperplasia and hemodynamic factors in arterial bypass and arteriovenous grafts: a review. J Artif Organs 6:227–235

Heethaar RM (1993) Atherosclerosis and blood flow. In: Strackee J, Westerhof N (eds) The physics of heart and circulation. Institute of Physics Publishing, Bristol/Philadelphia, pp S 321–S 334

Heise M, Husmann I, Grüneberg AK, Knobel A, Kirschner P, Heidenhain C (2011) Comparison of straight and Venaflo-type cuffed arteriovenous ePTFE grafts in an animal study. J Vasc Surg 53:1661–1667

Hofstra L, Bergmans DC, Leunissen KM, Hoeks AP, Kitslaar PJ, Daemen MJ, Tordoir JH (1995) Anastomotic intimal hyperplasia in prosthetic arteriovenous fistulas for hemodialysis is associated with initial high flow velocity and not with mismatch in elastic properties. J Am Soc Nephrol 6:1625–1633

Hofstra L, Bergmans DCJJ, Leunissen KML, Hoeks APG, Kitslaar PJEHM, Tordoir JH (1996) Prosthetic arteriovenous fistulas and venous anastomotic stenosis: influence of a high flow velocity on the development of intimal hyperplasia. Blood Purif 14:345–349

Huber TS, Carter JW, Carter RL, Seeger JM (2003) Patency of autogenous and polytetrafluoroethylene upper extremity arteriovenous hemodialysis accesses: a systematic review. J Vasc Surg 38:1005–1011

Huhle A (2002) Die Flussdynamik in der arteriellen Anastomose arterio-venöser Interponate in Abhängigkeit von der Anastomosenmetrik und der arteriellen Speisung. Dissertation, Medizinischen Fakultät Charité der Humboldt-Universität zu Berlin

Huhle A, Krüger U, Scholz H (2002) Die Hämodynamik in der arteriellen Anastomose arterio-venöser (av) Interponate in Abhängigkeit von der Anastomosenmetrik (eine in vitro Untersuchung). Zentralbl Chir 127:374–375

Jean-Baptiste E, Hassen-Khodja R, Haudebourg P, Declemy S, Batt M, Bouillanne PJ (2008) Axillary loop grafts for hemodialysis access: midterm results from a single-center study. J Vasc Surg 47:138–143

Kan CD, Wu HY, Wang JN, Wu JM, Yang YJ (2009) Improved pulmonary artery geometry after a Norwood procedure by using a Venaflo II graft as an RV-MPA conduit. Ann Thorac Surg 88:690–691

Kannan RY, Salacinski HJ, Butler PE, Hamilton G, Seifalian AM (2007) Current status of prosthetic bypass grafts: a review. J Biomed Mater Res B Appl Biomater 74:570–581

Kao CL, Chang JP (2004) The reverse upper arm curved graft with ringed PTFE graft as an alternative vascular access procedure for hemodialysis. J Cardiovasc Surg (Torino) 45:55–57

Kleinstreuer C (2006) Biofluid dynamics: principles and selected applications. Taylor Francis Inc, Boca Raton

Ko PJ, Liu YH, Hung YN, Hsieh HC (2009) Patency rates of cuffed and noncuffed extended polytetrafluoroethylene grafts in dialysis access: a prospective, randomized study. World J Surg 33:846–851

Kolakowski S Jr, Dougherty MJ, Calligaro KD (2003) Salvaging prosthetic dialysis fistulas with stents: forearm versus upper arm grafts. J Vasc Surg 38: 719–723

Krueger U, Heise M, Huhle A (2001) Effects of arterial and venous anastomotic design on hemodynamics in arteriovenous prosthetic grafts. In: Henry ML (ed) Vascular access for hemodialysis VII. W.L. Gore & Associates, Inc., and Precept Press, Chicago, pp S 177–S 191

Krueger U, Zanow J, Scholz H (2002) Computational fluid dynamics and vascular access. Artif Organs 26:571–575

Krueger U, Huhle A, Krys K, Scholz H (2004) Effect of tapered grafts on hemodynamics and flow rate in dialysis access grafts. Artif Organs 28:623–628

Krüger U, Scholz H (2008) Der Einstromradius arteriovenöser Schlingen. Gefäßchirurgie 13:45–50

Krueger U, Zanow J, Scholz H (2009) An attempt at explanation for etiology of stenotic lesions proximal of the venous anastomosis at arteriovenous vascular grafts. In: Proceedings of World Congress on Medical Physics and Biomedical Engineering, Munich, 7–12 Sept 2009

Lau KK, Jones DP, Gaber O, Nezatkatgoo N (2007) Use of a "composite" vascular access graft in a young child on hemodialysis. Hemodial Int 11:190–192

Lemson MS, Tordoir JH, Daemen MJ, Kitslaar PJ (2000) Intimal hyperplasia in vascular grafts. Eur J Vasc Endovasc Surg 19:336–350

Liu YH, Hung YN, Hsieh HC, Ko PJ (2006) Impact of cuffed, expanded polytetrafluoroethylene dialysis grafts on graft outlet stenosis. World J Surg 30:2290–2294

Liepsch D (1989) Pulsierende Strömung von nicht-Newtonschen Fluiden in starren und elastischen Modellen der menschlichen Arterien. Hamostaseologie 9:82–107

Liepsch D (1998) Biofluid mechanics. Biomed Tech 43:94–99

Longest PW, Kleinstreuer C (2000) Computational haemodynamics analysis and comparison study of arteriovenous grafts. J Med Eng Technol 24:102–110

Matsuda H, Miyazaki M, Oka Y, Nakao A, Choda Y, Kokumai Y, Kunitomo K, Tanaka N (2003) A polyurethane vascular access graft and a hybrid polytetrafluoroethylene graft as an arteriovenous fistula for hemodialysis: comparison with an expanded polytetrafluoroethylene graft. Artif Organs 27:722–727

Modarai B, Dasgupta P, Taylor J, Koffman G, Khan MS (2005) Follow-up of polytetrafluoroethylene arteriovenous fistulae for haemodialysis. Int J Clin Pract 59:1005–1007

Munson BR, Young DF, Okiishi TH (1994) Fundamentals of fluid mechanics. Wiley, New York

Niyyar VD (2008) Anterior chest wall arteriovenous grafts: an underutilized form of hemodialysis access. Semin Dial 21:578–580

Noack L, Tamaschke C (1988) Arteriovenous subclavio-subclavian Collier shunt - a further possibility in chronic hemodialysis. Zentralbl Chir 113:1359–1361

Nyberg SL et al (2001) Prelimary experience with a cuffed ePTFE graft for hemodialysis vascular access. ASAIO J 47:333–337

Ojha MJ, Cobbold RS, Johnston KW (1995) Flow and shear stress patterns at proximal and distal ends of bypass grafts: Implications for the development of intimal hyperplasia. In: Callow AD, Ernst EB (eds) Vascular surgery - theory and practice. Prentice-Hall, Appleton & Lange, Stamford, pp 1231–1236

Opitz H, Pfeiffer C (1984) Das kardiovaskuläre System. VEB Georg Thieme, Leipzig

Petzold K (2001) Experimentelle und klinische Untersuchungen zur Beeinflussung der subendothelialen Intimahyperplasie im Bereich der venösen Anastomose gerader arteriovenöser Interponate am Oberarm. Dissertation, Medizinischen Fakultät Charité der Humboldt-Universität zu Berlin

Ravari H, Kazemzade GH, Modaghegh MH, Khashayar P (2010) Patency rate and complications of polytetrafluoroethylene grafts compared with polyurethane grafts for hemodialyis access. Ups J Med Sci 115:245–248

Reddemann P (2010) Der Einfluss der Lokalisation der arteriellen Anastomose und des Flussminutenvolumens von arterio-venösen Gefäßzugängen auf den peripheren Perfusionsdruck bei in vitro Untersuchungen am Kreislaufmodell. Dissertation, 2010, Medizinische Fakultät Charité – Universitätsmedizin Berlin

Richman P, Wilson SE (1991) Bridge grafts for angioaccess. In: Ernst CB, Stanley JC (eds) Current therapy in vascular surgery. B.C.Decker Inc, Philadelphia/Toronto, pp S 927–S 932

Rotmans JI, Pasterkamp G, Verhagen HJ, Pattynama PM, Blankestijn PJ, Stroes ES (2005) Hemodialysis access graft failure: time to revisit an unmet clinical need? J Nephrol 18(1):9–20

Salam TA, Lumdsden AB, Suggs WD, Ku DN (1996) Low shear stress promotes intimal hyperplasia thickening. J Vasc Invest 2:12–22

Salimi J, Zafaghandi MR (2008) The patency rate and complication of polytetrafluoroethylene vascular access grafts in hemodialysis patients: a prospective study from Iran. Saudi J Kidney Dis Transpl 19:280–285

Santoro TD, Cambria RA (1997) PTFE shunts for hemodialysis access: progressive choice of configuration. Semin Vasc Surg 10:166–174

Scher LA, Katzman HE (2004) Alternative graft materials for haemodialysis access. Semin Vasc Surg 17:19–24

Schild AF (2008) Arteriovenous fistulae vs. arteriovenous grafts: a retrospective review of 1,700 consecutive vascular access cases. J Vasc Access 9:231–235

Schild AF, Schuman ES, Noicely K, Kaufman J, Gillaspie E, Fuller J, Collier P, Ronfeld A, Nair R (2011) Early cannulation prosthetic graft (Flixene™) for arteriovenous access. J Vasc Access 12:248–253

Schmidt RF, Thews G (2000) Physiologie des Menschen. Springer, Berlin

Scholz H, Naundorf M, Matthes G, Precht K, Röseler R, Schulze BD, Schoepke W (1988) Untersuchungen zum Einsatz formaldehydkonservierter, innenflächensilikonierter und formfixierter boviner Gefäße als Gefäßtransplantate. Zbl Chir 113:441

Scholz H, Zanow J, Petzold M, Petzold K (1999a) Desparate access. Prepectorial bridge grafts. Dialyse J 16:266

Scholz H, Zanow J, Petzold K, Krueger U, Settmacher U, Petzold M (1999b) Five years experience with arteriovenous patch prosthesis (AVP) as access for hemodialysis. In: Henry ML (ed) Vascular access for hemodialysis VI. W.L. Gore & Associates, Inc. and Precept Press, Chicago, pp 241–254

Scholz H, Simba A, Bürger K, Settmacher U (1995) Perioperative Antibiotikaprophylaxe in der Dialyseshuntchirurgie. Int J Exp Clin Chemother 7:25–35

Scholz H, Mauendor M, Precht K, Schulze BD, Rössler E, Buder HW, Matthes G, Scoepke W (1990) Subclavio-jugularer av-shunt (Colliershunt) für die Hämodialyse. Angio 1990(12):151–154

Scott JD, Cull DL, Kalbaugh CA, Carsten CG, Blackhurst D, Taylor SM, Snyder BA, York JW, Langan EM (2006) The mid-thigh loop arteriovenous graft: patient selction, technique, and results. Am Surg 72: 825–828

Shu MC, Hwang NH (1991) Haemodynamics of angioaccess venous anastomoses. J Biomed Eng 13:103–112

Sivanesan S, How TV, Black RA, Bakran A (1999) Flow patterns in the radiocephalic arteriovenous fistula: an in vitro study. J Biomech 32:915–925

Slayden GC, Spergel L, Jennings WC (2008) Secondary arteriovenous fistulas: converting prosthetic AV grafts to autogenous dialysis access. Semin Dial 21:474–482

Sorom AJ et al (2002) Prospective, randomized evaluation of a cuffed expanded polytetrafluoroethylene graft for hemodialysis vascular access. Surgery 132:135–140

Sottiurai VS (1990) Biogenesis and etiology of distal anastomotic intimal hyperplasia. Int Angiol 9:59–69

Staalsen NH, Ulrich M, Winther J, Pedersen EM, How T, Nygaard H (1995) The anastomosis angle does change the flow fields at vascular end-to-side anastomoses in vivo. J Vasc Surg 21:460–471

Staramos DN, Lazarides MK, Tzilalis VD, Ekonomou CS, Simopoulos CE, Dayantas JN (2000) Patency of autologous and prosthetic arteriovenous fistulas in elderly patients. Eur J Surg 166:777–781

Thubrikar MJ (2007) Vascular mechanics and pathology. Springer Science + Business Media, LLC, New York

Tordoir JH (1999) Hemodynamic causes for chronic access failure. Dialyse J Heft 66:230–231

Tsoulfas G, Hertl M, Ko DSC, Elias N, Kawai T (2008) Long-term outcome of cuffed expanded PTFE graft for hemodialysis vascular access. Vascular Access XI Symposium, Orlando

Vega D, Polo JR, Polo J, López Baena JA, Pacheco D, García-Pajares R (2001) Brachial-jugular expanded PTFE grafts for dialysis. Ann Vasc Surg 15:553–556

Wijeyartne SM, Kannangara L (2011) Safety and efficacy of electrospun polycarbonate-urethane vascular graft for early hemodialysis access: first clinical results in man. J Vasc Access 12:28–35

Zarins CK, Bassionuny HS, Glagov S (1996) Intimal hyperplasia. In: Haimovici H (ed) Haimovici's vascular surgery. Blackwell Science, Cambridge, MA, pp S 678–S 687

5 Arterioarterial Grafts

W.D. Brittinger had the basic idea for this kind of hemodialysis access. He was the first to publish the superficialization of the superficial femoral artery for puncture (Brittinger et al. 1969), which was abandoned because of frequent microembolisms. In 1994 the access described below was developed for a patient in whom all large deep veins were occluded.

Principle

Interposition of a prosthetic loop graft into the infraclavicular axillary artery or common femoral artery.

Indication

An arterioarterial graft for hemodialysis is only rarely indicated. There are four indications:

1. All six large deep veins (femoral, jugular, and subclavian) are occluded or not suitable due to septic complications.
2. Only one of the six large deep veins is patent, which has to be preserved as an emergency access.
3. With heart failure refractory to therapy, the increased cardiac output induced by an AV access would impair the preexisting dysfunction even further.
4. Peripheral vascular disease with inadequate limb perfusion:
   - Already without an AV access of the extremity and/or
   - After proximalization of the arterial inflow into an AV shunt from the feeding infraclavicular axillary artery

5.1 Physiology of Arterioarterial Grafts

To guarantee a sufficient flow for effective dialysis, the following requirements have to be fulfilled:

- Always insert the loop graft into the course of the artery and not just as a bypass to a patent artery, for then the flow in the prosthetic graft would be relatively low due to the flow distribution. Dialysis could be ineffective with a high risk of thrombosis.
- Only choose a large artery with a high flow volume. Thus only the infraclavicular axillary artery and the common femoral artery are practicable options.

Definite physiologic advantages of arterioarterial interpositon grafts include their lack of influence on:

- Cardiac output
- Peripheral perfusion

Take care to add only drugs to the dialysate which are approved for *intraarterial administration*.

Due to the flow rate (typically around 150–250 mL/min), which is significantly lower than in

H. Scholz, *Arteriovenous Access Surgery*,
DOI 10.1007/978-3-642-41139-7_5, © Springer-Verlag Berlin Heidelberg New York 2015

AV shunts, the time required for a dialysis session is longer (frequently 5–6 h). Large surface area dialyzers increase the efficiency of hemodialysis.

5.2 Infraclavicular Arterioarterial Graft

Indication
Preferred to femoral position.

Prerequisite
Patent arterial vasculature of the upper extremity.

Contraindication
Amputation of the ipsilateral arm (with low flow perfusion).

Approach
Exposure of the artery via an infraclavicular transverse incision and placement of the prosthetic graft into a looped subcutaneous tunnel of the ventral thoracic wall (Fig. 5.1).

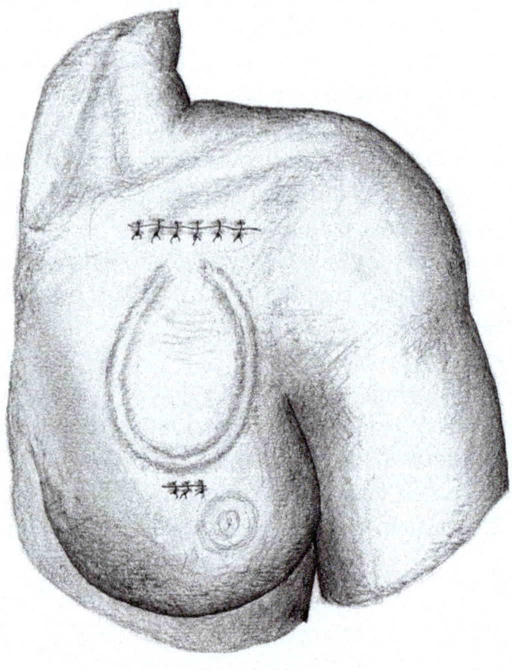

Fig. 5.1 Subclavian arterioarterial graft

Technical hints
Clamping of the axillary artery after systemic heparinization, transverse severance of the artery, and terminoterminal anastomoses to the prosthesis (Fig. 5.2). The diameter of the graft should match the diameter of the artery. Seven millimeter grafts seem to be suitable.

Prognosis
When thrombosis occurs, patients almost always only complain of a cold sensation in the arm.

Evaluation
Effective and safe vascular access for many years when taking into account its particularities.

5.3 Femoral Arterioarterial Graft

Indication
Infraclavicular graft not possible.

Prerequisite
Patent arterial vasculature of the lower extremity.

Contraindication
Insufficient flow in the common femoral artery (e.g., after above knee amputation).

Approach
Exposure of the common femoral artery via a longitudinal groin incision. Due to the path of the artery, the graft should be placed laterally for practical reasons (Fig. 5.3).

Technical hints
Clamping of the common femoral artery after systemic heparinization, transverse severance of the artery, and terminolateral anastomoses of the prosthesis (Fig. 5.4). The diameter of the graft should match the diameter of the artery. Seven millimeter grafts seem to be suitable.

Prognosis
Satisfactory function for years. More often than with AV grafts, false aneurysms at puncture sites require repair. When thrombosis occurs, acute insufficient peripheral perfusion leads to rest pain.

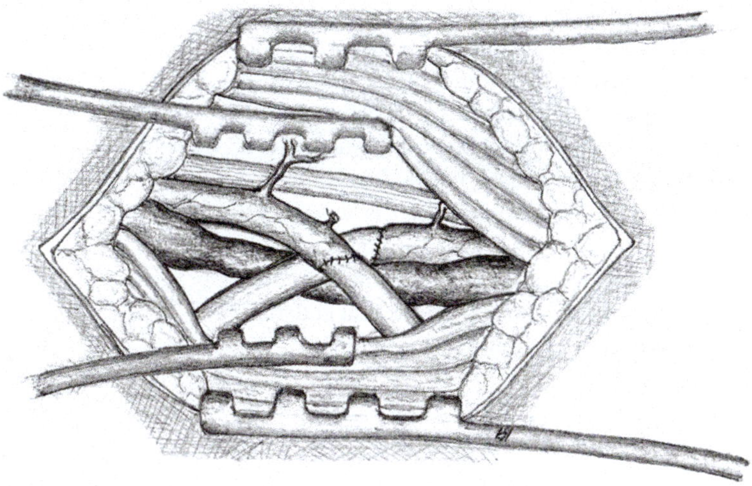

Fig. 5.2 Anastomoses of a subclavian arterioarterial graft

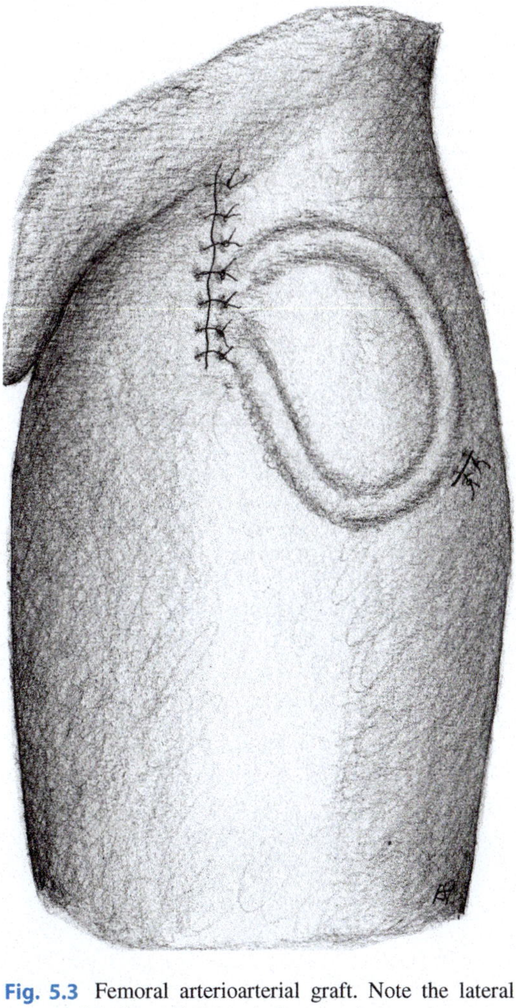

Fig. 5.3 Femoral arterioarterial graft. Note the lateral course of the loop (for practical reasons)

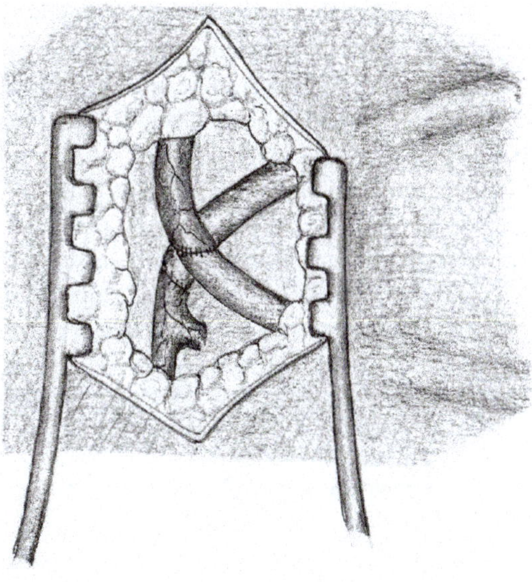

Fig. 5.4 Anastomoses of a femoral arterioarterial graft

Evaluation
Effective and safe vascular access for many years when taking into account its particularities.

5.4 Repair of Arterioarterial Grafts

Due to the small number of cases, our experience with femoral arterioarterial grafts is limited in contrast to that with infraclavicular arterioarterial grafts. The most frequent complications are false aneurysms at puncture sites, which may be corrected by inserting a new prosthetic segment (also long, if needed) to replace the function of the faulty segment. We place the new segment into a new subcutaneous tunnel mostly lateral to the existing loop. Thrombosis, which is most often caused by a stenosis of the distal anastomosis, rarely occured. If so, hard tissue proliferates could be found at the anastomotic ring. Local endarterectomy proves successful.

5.5 Clinical Observations

Because of isolated observations of microcembolisms under single antiplatelet therapy (acetyl salicylic acid), all patients received oral vitamin K antagonists (desired international normalized ratio (INR): 3–4). In a patient with a low flow in an infraclavicular graft (80 mL/min), which was due to a high peripheral resistance, we created an additional femorofemoral loop.

The arterial pressure in the graft increases the risk of hematomas and false aneurysms at frequent puncture sites. This should be taken into account with sufficiently long postpuncture compression and by choosing different puncture sites.

5.6 Hints for Handling Arterioarterial Interposition Grafts

As arterioarterial grafts are rare, both dialysis staff and patients need to know about the specific peculiarities. A leaflet that we distribute (see Appendix) explains what to expect, such as not to feel a thrill as in AV accesses but a pulse. We recommend waiting for at least 2 weeks for the first puncture after surgery if possible.

Literature

Brittinger WD, Strauch M, Huber W, von Henning GE, Twittenhoff WD, Schwarzbeck A, Wittenmeier KW, Vogel G (1969) Shuntlose Hämodialyse durch Punktion der subkutan fixierten Arteria femoralis superficialis. Klin Wochenschr 47:824–826

Bünger CM, Kröger J, Kock L, Henning A, Klar E, Schareck W (2005) Axillary-axillary interarterial chest loop conduit as an alternative for chronic hemodialysis access. J Vasc Surg 42:290–295

Krisper P, Martinelli E, Zierler E, Schilcher G, Tiesenhausen K, Schneditz D (2011) More may be less: increasing extracorporeal blood flow in an axillary arterio-arterioal access decreases effective clearance. Nephrol Dial Transplant 26:2401–2403

Salgado OJ (2008) Subcutaneous transposition of the superficial femoral artery for arterioarterial hemodialysis: techniques and results. Artif Organs 32: 969–973

Scholz H (2002) Der adäquate AV-Gefässzugang für die Hämodialyse. Bard, Impra München. ISBN 3-00-002561-8

Scholz H, Zanow J (1999) Arterio-arterial interposition as access for hemodialysis. In: Henry ML (ed) Vascular access for hemodialysis VI. Gore& Associates, Precept Press, Chicago, pp 255–262

Scholz H, Petzold K, Petzold M, Zanow J, Miller H, Krüger U (2007) Das arterioarterielle Interponat für die Hämodialyse. Gefässchirurgie 12:167–171

Settmacher U, Heise M, Scholz H (1998) Das arterioarterielle Interponat als Dialysezugang. Gefässchirurgie 3:11–13

Zanow J, Kruger U, Petzold M, Petzold K, Miller H, Scholz H (2005) Arterio-arterial prosthetic loop: a new approach for hemodialysis access. J Vasc Surg 41:1007–1012

6 Redo Surgery with Prosthetic Grafts

Thrombosis, aneurysms, stenoses, and infections are possible causes for redo surgery. In the previous chapters we presented the typical procedures for the correction of stenoses of venous anastomoses and draining veins of different AV access variants. The same principles apply to thrombectomies and reconstructions of long segment stenoses of prosthetic grafts. A special extra chapter deals with infections.

6.1 Thromboses

Thrombectomies of a prosthetic graft are similar to those of AV fistulas. They entail:

- Removal of a thrombus
- Investigation into its cause

6.1.1 Finding the Cause of Thrombosis

This is a three-stage procedure involving history, clinical examination, and intraoperative findings.

History

Signs of impaired venous drainage are:

- Prolonged bleeding after puncture
- Raised pressure of venous line during dialysis
- Decrease of thrill and increased pulsation

Signs of diminished arterial inflow are:

- Decreased thrill
- Low flow during dialysis

Arterial hypotension or hypotensive episodes may also be contributing factors.

Hypercoagulability for infectious or other reasons leads to an increased risk for thrombosis.

Clinical Examination

- Stenoses or occlusions of draining veins may show by distended superficial veins.
- A tightly filled shunt prosthesis is typical for a stenosis of the venous anastomosis.
- Large aneuryms with thrombi that are adherent to the walls may cause occlusions.
- Infections of the shunt may also favor thrombosis.

Intraoperative Findings

Catheter Thrombectomy

During thrombectomy procedures using a Fogarty catheter, an experienced surgeon can evaluate the lumen of grafts and anastomoses.

Intraoperative Angiography

Routine intraoperative angiography showing both anastomoses after thrombectomy is desirable. It should be performed if stenoses of the prosthesis, the anastomoses, or the feeding or draining vessels are suspected

Evaluation of the Thrombi

- With predominantly red thrombi, a hypercoagulable state is unlikely.
- With hypercoagulability, thrombi are mixed or predominantly white.

H. Scholz, *Arteriovenous Access Surgery*,
DOI 10.1007/978-3-642-41139-7_6, © Springer-Verlag Berlin Heidelberg New York 2015

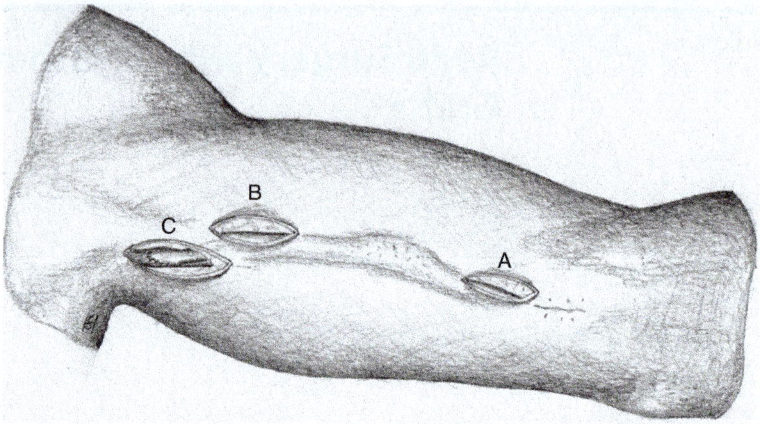

Fig. 6.1 Incisions for thrombectomies of straight grafts. If there is no suspicion of a stenosis close to the venous anastomosis, the puncturable segment should be spared (*A* or *B*). Otherwise isolate the venous anastomosis (*C*)

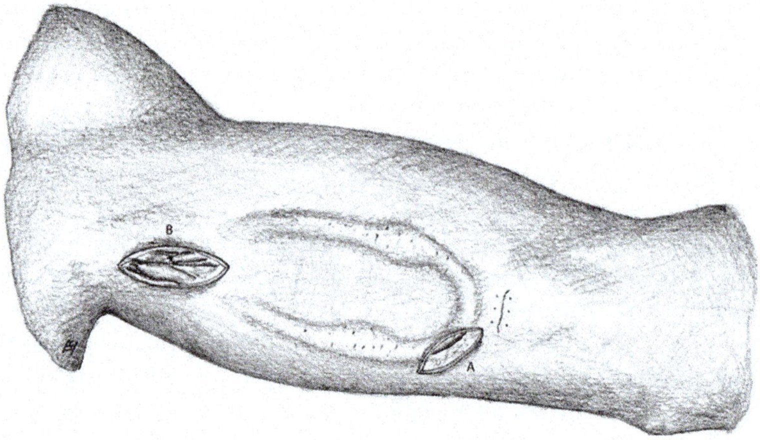

Fig. 6.2 Incisions for thrombectomies of loop grafts. If there is no suspicion of a stenosis close to the venous anastomosis, the graft is exposed near its apex (*A*). Otherwise isolate the venous anastomosis (*B*)

- Whitish circular adhesions to the prosthetic wall which look like tubes when they are removed by the thrombectomy catheter and occur when hypotension, venous or arterial stenoses, or hypercoagulability cause low flow.

6.1.2 Choice of the Thrombectomy Site

Three aspects deserve attention:

- Preservation of puncturable segments.
- Opportunity to repair an underlying stenosis.
- Chance to reach both anastomoses with the catheter.

The incision is different for straight and looped grafts.

Straight Grafts

If there is no suspicion of a stenosis of the venous anastomosis, the graft should be exposed near the venous or arterial anastomosis where it is not punctured (Fig. 6.1, incisions A or B). If you suspect a stenosis of the venous anastomosis, you should expose it (incision C).

Loop Grafts

If there is no suspicion of a venous stenosis, the graft should be exposed near its apex, which is equidistant from both anastomoses (Fig. 6.2, incision B). If you suspect a stenosis

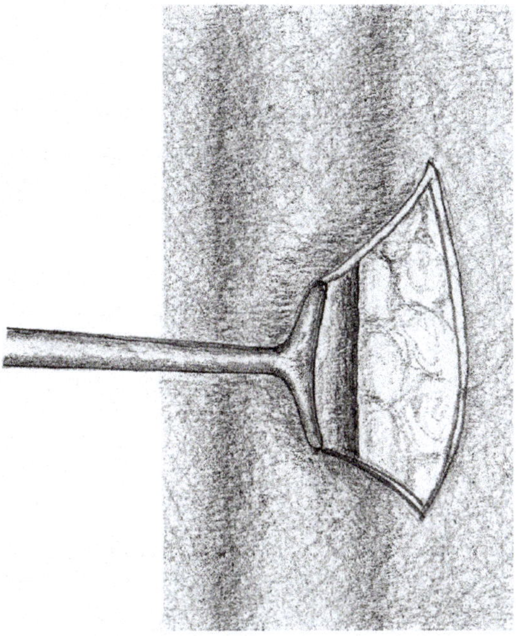

Fig. 6.3 Exposure of the prosthesis via a lateral longitudinal incision

of the venous anastomosis, you should then expose it (incision A).

6.1.3 Incision

Except for the areas directly adjacent to the anastomoses, the graft lies in a subcutaneous tunnel. In order to avoid wound infections, the incision for thrombectomy should be parallel to the prosthesis, leaving enough subcutaneous tissue to cover the prosthesis when closing the wound (Fig. 6.3). The skin incision should be long enough to be able to complete the suture of the clamped vessel (mostly 2.5–3.5 cm). A lateral graft incision helps hide the knotted ends of the suture in the subcutaneous tissue so that they don't pierce the skin surface. This might lead to a cutaneous fistula and subsequent graft infection (Fig. 6.4a, b).

6.1.4 Technique for Thrombectomy

After the sufficient circular exposure of the prosthesis, a lateral transverse incision is made to

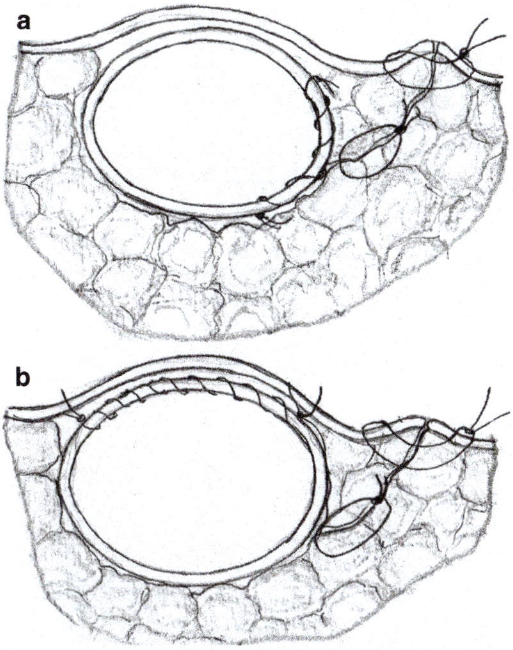

Fig. 6.4 Different options for graft incisions: (**a**) lateral and (**b**) towards the skin surface with a risk of a thread perforating the skin

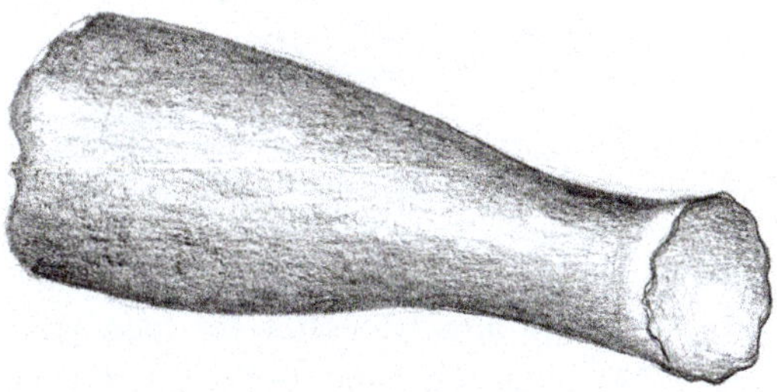

Fig. 6.5 Typical shape of the thrombus at the arterial anastomosis

open it. We recommend performing thrombectomy of the venous side first. Care should be taken to remove the end of the thrombus (Fig. 6.5) from the anastomosis. It is characterized by its concave and lighter surface. If you have not found it, you should continue with the thrombectomy maneuver. During the clamping period, the sides which have already been freed of thrombi should be filled with heparin solution (e.g., 5,000 I.U. of heparin per 100 mL normal saline). Frequently it proves difficult to remove adherent white thrombi. Then flexible remote annular cutters (e.g., Fehling

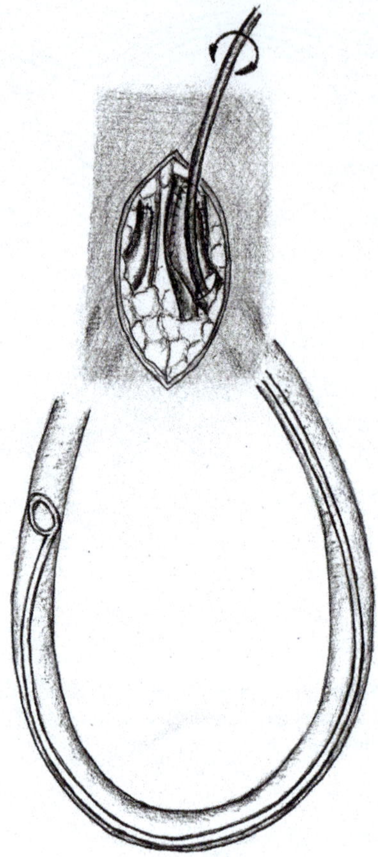

Fig. 6.6 Removal of wall-adherent thrombi from the graft using a flexible annular cutter

company) may also be useful for loop grafts (Fig. 6.6). A titanium spiral probe (e.g., Fehling company) may also prove helpful when cleaning off strongly adherent material (Fig. 6.7).

6.1.5 Closure of the Graft

It is important to pay particular attention to the closure of the graft. Implanted prostheses tend to become quite hard over the course of time. We recommend the following course of action:

- Pushing down on the far sides of both clamps opens the edges of the cut.
- We begin suturing from both edges with 6-0 mattress sutures to the middle (Fig. 6.8a).
- Raising the clamps approaches the wound edges. The threads may then be tightened and the knots completed (Fig. 6.8b).

If bleeding from the suture canals persists, two-component fibrin glue can effectively solve this problem using the following technique:

- Clamp the prosthesis and compress the clamped segment for relief of the intraluminal pressure.
- Apply and massage the fibrin component of the glue into the sutureline with your gloved fingers.
- Do the same with the thrombin component.
- Release the blood flow after a 1-min break. This technique helps achieve hemostasis.

6.1.6 Wound Closure

Before the wound can be closed, any bleeding should have stopped. It seems important to close the subcutaneous tissue (Fig. 6.9a) as well as the skin in order to avoid empty spaces which might favor hematomas and infections (Fig. 6.9b).

6.2 Repair of Graft Aneurysms

Aneurysms are mainly caused by the destruction of wall structures due to frequent punctures. A false aneurysm rarely occurs.

6.2.1 False Aneurysm

Indication

The indication for surgery depends on size, skin cover, danger of rupture, site, and progress. Small size aneurysms may be observed to see how they develop. A small aneurysm which is occluded by a thrombus does not require surgery.

Technical hint

The treatment of a false aneurysm usually does not cause major problems. There are two possibilities.

- A small hole (isolated puncture site) may be repaired if the assistant compresses both sides of the prosthesis with his hands while the surgeon closes the hole with a suture.
- Larger defects may also temporarily be occluded by finger compression. After the

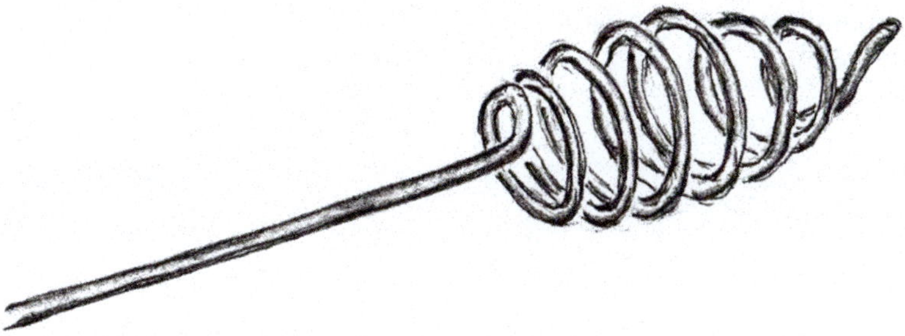

Fig. 6.7 Spiral-shaped instrument to remove adherent linings from the prosthesis

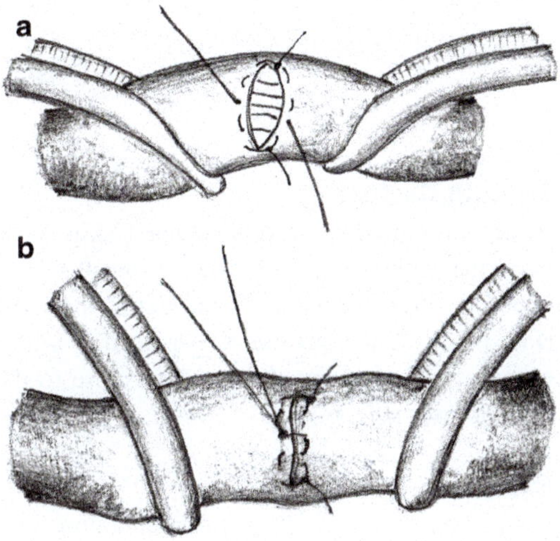

Fig. 6.8 Closure of the graft. (**a**) Suturing while pushing down on the far sides of the clamps. (**b**) Tightening the threads and tying the knots

prosthesis has been exposed sufficiently for clamping both sides, the surgeon deals with the damage as required.

- As false aneurysms are mostly only covered by sparse subcutaneous tissue, all bleeding should have stopped before closing the wound.

6.2.2 Puncture Site Aneurysms

Indications

Indications for repair include:

- Rapid progress
- Relevant skin changes over the aneurysm
- Prolonged required compression time after dialysis
- Wall-adherent thrombi

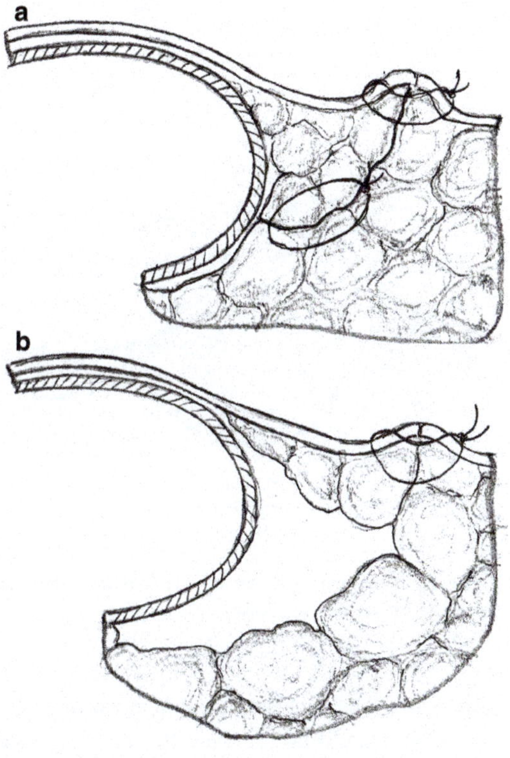

Fig. 6.9 (**a**) Closure of the incision after thrombectomy with approximation of the subcutaneous tissue by suturing. (**b**) Cavity formation when not suturing the subcutaneous tissue

Technical hints

Large aneurysms require special attention. Their repair should also maintain prosthetic material for immediate postoperative puncture if possible. The extent of the aneurysm and the kind of prosthesis are important criteria when planning surgery.

Short Aneurysms

With small aneurysms we advocate the resection of the aneurysmatic segment and the reestablishment of continuity by inserting a vascular graft

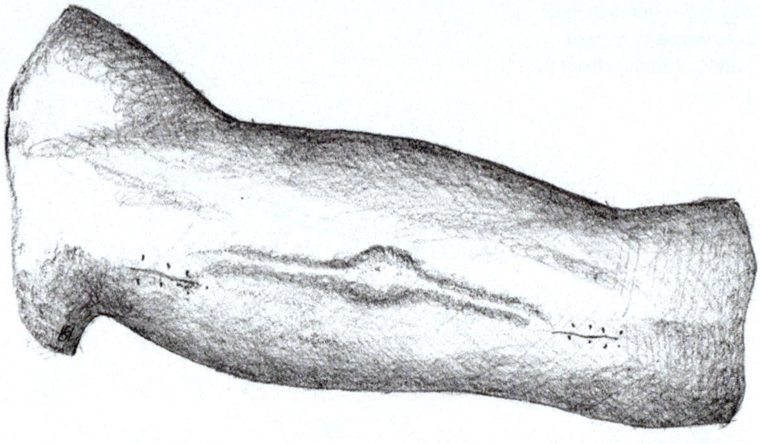

Fig. 6.10 Isolated aneurysm of a graft

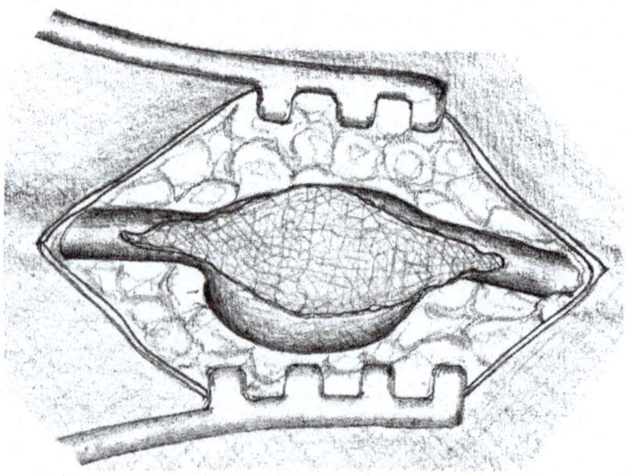

Fig. 6.11 Elliptical excision of the skin covering an aneurysm before its resection

(Fig. 6.10). The superfluous skin and subcutaneous tissue should be removed in order to avoid cavity formation (Fig. 6.11). Postoperatively the graft segments which lie outside the wound area may be punctured immediately.

Long Aneurysms

There are two particularities concerning the treatment of a long and vast aneurysm:

- After its exclusion from the blood stream, the aneurysm should be totally excised in order not to favor microbial colonization and infection.
- The space left behind should not be used to accommodate the new prosthesis. The new graft should be placed separately in a curved subcutaneous tunnel that avoids the old path.

Straight Grafts

After a longitudinal spindle-shaped skin excision, the aneurysmatically altered prosthesis is exposed circumferentially via extra incisions (Fig. 6.12). A new prosthesis is placed in a new tunnel which connects the incisions close to the anastomoses (Fig. 6.13).

Evaluation

Depending on the lengths of the remaining segments of the old prosthesis, it may be necessary to insert a temporary catheter for hemodialysis.

Looped grafts

Isolated aneurysms which involve only one side of the prosthesis may be repaired as shown in Figs. 6.10 and 6.11. If the aneurysmatic changes concern the whole loop, we prefer a two-stage procedure (Fig. 6.14a). First one side of the aneurysmatic loop is resected and replaced by a new graft whose new subcutaneous tunnel avoids the former path (Fig. 6.14b). During a second procedure, the same is done for the remaining half (Fig. 6.14c). During the healing process after the first stage, the remaining aneurysmatic side of the loop is used for hemodialysis (Fig. 6.14c).

Evaluation

As the remaining half of the aneurysmatic prosthesis may be still be used for hemodialysis, there is no need for a temporary catheter with a two-stage procedure.

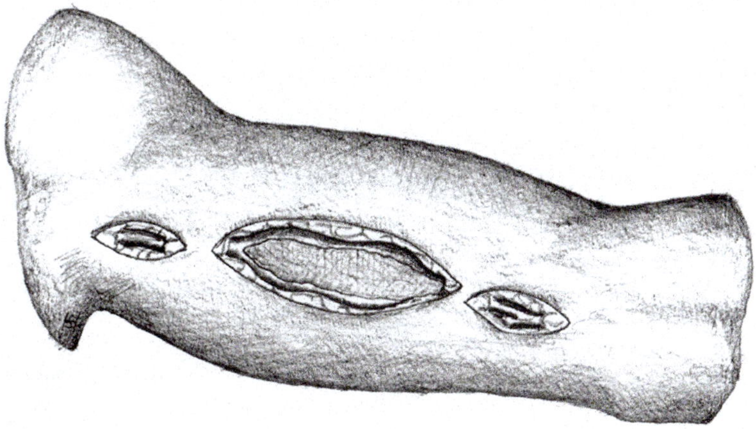

Fig. 6.12 Incisions and dissection for resection of a long graft aneurysm

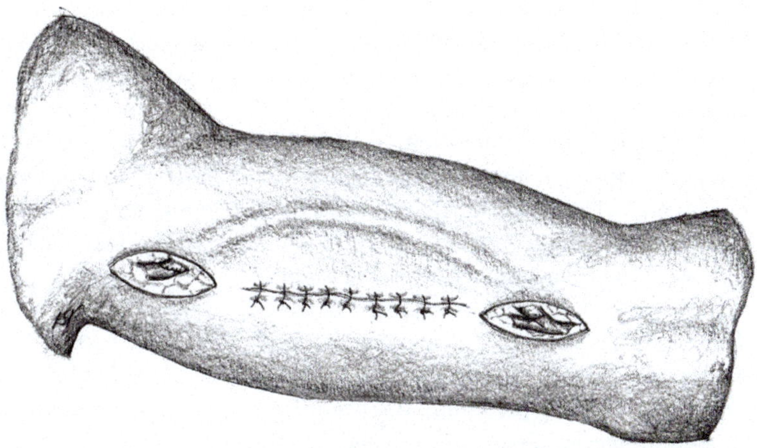

Fig. 6.13 Surgical field of Fig. 6.12 after aneurysm resection and graft interposition

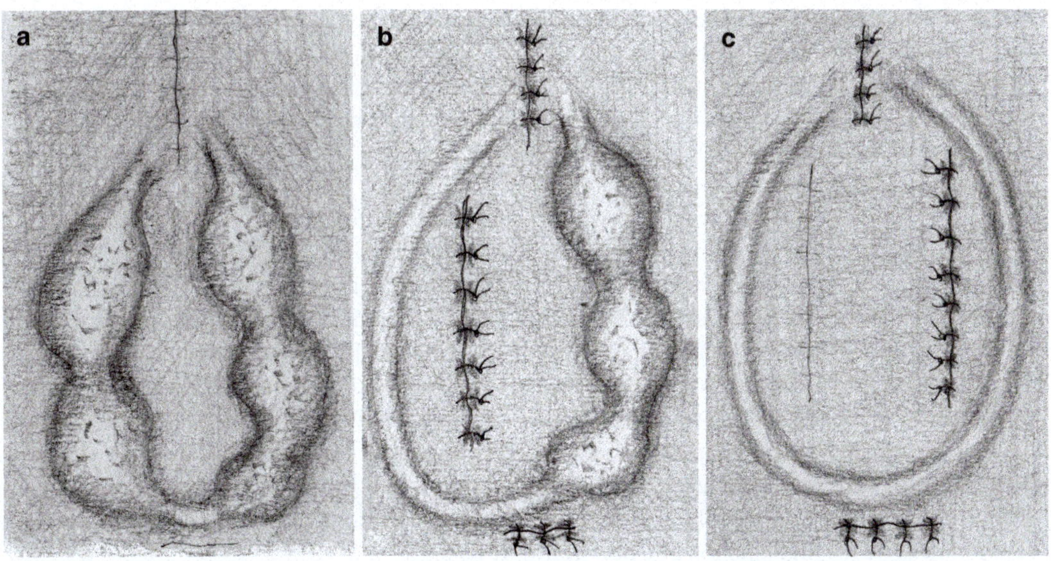

Fig. 6.14 Resection and exchange of graft with aneurysmatic dilation of the whole graft loop. (**a**) Baseline status. (**b**) After exchange of one side of the graft. (**c**) After delayed exchange of the other side

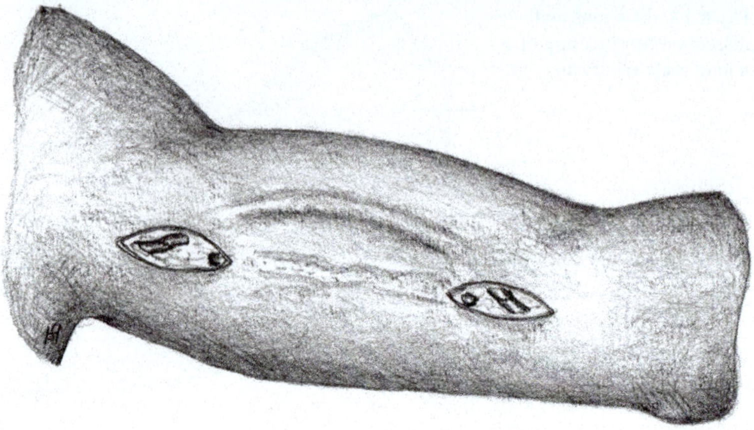

Fig. 6.15 Repair of a long graft stenosis with exclusion of the old graft and implantation of a new graft

6.3 Repair of Graft Stenoses

Stenoses of grafts can be caused by:

- Suture lines after thrombectomy
- Residual thrombi after thrombectomy
- Chronic white thrombi (mostly seen with hypercoagulability or low flow)
- Transmural connective tissue proliferation

Stenoses after sutures mostly require the resection of the affected segment and the interposition of a new prosthetic graft. *Residual thrombi* require a new thrombectomy procedure. If *circular white thrombi line the prosthetic wall*, an annular remote cutter may help remove them completely. If there are no hemodynamically siginificant stenoses of the inflow or outflow regions which might have led to fibrin lining of the graft, we prophylactically prescribe oral anticoagulants.

Transmural proliferation of connective tissue into the lumen of a graft can often be observed – particularly in younger patients and a long time after the graft has been implanted. This phenomenon mostly occurs near puncture sites. The tissue consists of fibrocytes, fibroblasts, and hyaline matter. Near puncture sites, sprouting capillaries can frequently be found. Intraoperatively this material appears as hard, grayish white tissue that cannot be separated from the prosthetic wall. With this kind of hemodynamically significant short stenoses, the resection of the relevant segment followed by the implantation of a new graft segment should be performed as necessary. If the entire graft is affected, a complete replacement may be necessary. In contrast to aneurysmatically-altered prostheses, the risk of infection is much lower if the stenosis is due to connective tissue proliferation. Therefore the removal of the whole prosthesis is not always indicated.

Indications for a Complete Graft Replacement

It is indicated if:

- The whole prosthesis is involved.
- The flow is not sufficient for hemodialysis.
- Puncturing is too difficult because of the narrowed lumen.

If the anastomoses are concerned as well, they should be reconstructed simultaneously. The procedure is different for either straight or looped grafts.

Technical Hints for Straight Grafts

The prosthesis is freed via two longitudinal incisions near the anastomoses. Then the prosthesis is isolated towards its center. After clamping near the anastomoses, the prosthesis is resected. The former canal is closed with subcutaneous sutures. After the creation of a new curved subcutaneous tunnel and placement of the new prosthesis, continuity is re-established by anastomosing the new prosthesis to the anastomotic stumps of the old prosthesis (Fig. 6.15).

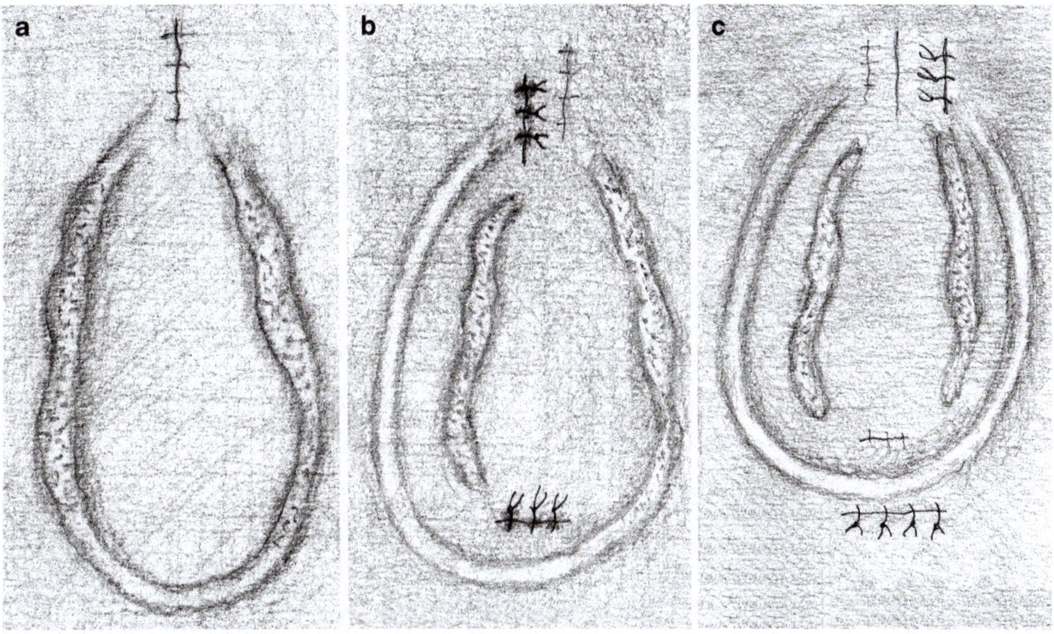

Fig. 6.16 Stenosis of almost the entire loop graft. (**a**) Baseline status. (**b**) After exclusion and implantation of one side. (**c**) After delayed exclusion and implantation of the new other side

Evaluation
A safe method for the preservation of the native vessels. A temporary catheter is needed till healing is finished.

Technical hints for looped grafts
With stenoses involving the entire graft (Fig. 6.16a), we replace only one side during the first session in a similar way to straight grafts (Fig. 6.16b). After healing is completed and the new side punctured, we replace the remaining side (Fig. 6.16c).

Evaluation
A safe method for continuous hemodialysis use of the vessel by a two-stage procedure.

7 Infections

An infection of a vascular access for hemodialysis constitutes a serious complication which particularly occurs in immuno-compromised patients. Many infections are avoidable. The influence of puncture techniques on infections is discussed in Chap. 17.

7.1 Prevention of Infections

Infections occuring directly after surgery have other causes than later ones. Therefore they are discussed separately.

7.1.1 Prevention of Perioperative Infections when Creating a Vascular Access

An infection arises with contamination and supporting local factors.

The microbial contamination of a wound may be minimized by:

- A thorough shave of the operative and prepped fields.
- Covering the field with incise film when using vascular prosthetic grafts.

Other Influences That Favor Infections Which Can Be Influenced

1. *Correct timing of surgery*. For obvious reasons do not operate during septicemia.
2. *Potential catheter locations*. If you operate on an upper extremity, preferably use the side that is contralateral to a catheter, as otherwise (increased flow velocities after AV access surgery) this might facilitate bacteremia if there is bacterial colonization of the catheter.
3. *Choose the correct incision*. The skin incision should be placed directly over the vessels which were selected for anastomoses to avoid large cavities. With a few exceptions (incision at the apex of a looped graft, creation of a distal cephalic fistula), choose longitudinal incisions only.
4. *Use atraumatic operative techniques*. Use bipolar diathermy with a fine forceps only. Don't pull apart the wound edges more than necessary.
5. *Maintain careful hemostasis*. It should not be necessary to place a drain except for special cases.
6. *Close wounds in layers* in order to avoid subcutaneous cavities.

H. Scholz, *Arteriovenous Access Surgery*,
DOI 10.1007/978-3-642-41139-7_7, © Springer-Verlag Berlin Heidelberg New York 2015

7. *Perform redo surgery in time* if a hemotoma requires this step.
8. *Consider the intraoperative administration of antibiotics* when using prosthetic grafts.

7.1.2 Prevention of Perioperative Infections in Redo Surgery

Redo surgery sometimes necessitates the exposure of the vessels in places where they are covered by only a thin layer of subcutaneous tissue. Thus the risk of a wound infection is increased. As mentioned above, a longitudinal incision parallel to the vessel, meticulous hemostasis, and exact wound closure including the subcutaneous tissue are important factors.

7.2 Therapy of Infections of AV Fistulas

7.2.1 Early Postoperative Infections

Early postoperative infections are extremely rare after the creation of AV fistulas (0.1 % in our patients over the last 13 years). Long operations, large wound areas, and hemotomas favor infections. With slight superficial soft tissue infections, the administration of antibiotics and additional cooling may be sufficient. Redo surgery is necessary with deep infections reaching the vessels in order to remove necrotic and infected tissue. After thorough flushing and drain placement, the wound is closed completely. In the few such cases that we have observed, the evacuation of hematomas or abscesses, wound debridement, and additional administration of antibiotics have led to complete restitution while preserving functioning fistulas.

7.2.2 Late Postoperative Infections

Late postoperative infections are much more frequent than early infections. In the majority of cases they involve frequent punctures sites which lie close to each other. From a clinical point of view there are three kinds of late infections:

- Inflammatory infiltration of the skin and subcutaneous tissue over the vein
- Isolated necroses at puncture sites
- Extended soft tissue infections of the punctured vein

Inflammatory Infiltration Of The Skin And Subcutaneous Tissue Over The Vein

Characteristics are erythema, edema, and painfulness.

Therapy

Antibiotics, local cooling, and immobilization.

Isolated Necroses at Puncture Sites

Isolated, mostly 2–8 mm slough and necrosis cover the puncture site with or without inflammation of the surrounding tissue.

Frequently there is a tissue defect corresponding in size to the crust which extends through the tissue to the vessels. Only the existence of an intraluminal thrombus adjacent to the wall prevents bleeding. Mostly there are no inflammatory signs of the surrounding tissue.

Therapy

Depending on morphological conditions (subcutaneous position, mobility of the vein, topographical considerations), the surgical therapy varies.

Local Excision

While the assistant manually compresses the vein, the surgeon transversally excises the affected tissue and vascular defects, closes the vessel, the subcutaneous tissue, and the skin. This is only possible in a few cases (Fig. 7.1a, b).

Resection of a Segment

Also under manual compression, the infected puncture site is exposed via a transverse incision. After the oval excision of the infected puncture site, the afferent and efferent sides of the vein are mobilized (if possible) and reunited after resection of the affected segment. It is important to cover the anastomosis sufficiently (Fig. 7.2a, b). Antibiotics are selected according to bacterial sensitivity.

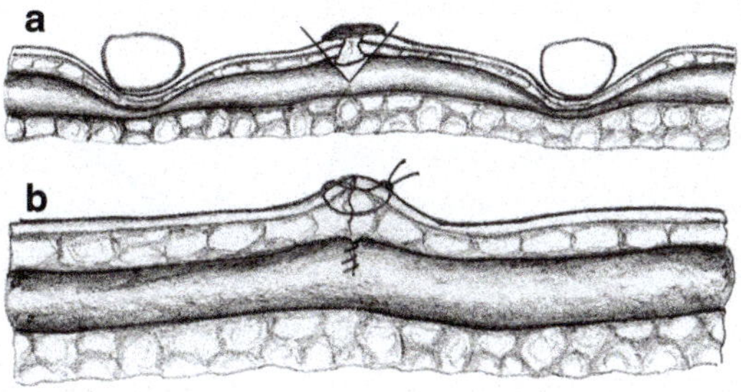

Fig. 7.1 Treatment of infected puncture site of a fistula. (**a**) Excision of the infected tissue under manual compression of the vein. (**b**) After completion

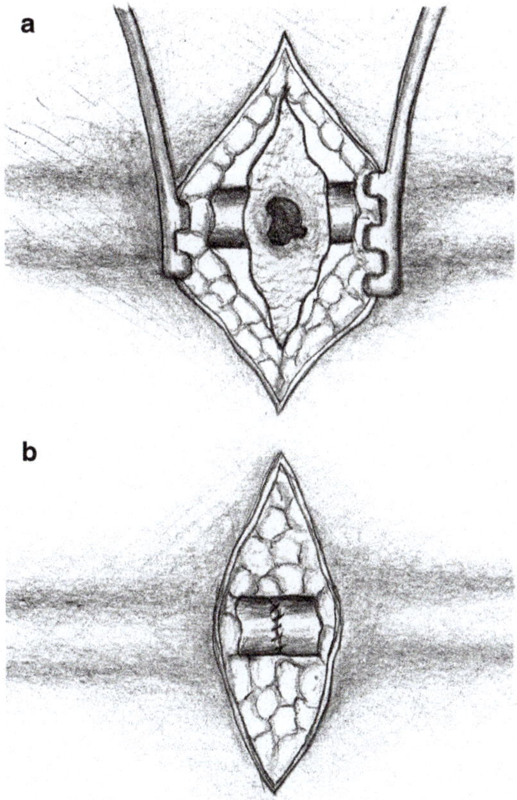

Fig. 7.2 Segmental resection of the infected puncture site of a fistula. (**a**) After isolation of the relevant segment. (**b**) After completion

Extended Soft Tissue Infections Of The Punctured Vein

Extended soft tissue infections of the punctured vein frequently also show intracutaneous bullae and skin necroses.

Therapy

Depending on the state of the vein proximal to the infected site.

Vein Proximal to the Infection Suitable for Punctures (Fig. 7.3)

- Apply incise film.
- Isolate the vein and the corresponding artery in an area which is definitely not infected, make a longitudinal incision, transect the vein and anastomose the proximal stump to the corresponding artery (Fig. 7.3b).
- After closing the first wound, cover it with incise film to prevent microbial spread.
- Make a spindle-shaped incision circumscribing the infected vein and free the vein up to the anastomosis (Fig. 7.3c).
- Ligate the anastomosis, resect the infected vein, insert a drain, and close the wound (Fig. 7.3d).
- Administer adequate antibiotics according to the resistogram.

Vein Proximal to the Infected Site Not Suitable for Punctures

If the segment suitable for puncture is too short, or is drained by unsuitable collaterals only, the vascular access has to be abandoned.

- Make a spindle-shaped incision circumscribing the skin over the infected vein, and free the vein up to the anastomosis.
- Ligate the anastomosis, resect the infected vein, insert a drain, and close the wound.

Administer adequate antibiotics according to the resistogram.

7.2.3 Infections of Thrombosed AV Fistulas

Relatively often, some days to weeks after thrombosis of an old AV fistula, an infection of the vein arises. It is mainly frequently-punctured segments of already dilated veins that are concerned. Thrombosis seems to favor the growth of microorgansisms. There are two different clinical forms of these infections:

1. Acute local erythema, pain, and edema over the thrombosed vein

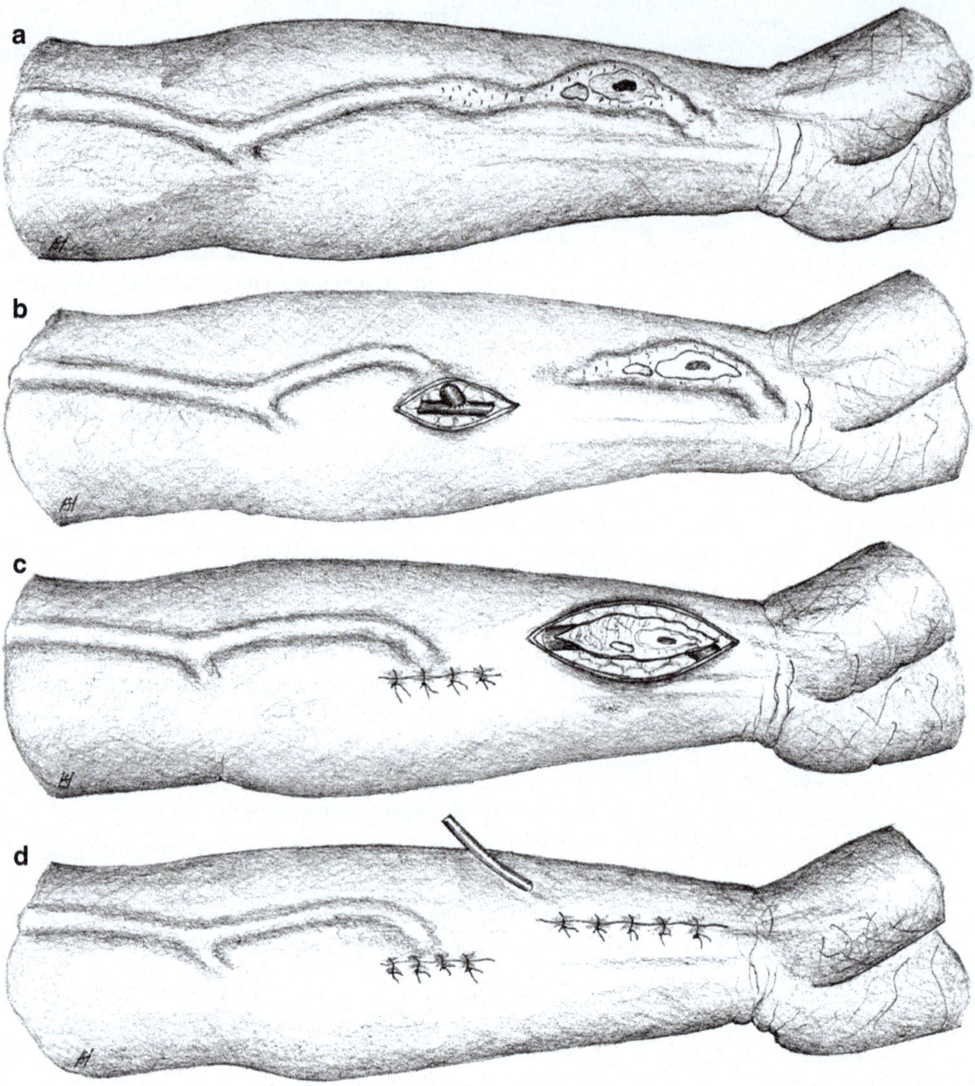

Fig. 7.3 Course of action for extended distal infection of a fistula whose proximal segment is suitable for puncturing. (**a**) Baseline status. (**b**) After proximal new anastomosis. (**c**) Isolation of the infected venous segment. (**d**) Final result

2. Erythema, pronounced pain, edema, and intracutaneous bulla formation over the thrombosed vein

Therapy for Variant 1

Cooling, systemic antibiotics, and immobilization if possible. If there is no improvement after 3–4 days, or there is a change for the worse, the entire affected venous segment should be resected.

Therapy for Variant 2

- Start sytemic antibiotic therapy.
- Resect the infected venous segment along with the infected skin areas via a longitudinal incision.
- Take a wound swab for microbiological investigation and antibiogram.
- Insert a drain and close wound as appropriate.

Continue with antibiotics according to antibiogram test results.

7.3 Infections of Prosthetic AV Grafts

Etiology, clinical presentation, and therapy of postoperative early and late infections are different. Therefore they are discussed separately.

7.3.1 Early Postoperative Infections

Following the intraoperative administration of antibiotics, we observed four perioperative infections in 1,031 prosthetic AV grafts (0.39 %) over a 10-year period (January 2000 through December 2009). One of these infections entailed extensive tissue necrosis caused by calciphylaxis (not preventable). Two patients had hematomos which were not evacuated in time (preventable). The etiology of the remaining infection remained unclear. Perioperative infections are likely to be due to surgical mistakes. There are three different pathogenetic pathways:

1. Primary contamination of the prosthesis
2. Secondary hematogenous contamination caused by preexisting septic foci
3. Secondary contamination with delayed wound healing

The clinical presentation of primary and secondary contamination is the same: inflammatory erythema and pain over the graft's path as well as raised inflammatory markers. Pay attention not to confound it with the edematous swelling and possible erythema observed with perigraft seroma or the lymphematous swelling observed in the tissue that is surrounded by a U-shaped loop.

Therapy

If major parts of the prosthesis or the entire prosthesis are infected, it must be removed completely.

If possible the artery and vein concerned should be preserved by closing the arteriotomy/venotomy at the anastomoses with running sutures. An infection may also result in the rupture of an anastomosis with bleeding. Both of the following techniques have proved useful under general anesthesia.

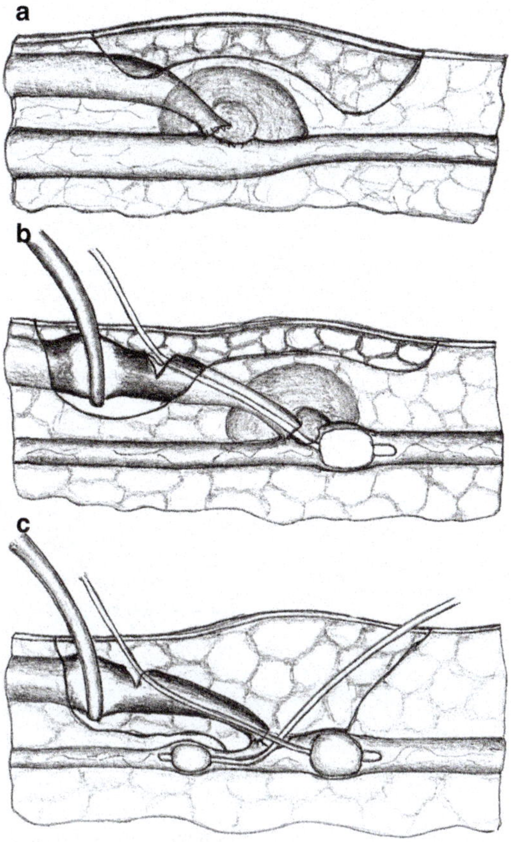

Fig. 7.4 Course of action for completely infected shunt graft with insufficient deep arterial anastomosis. (**a**) Isolation of the graft away from the false aneursm. (**b**) Clamping the graft to the venous side, then insertion and inflation of a Fogarty catheter in the proximal artery. (**c**) Control of the distal artery with the help of a Fogarty catheter, then suture for closure of the arteriotomy after removal of the graft

Deep Arterial Anastomosis (e.g., Infraclavicular or Femoral Loop)

- Expose the graft away from the arterial anastomosis (Fig. 7.4a) and insert a Fogarty catheter into the proximal artery for control (Fig. 7.4b).
- Clamp the venous side of the graft.
- Separate the graft from the artery.
- Insert a Fogarty catheter into the distal artery to prevent arterial backflow (Fig. 7.4c).
- Close the arteriotomy as appropriate (see below).

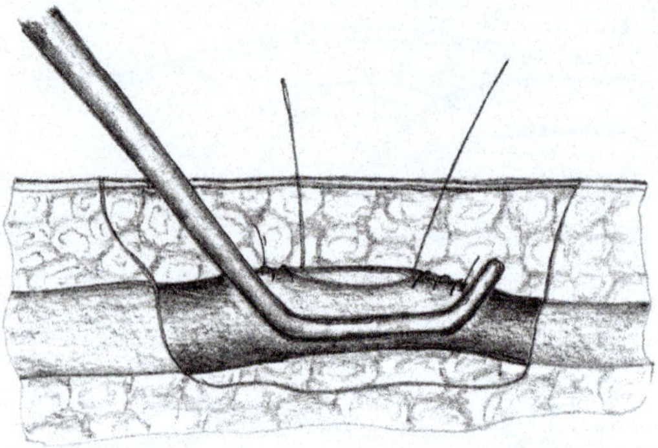

Fig. 7.5 Closure of the venotomy after removal of the graft

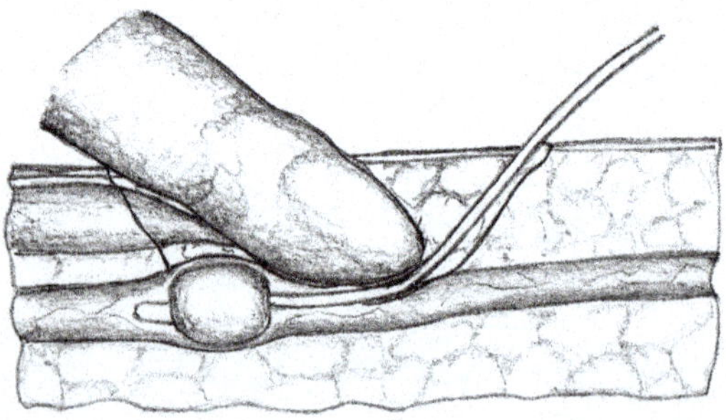

Fig. 7.6 Course of action for completely infected shunt prosthesis with insufficient superficial arterial anastomosis. Insertion of a Fogarty catheter under manual compression in the proximal artery after opening the false aneurysm

- Dissect the venous anastomosis, clamp the vein, separate the graft from the venous anastomosis, and use a longitudingal running suture to close the venotomy site (Fig. 7.5).
- Remove the entire graft. Insert a drain into its former tunnel. Leave antibiotic sponges at former anastomoses.
- Close wounds as appropriate.
- Administer systemic antibiotics according to antibiogram results.

Superficial Arterial Anastomosis

- Prepare two Fogarty catheters with stopcocks. Have suction machine ready.
- Incise skin and subcutaneous tissue down to the false aneurysm and manually compress the infected anastomosis.
- Insert one Fogarty catheter each into the distal and proximal sides of the artery to control bleeding (Fig. 7.6).
- Continue as described above.

Surgical Care of the Arteriotomy Site as Dictated by Circumstances

You should always seek to preserve the continuity of the artery. Depending on the wall defects of the artery caused by infection, this is not always possible.

Suturing of the Arteriotomy Site While Maintaining the Vascular Continuity

There needs to be sufficient material. It is almost always possible to close a longitudinal arteriotomy using a running suture. The closure of large diameters such as the common femoral artery does not cause problems although luminal narrowing may result from this procedure. Vein patch closure or a venous graft may also be useful.

Closure of the Arteriotomy Site by Bilateral Ligation of the Artery

If an infection has completely destroyed the arterial wall near the former anastomosis, it may not be feasible to preserve its continuity. Then we ligate the artery proximal and distal to the former anastomosis. From February 1980 through May 2011 we ligated the brachial arteries in the cubital fossa proximal to their bifurcations in 19 patients, and in 2 patients we ligated the infraclavicular brachial arteries. None of these patients developed noteworthy peripheral ischemia. The axillary and cubital collaterals were sufficient.

Healing by Second Intention and Only Limited Local Infection

With secondary wound healing and questionable or rather definitely only localized graft infections, attempts at purely conservative treatments may be justified with:

- Effective systemic antibiotics
- Local wound care (including vacuum assisted closure)

7.3.2 Late Infections

Late infections involving the entire graft are extremely rare. They mostly result from a delayed start of treatment. Just as in early infections, the whole graft needs to be removed.

Segmental Graft Infection

A localized infection of the soft tissue over the prosthesis at puncture sites characterized by a localized erythema and edema often resolves under antibiotic therapy. If the graft itself is concerned, the respective segment has to be taken out (Fig. 7.7a).

Our aim is to preserve the AV shunt by interposing a new prosthesis whose path avoids the infected area.

We proceed as follows:

- Cover the entire surgical field with incise film.
- Expose the graft proximally and distally sufficiently far away from the infected segment (Fig. 7.7b).
- Prepare a subcutaneous tunnel that connects both incisions for the new prosthesis while bypassing the infected area.
- Clamp the proximal and distal sides of the old prosthesis after systematic heparinization. Ligate the sides of the old prosthesis which have to be excluded (Fig. 7.7c).
- Close the old tunnel on the sides of the ligated segments by subcutaneous sutures (Fig. 7.7d).
- Re-establish the continuity by creating the anastomoses between the old and the new grafts (Fig. 7.7e).
- Administer systemic protamine, remove the vascular clamps, and close both incisions with subcutaneous and skin sutures (Fig. 7.7f).
- Use new incise film to cover both wounds.
- Make an extra incision to excise the infected graft. Continue with local wound care as appropriate (Fig. 7.7g, h).
- Administer appropriate antibiotics.

Infection After Thrombectomy

Local infections at thrombectomy sites mostly result from intraoperative surgical errors such as an insufficient subcutaneous wound closure, an inadequate incision crossing the graft, insufficient surgical hemostasis, and a delayed surgical revision if indicated. The treatment corresponds to that of segmental infections.

Local Infection at a Puncture Site

It is mainly observed with repetitive punctures which are situated close to each other. Clinically you may observe a prominent darkish crust with surrounding erythema (Fig. 7.8). The removal of this slough can lead to massive bleeding if there is a wall defect of the graft underneath. If the infection is definitely limited to the puncture site, the resection of a short segment of the graft along with the involved soft tissue may still be sufficient and allow for a terminoterminal anastomosis of both ends of the grafts.

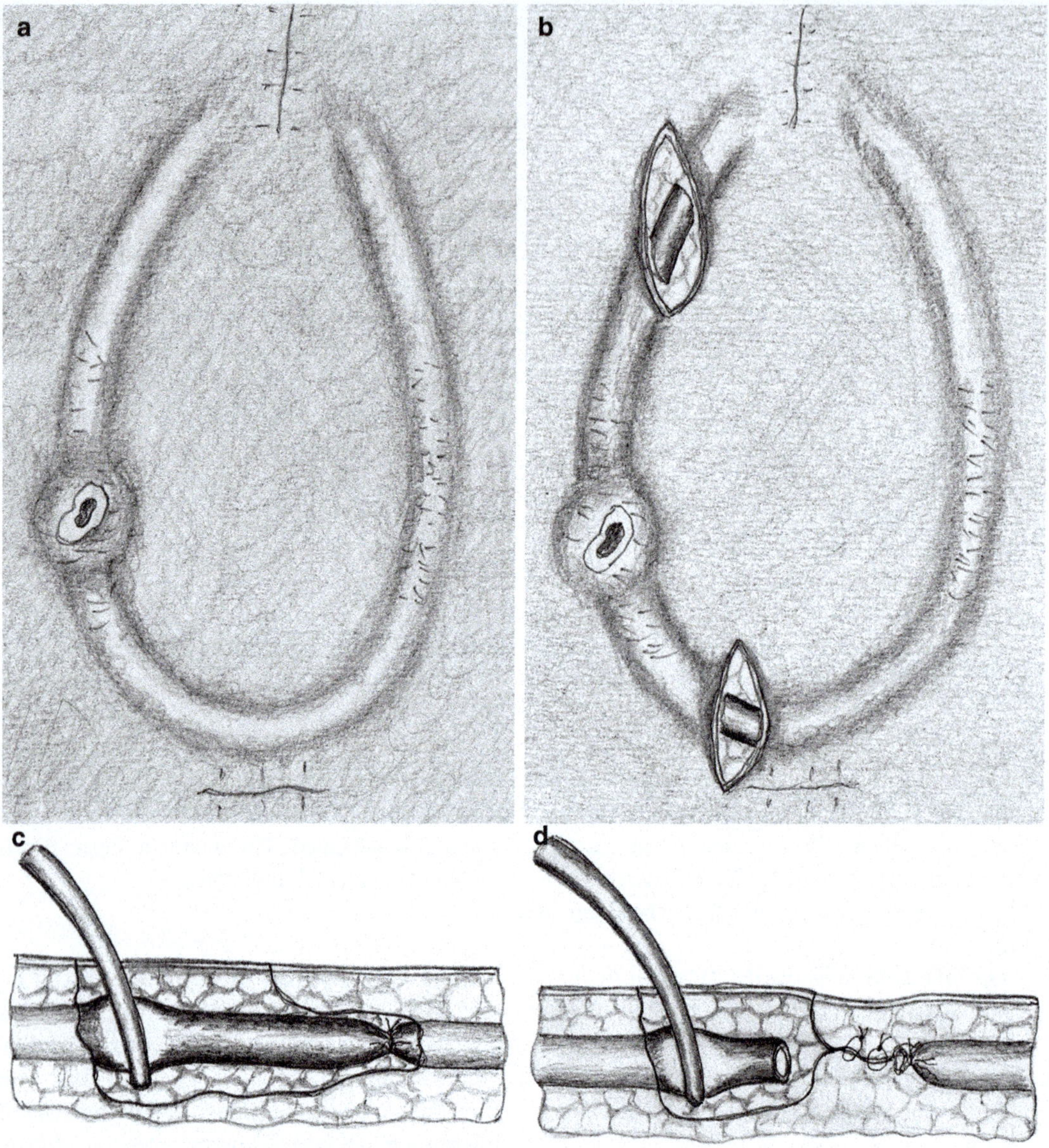

Fig. 7.7 Course of action for a segmental infection of a shunt prosthesis. (**a**) Baseline situation. (**b**) Exposure of the prosthesis in definitely not infected areas on both sides of the infection. (**c**) Ligation of both ends of the prosthesis that lead to the infection in the subcutaneous tunnel. (**d**) Resection of the prosthesis from both sides and subcutaneous closure of the tunnel. (**e**) Re-establishment of the graft continuity by implanting a new prosthesis into a new tunnel which circumvents the infected area. (**f**) Site after creating the anatomoses. (**g**) Removal of the infected graft segment. (**h**) Completion

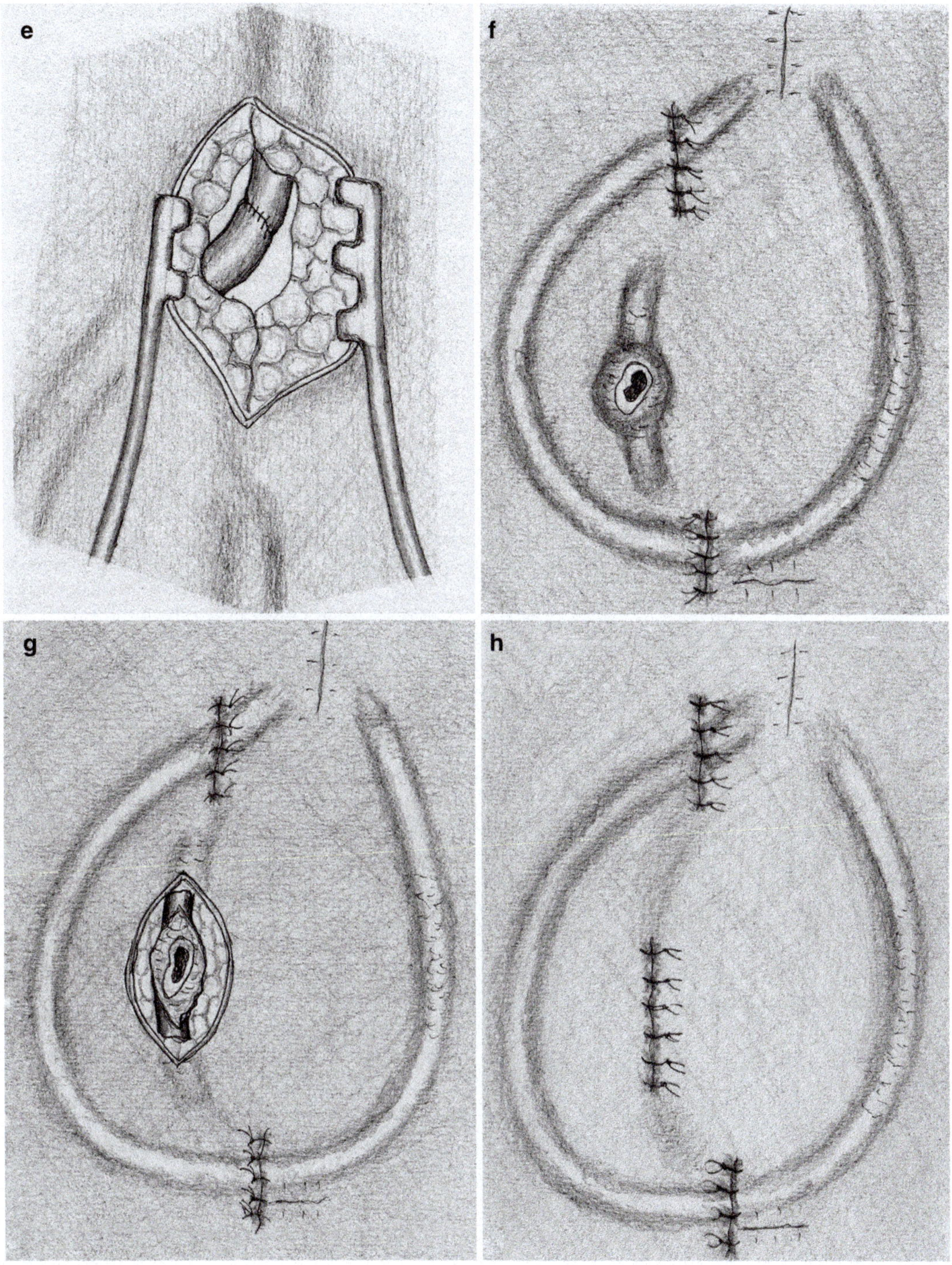

Fig. 7.7 (continued)

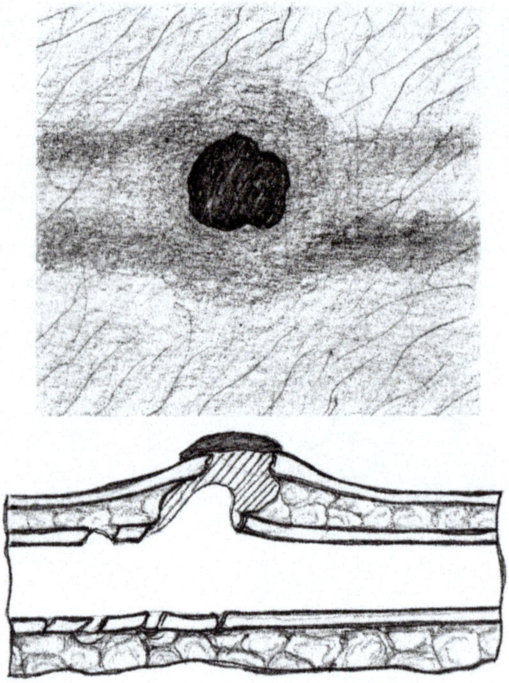

Fig. 7.8 Infected puncture site/longitudinal section

Literature

Akoh JA, Patel N (2010) Infection of hemodialysis arteriovenous grafts. J Vasc Access 11:155–158

Claeys LG, Matamoros R (2002) Anaerobic cellulitis as the result of clostridium perfringens: a rare cause of vascular access graft infection. J Vasc Surg 35:1287–1288

Fong IW, Capellan JM, Simbul M, Angel J (1993) Infection of arterio-venous fistulas created for chronic haemodialysis. Scand J Infect Dis 25:215–220

Gulati S, Sahu KM, Avula S, Sharma RK, Ayyagiri A, Pandey CM (2003) Role of vascular access as a risk factor for infections in hemodialysis. Ren Fail 25:967–973

Maya ID, Weatherspoon J, Young CJ, Barker J, Allon M (2007) Increased risk of infection associated with polyurethane dialysis grafts. Semin Dial 20: 616–620

Nassar MN, Ayus JC (2001) Infectious complications of the hemodialysis access. Kidney Int 60:1–13

Nassar MN, Ayus JC (2002) Infectious complications of old nonfunctioning arteriovenous grafts in renal transplant recipients: a case series. Am J Kidney Dis 40:832–836

Rodríguez Guardado A, Carton JA, López Ponga B, Casado L, Pérez F, Aguado S (1997) Bacteremia in patients undergoing chronic hemodialysis in a 16-year period. Rev Clin Esp 197:484–489

Ryan SV, Calligaro KD, Scharff J, Dougherty MJ (2004) Management of infected prosthetic dialysis arteriovenous grafts. J Vasc Surg 39:73–78

Saxena AK, Panhotra BR, Naguib M, Sundaram DS, Venkateshhappa CK, Uzzaman W, Al-Mulhim K (2002) Vascular access related septicemia in hemodialysis: a focus on bacterial flora and antibiotic access slavage. Saudi J Kidney Dis Transpl 13:29–34

Schild AF, Perez E, Gillaspie E, Seaver C, Livingstone J, Thibonnier A (2008) Arteriovenous fisulae vs. arteriovenous grafts: a retrospective review of 1,700 consecutive vascular access cases. J Vasc Access 9:231–235

Scholz H, Simba A, Bürger K, Settmacher U (1995) Perioperative Antibiotikaprophylaxe in der Dialyseshuntchirurgie. Int J Exp Clin Chemother 7: 25–35

Stevenson KB, Hannah EL, Lowder CA, Adcox MJ, Davidson RL, Mallea MC, Narasimhan N, Wagnild JP (2002) Epidemiology of hemodialysis vascular access infections from longitudinal infection surveillance data: predicting the impact of NKF-DOYI clinical practice guidelines for vascular access. Am J Kidney Dis 39:549–555

Venous Congestion After the Creation of AV Accesses

8

Stenoses and/or occlusions of the venous runoff do not automatically cause thrombosis of the AV access. If there are venous side branches distal to the occlusion whose valves do not function properly, venous drainage is still possible via these collaterals. Regarding these collaterals, there are two clinical entities:

- Venous congestive syndrome
- Syndrome of retrograde venous arterialization

The impressive and unique clinical presentation already allows for a quick visual diagnosis.

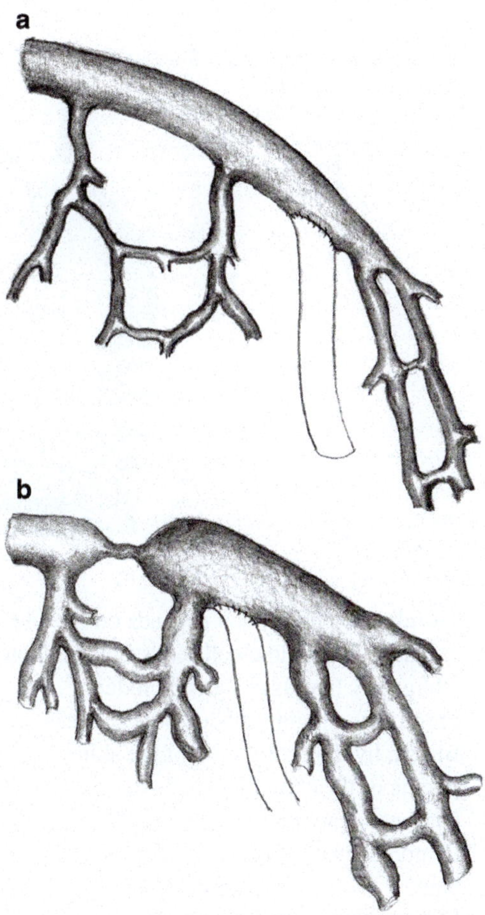

Fig. 8.1 Pre-existing venous collaterals (**a**) are more pronounced with venous congestion (**b**)

8.1 Venous Congestive Syndrome

8.1.1 Pathophysiology

With a proximal venous stenosis or occlusion, proximal venous drainage of an AV shunt is maintained by a web of (varying) large or medium size collateral veins (Fig. 8.1).

Because of the increased resistance in these collaterals, the raised pressure impairs drainage from the extremity. Therefore in the respective extremity, there will be:

- Numerous enlarged veins
- Venous edema
- Worsening of the edema by secondary decompensation of the lymphatic drainage

H. Scholz, *Arteriovenous Access Surgery*,
DOI 10.1007/978-3-642-41139-7_8, © Springer-Verlag Berlin Heidelberg New York 2015

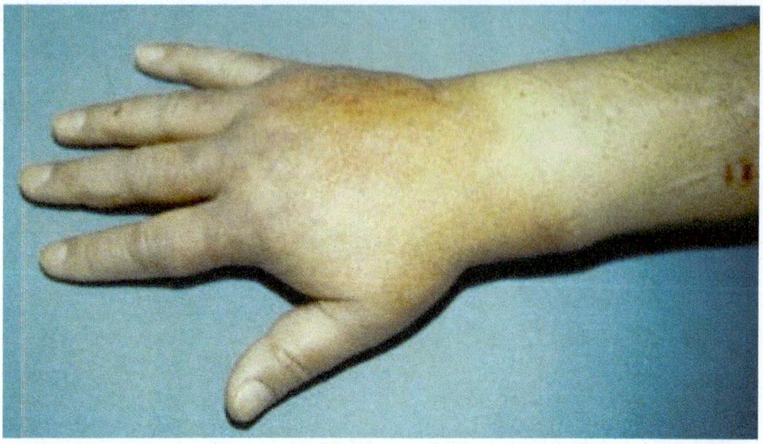

Fig. 8.2 Venous congestion. Edema of the hand after distal cephalic fistula with occlusion of the cephalic vein in the middle of the forearm

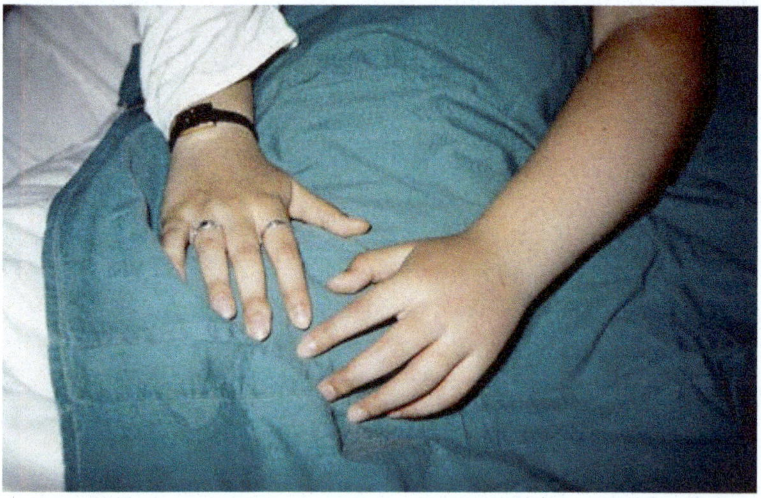

Fig. 8.3 Venous congestive syndrome. Edema of the forearm after cephalic elbow fistula and occlusion of the cephalic vein in the distal upper arm

The clinical presentation depends on the site of the occlusion, shunt flow, collaterals, and duration.

Obligatory (varying) signs include:

- Prominent, bulging subcutaneous veins
- Bluish, livid discoloration of the skin
- Edema of the extremity

Optional signs are:

- Lymph edema
- Pain
- Hemosiderin deposits in the skin
- A decreased range of motion of the joints

Indication

We see an indication for treatment if:

- The function of the AV access is at risk
- Patients suffer

Frequently wait-and-see is a valid tactic, as clinical symptoms decrease with the formation of further effective collaterals. Sometimes we merely perform flow reduction when there is:

- A high flow AV access
- No way to improve venous drainage
- Only limited options for other new potential vascular accesses

8.1.2 Occlusions/Stenoses of the Forearm Cephalic Veins with Distal AV Anastomoses

Clinical features distal to the occlusion may be discrete (Fig. 8.2). Collateral drainage mostly

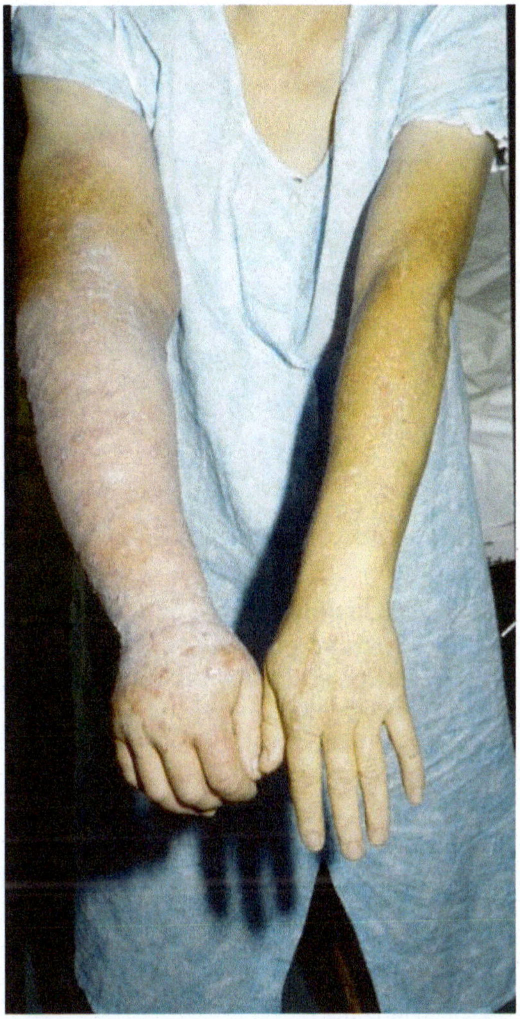

Fig. 8.4 Venous congestive syndrome. Chronic lymph edema with secondary chages after elbow cephalic fistula and occlusion in the distal upper arm 5 years earlier

happens into the basilic veins, or less often into deep veins.

Therapy

The whole armamentarium of endovascular (PTA/stenting) and surgical techniques may be used for short stenoses or occlusions. Long occlusions require a prosthetic graft to a suitable proximal vein for improved drainage. Rarely the basilic vein may be used for puncture after its arterialization via a side branch of the cephalic vein.

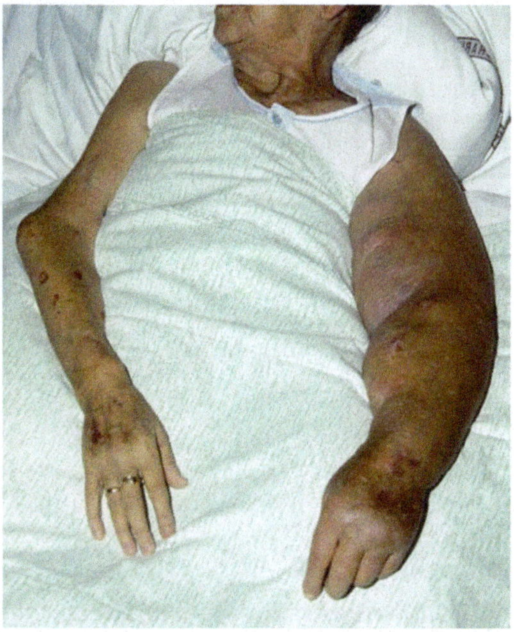

Fig. 8.5 Venous congestive syndrome. Edema of the entire arm after cephalic elbow fistula with occlusion of the axillary veins

8.1.3 Occlusions/Stenoses of the Cubital Veins with Distal AV Anastomoses

Clinical features are usually more pronounced (Fig. 8.3). They generally involve the whole forearm. Collaterals drain into the basilic vein and deep veins, and seldom into the cephalic vein. We have witnessed the development of chronic lymph edema with secondary changes several times (Fig. 8.4).

Therapy

As endovascular interventions usually offer only short-term improvement, we see the indication for surgical correction with grafts.

8.1.4 Occlusions/Stenoses of the Axillary Veins with Infraaxillary AV Anastomoses

Symptoms may be extreme and involve the whole arm distal to the axilla (Fig. 8.5). Typical features

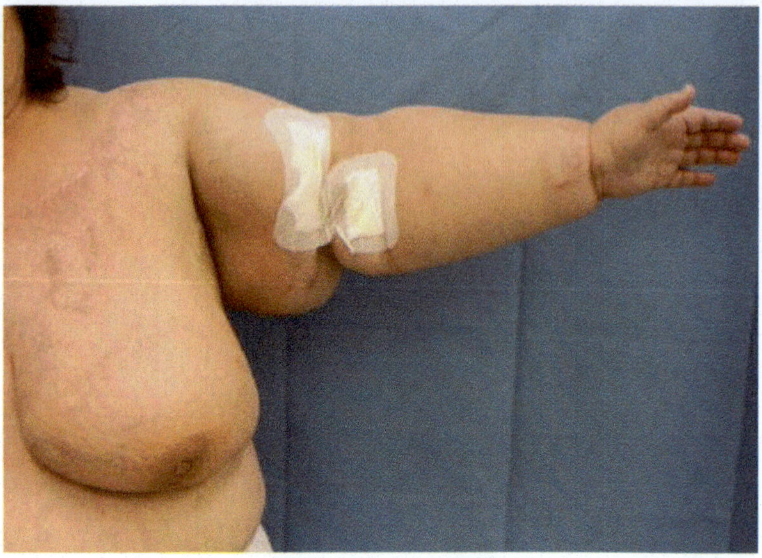

Fig. 8.6 Venous congestive syndrome. Edema of the arm, the shoulder, the left ventral thorax wall, and the breast with a cephalic elbow fistula and an occluded subclavian vein

are visible venous subcutaneous collaterals of the shoulder and ventral thorax.

Therapy
Unlike surgery, endovascular treatment does not promise good results.

8.1.5 Occlusions/Stenoses of the Axillary Veins or Subclavian Veins with Infraclavicular AV Anastomoses

Usually extreme symptoms involve the entire arm, the shoulder, and the mamma (Figs. 8.6 and 8.7). Subcutaneous collaterals cross to the other side of the thorax. Due to the extreme swelling, the arm cannot be used, and even hand closing is impossible. Patients often suffer from severe pain.

Therapy
Endovascular treatment with PTA and stent placement can offer instant relief. From our own observations, reocclusions frequently occur within a few months. Therefore we prefer open surgery. Depending on findings, local repair or a bypass to the internal jugular vein may be indicated.

8.1.6 Occlusions/Stenoses of the Brachiocephalic Vein with Peripheral AV Anastomosis and Occlusions/Stenoses of the Contralateral Internal Jugular Vein

Shoulder and arm symptoms are pronounced but usually not extreme. At first sight you notice a swelling of the head with eyelid edema and conjunctival hyperemia (Fig. 8.8). Patients complain of headaches and sometimes also of neurological symptoms.

Therapy
In all patients that we have treated, ligation of the AV anastomosis was the only viable solution.

8.1.7 Occlusions/Stenoses of the Femoral or Iliac Veins with Femoral AV Anastomoses

Apart from an increase in volume of the entire lower extremity and partly also of the hip region, which may be extreme, there are also subcutaneous collaterals of the lower abdomen.

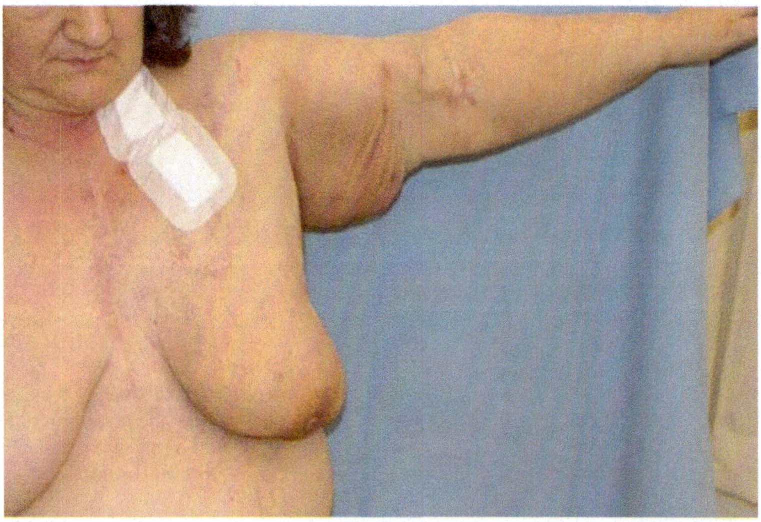

Fig. 8.7 Venous congestive syndrome. Patient from Fig. 8.6 after creation of an axillojugular bypass and withdrawal of 8 L by ultrafiltration

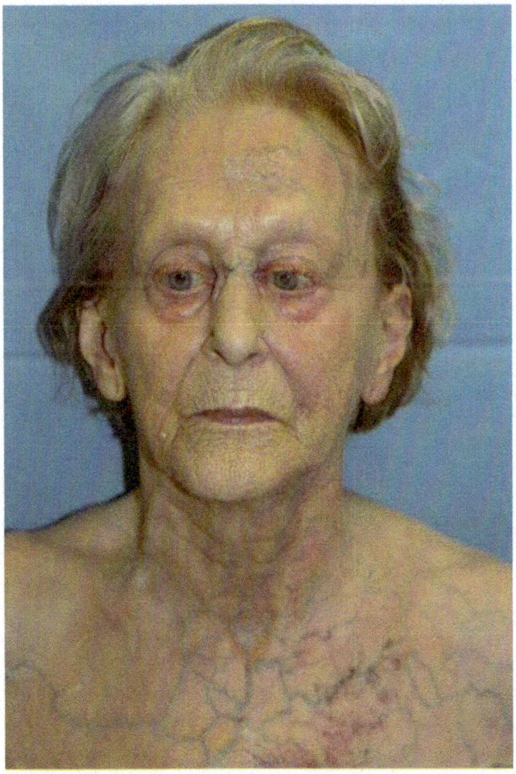

Fig. 8.8 Venous congestive syndrome. Pronounced collaterals and edema of the ventral thorax wall after AV access of the left arm and occlusion of the left brachiocephalic vein and the right internal jugular vein

Therapy

In the case of an infrainguinal stenosis of the draining femoral vein, we prefer surgical reconstruction. In a suprainguinal position we prefer PTA and stent placement. With a long stenosis (e.g., after irradiation) in which PTA fails, we close the AV anastomosis. After its ligation, large fluid volumes may enter the circulatory system within a few minutes, potentially resulting in lung edema. We observed such a case with manifest lung edema only 25 min after the anastomosis had been ligated. The patient needed immediate dialysis treatment, during which 5.5 L were withdrawn. Since then, we plan dialysis treatment for volume reduction directly after each ligation or drainage operation for venous congestion with distinct soft tissue swelling.

8.1.8 Clinical Symptoms After Curing Venous Congestion

After correcting the causes of venous congestion, clinical symptoms resolve within hours or rarely days. The subcutaneous venous collaterals, however, remain visible even after months. Chronic edemas are mostly due to damage to the lymphatic system.

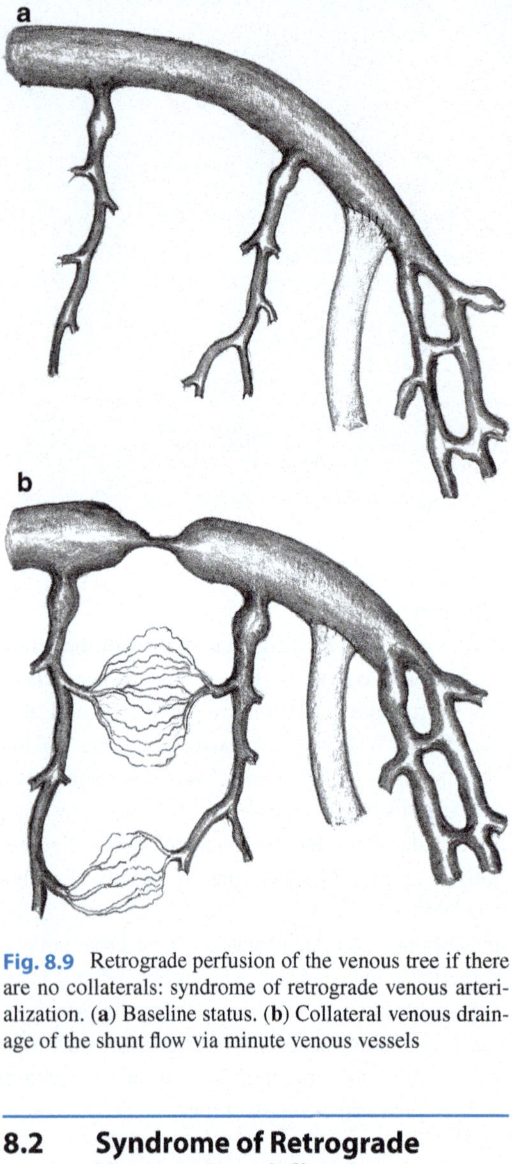

Fig. 8.9 Retrograde perfusion of the venous tree if there are no collaterals: syndrome of retrograde venous arterialization. (**a**) Baseline status. (**b**) Collateral venous drainage of the shunt flow via minute venous vessels

8.2 Syndrome of Retrograde Venous Arterialization

The characteristics of this clinical presentation and its pathophysiology justify the definition of a diagnosis in its own right (Scholz et al. 1988).

8.2.1 Pathophysiology

Retrograde venous arterialization only develops if there are inadequate or lacking venous collaterals for centrally-directed drainage. In the case of a venous occlusion or stenosis proximal to the AV shunt, drainage is mainly secured by numerous small superficial veins. Their entire vascular tree back to the venules is perfused retrogradely. Only there are they connected to a centrally-draining vein (Fig. 8.9).

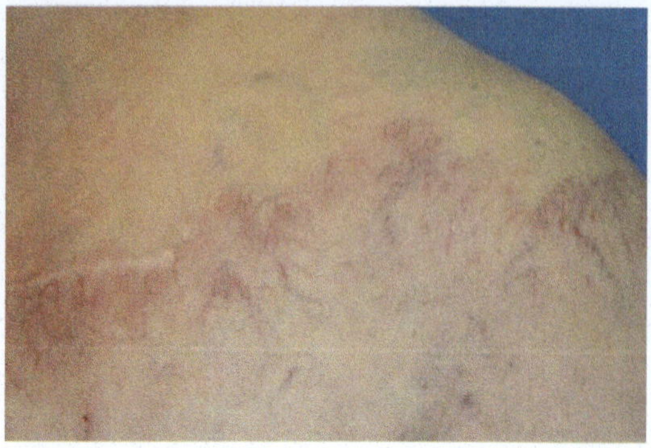

Fig. 8.10 Syndrome of retrograde venous arterialization. Note the brightly red, sickle-shaped arrangement of minute veins in the shoulder region with a cephalic elbow fistula and occlusion of the axillary veins

8.2.2 Clinical Signs

The typical signs and symptoms include:

- Minuscule light red spider or reticular veins without any recognizable feeding vessel arranged in a segmental sickle-shaped pattern (Fig. 8.10), which
  - Pulsate (visible when inspected under magnification)
  - Refill immediately after pressure is released
- Hard, possibly painful edema
- Feeling of heat in the respective extremity
- Rarely ulcerations

We most often observe the syndrome of retrograde venous arterialization with occlusions in the upper arm and shoulder regions. It is less frequent than mere venous congestion. Its treatment and the results are similar.

Literature

Scholz H, Naundorf M, Wolff H, Precht K, Röseler E, Schulze BD, Reinke P, Schoepke WD (1988) Syndrom der retrograden venösen Arterialisation nach arteriovenösen Gefässanschlüssen für die Hämodialyse. Z Urol Nephrol 81:675–679

Stenoses and Occlusions of the Central Veins

9

In this chapter, by central veins we mean the axillary segment of the brachial, the axillary, the subclavian, the internal jugular, the brachiocephalic, the common femoral, the iliac veins, and the superior vena cava.

9.1 Pathophysiology

The causes of stenoses and occlusions differ according to their sites. The most frequent causes are:

- Central venous catheters (subclavian, internal jugular, and femoral veins)
- Unphysiological hemodynamic conditions near venous anastomoses of AV shunts (brachial, axillary, and subclavian veins)
- Stents (cephalic and subclavian veins)
- Chemotherapy

From March 2007 through June 2011 (51 months), 297 arm venograms were performed at our institution for malfunctioning AV accesses. In 129 patients we found stenoses and occlusions of central veins. Their topographic distribution is shown in Fig. 9.1. The subclavian vein is concerned strikingly often (right 22.2 %, left 11.4 %). All these patients had had subclavian catheters weeks to years previously. The central segments of the axillary veins on both sides showed 25 (13.5 %) stenoses or occlusions (Fig. 9.1, segment 3). Of these, 18 were caused by catheters and 7 by venous anastomoses of AV shunts. All 25 stenoses and occlusions (13.6 %) of the axillary segment of the brachial vein (Fig. 9.1, segment 1) can be traced back to venous anastomoses of AV shunts.

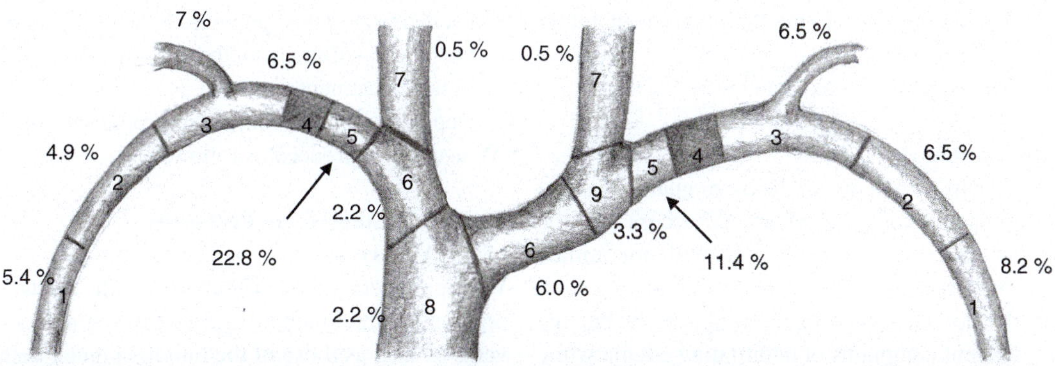

Fig. 9.1 Topographic distribution of stenoses and occlusions in 129 patients. *1* Axillary segment of the brachial vein, *2* peripheral segment of the axillary vein, *3* central segment of the axillary vein, *4* retroclavicular segment of the subclavian vein, *5* central segment of the subclavian vein, *6* brachiocephalic vein, *7* internal jugular vein, *8* superior vena cava, *9* confluence of the subclavian and left internal jugular veins

H. Scholz, *Arteriovenous Access Surgery*,
DOI 10.1007/978-3-642-41139-7_9, © Springer-Verlag Berlin Heidelberg New York 2015

9.2 Clinical Signs and Investigations

Central venous stenoses or occlusions manifest themselves as:

- *Venous congestion with a patent AV access or*
- *Thrombosis of the AV access*

As the process of developing a stenosis or occlusion usually takes some time, subcutaneous venous collaterals, which do not have to be tightly filled, are frequently present. Diagnostics should include color duplex studies. Except for retroclavicular and retrosternal venous segments, reliable results may be obtained. With confirmed or suspected stenoses or occlusions of central veins, we also order venograms. Without a digital subtraction technique, however, contrast medium dilution may lead to an insufficient depiction of the large veins if contrast medium is injected into a (still) high flow AV access. Temporary flow reduction may be achieved by manual compression of the AV access distal to the injection site.

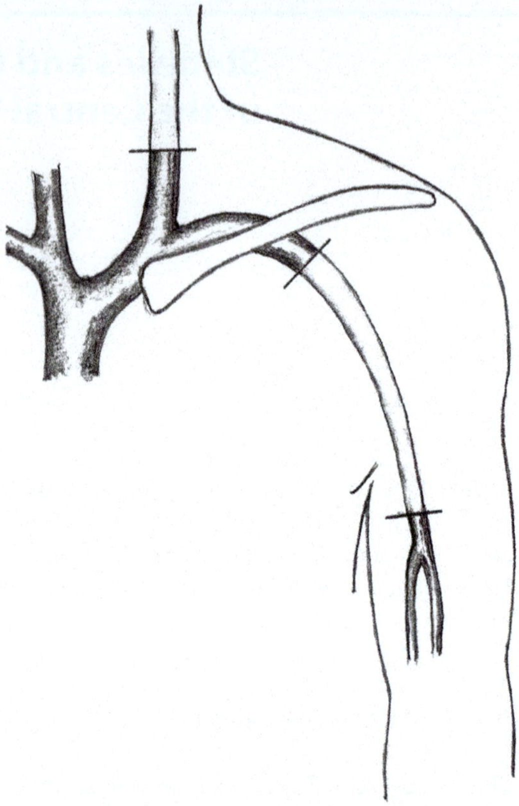

Fig. 9.2 Central veins in the upper part of the body which are relevant for AV access surgery. *Shaded areas* show segments which are amenable to endovascular treatment, whereas non-shaded segments seem to be more suitable for surgery

9.3 Therapy

The choice of treatment depends on:

- Clinical impact of the stenosis or occlusion
- Its location
- The long-term prognosis of the AV access
- Previous surgery in the region of the stenosis or occlusion
- Prospects of endovascular therapy
- Remaining options for the creation of future AV accesses
- The patient's life expectancy

Indications

- If sufficient collateralization guarantees the proper functioning of an AV access and the patient does not suffer, we will not initiate therapy.
- If the AV access functions properly but the patient complains of debilitating edema while options for the creation of a future AV access are limited, we will surgically reduce shunt flow provided it is high enough.
- If a stenosis or occlusion causes malfunctioning of the dialysis access by thrombosis, reduced shunt flow (recirculation), high pressure in the AV access (long compression needed to stop post puncture bleeding), and/or the patient suffers from the ensuing edema, we initiate treatment.

Depending on the long-term prognosis of the AV access we proceed as follows.

Favorable Long-Term Prognosis of the AV Access

We repair stenoses and occlusions of the axillary segment of the brachial vein and of the axillary veins as well as those of the internal jugular vein near anastomoses (Fig. 9.2, lightly hatched areas):

- Isolated stenoses or occlusions of the axillary segments of the brachial vein deserve patch plasty or interposition grafts (Fig. 9.3a).

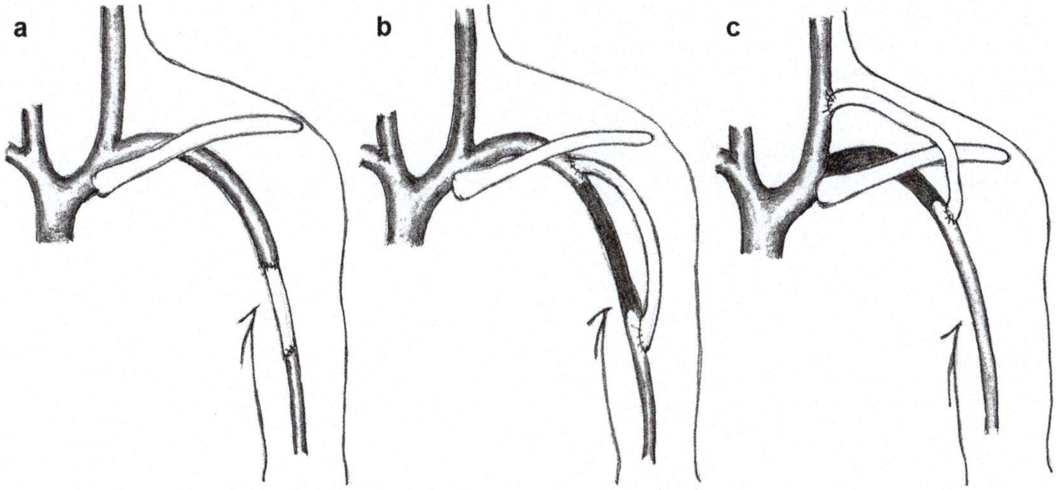

Fig. 9.3 Options for reconstructing occlusions of proximal veins of the upper extremities. (**a**) Interposition graft for infraaxillary occlusion. (**b**) Brachioaxillary bypass graft for axillary occlusion. (**c**) Axillojugular bypass graft for subclavian occlusion

- Long occlusions of the axillary vein are bypassed by extra-anatomic brachioaxillary ePTFE grafts (7- or 8-mm) (Fig. 9.3b).
- In occlusions of the subclavian vein which cannot be successfully treated by endovascular means, we create an axillojugular bypass (7–8 mm ePTFE) (Fig. 9.3c).

With stenoses and occlusions of the subclavian vein, the caudal part of the internal jugular vein, the brachiocephalic vein, and the superior vena cava (Fig. 9.2, darkly hatched areas) we prefer endovascular treatment, which may often be successfully repeated several times if necessary.

Lower Extremity

If possible we repair stenoses of the venous anastomosis with the common femoral artery by open surgery and patch plasty. More cranial stenoses proximal to the inguinal ligament including those of the iliac vessels are usually treated by endovascular means.

Poor Long-Term Prognosis of the AV Access with Alternative Options for Future Accesses

If the prognosis is poor anyway, you should avoid any disproportionate efforts to save it.

Literature

Agarwal AK, Patel BM, Haddad NJ (2007) Central vein stenosis: a nephrologist's perspective. Semin Dial 20:53–62

Anaya-Ayala JE, Smolock CJ, Colvard BD, Naoum JJ, Bismuth J, Lumsden AB, Davies MG, Peden EK (2011) Efficacy of covered stent placement for central venous occlusive disease in hemodialysis patients. J Vasc Surg 54:754–759

Bakken AM, Protack CD, Saad WE, Lee DE, Waldman DL, Davies MG (2007) Long-term outcomes of primary angioplasty and primary stenting of central venous stenosis in hemodialysis patients. J Vasc Surg 45:776–783

Criado E, Marston WA, Jaques PF, Mauro MA, Keagy BA (1994) Proximal venous outflow obstruction in patients with upper extremity arteriovenous dialysis access. Ann Vasc Surg 8:530–535

Gonsalves CF, Eschelman DJ, Sullivan KL, DuBois N, Bonn J (2003) Incidence of central vein stenosis and occlusion following upper extremity PICC and port placement. Cardiovasc Intervent Radiol 26: 123–127

Haage P, Vorwerk D, Piroth W, Schuermann K, Guenther RW (1999) Treatment of hemodialysis-related central venous stenosis or occlusion: results of primary Wallstent placement and follow-up in 50 patients. Radiology 212:175–180

Haskal ZJ, Trerotola S, Dolmatch B, Schuman E, Altman S, Mietling S, Berman S, McLennan G, Trimmer C, Ross J, Vesely T (2010) Stent graft versus balloon angioplasty for failing dialysis-access grafts. N Engl J Med 362:494–503

Suliman A, Greenberg JI, Angle N (2008) Surgical bypass of symptomatic central venous obstruction for arteriovenous fistula salvage in hemodialysis patients. Ann Vasc Surg 22:203–209

Tesio F, Panarello G, De Baz H, Canzi M, De Mattia T, Pasut R (2003) Central vascular access: rational and results. G Ital Nefrol 20(Suppl 22):30–34

Vanherweghem JL (1994) Thrombosis and stenosis of central venous access in hemodialysis. Nephrologie 15:117–121

Leakage of ePTFE Grafts (Perigraft Seroma)

10

10.1 Pathophysiology

The following experience is exclusively based on ePTFE prostheses. Their surface is uneven, fibrillary, and hydrophobic with pore sizes 50–70 μm, varying with the respective manufacturers. Only after exceeding a critical pressure may fluid permeate the wall. This pressure is called the hydrophobic barrier. According to manufacturers it is around 300 mmHg.

In practice, however, in some patients plasma leaks from grafts at much lower pressures. Our lab tests showed that the protein and electrolyte content of this leaking fluid corresponds to that of blood plasma. Consequently there is a filtration process rather than a tissue reaction to the prosthesis, but it may also be called perigraft reaction in so far as this filtration also leads to alterations of the surrounding tissue. This filtration is caused by the conversion of the ePTFE graft surface from a hydrophobic to a hydrophilic state brought about by plasma molecules.

Before 1992 when we started selective sequential fibrin sealing of the outer graft surface, we observed the intraoperative filtration of prostheses in almost a third of our dialysis patients. In patients who did not require hemodialysis, we could observe a clinically relevant filtration of non fibrin-sealed ePTFE grafts (peripheral bypass surgery) in around 1 %. Damage to the ePTFE wall and also to its potential fibrin coating (e.g., by clamping or grasping) favors filtration. As we take care to avoid this damage as much as possible, the experience reported here mostly refers to patients who had already been treated elsewhere.

The clinical presentation depends on the relation of the filtered volume (filtrate) to the absorptive capacity of the surrounding tissue and the duration of the filtration.

10.2 Clinical Presentation and Therapy

According to the clinical presentation and course we distinguish between five types of graft filtration.

10.2.1 Type I

Intraoperative filtration of small droplets (frequently only near the arterial anastomosis) (Fig. 10.1). After the wound closure, healing is usually not impaired as filtration tends to stop soon.

Frequency
Around 30 %.

10.2.2 Type II

Edema and slight erythema over the prosthesis lasting for days to weeks without (sonographic) proof of a fluid collection around the graft (Fig. 10.2).

H. Scholz, *Arteriovenous Access Surgery*,
DOI 10.1007/978-3-642-41139-7_10, © Springer-Verlag Berlin Heidelberg New York 2015

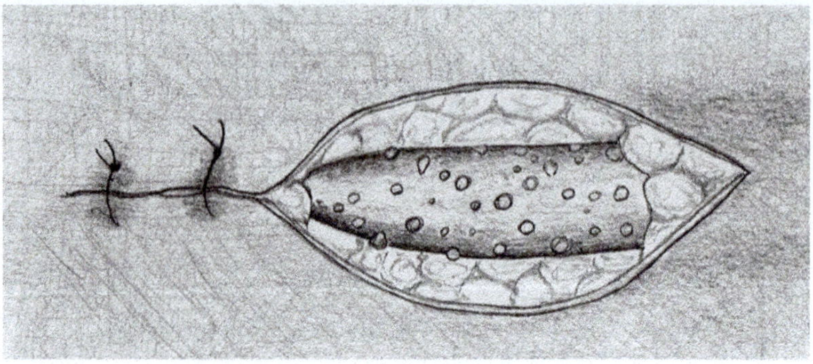

Fig. 10.1 Intraoperative findings. Loss of clear fluid through the graft surface

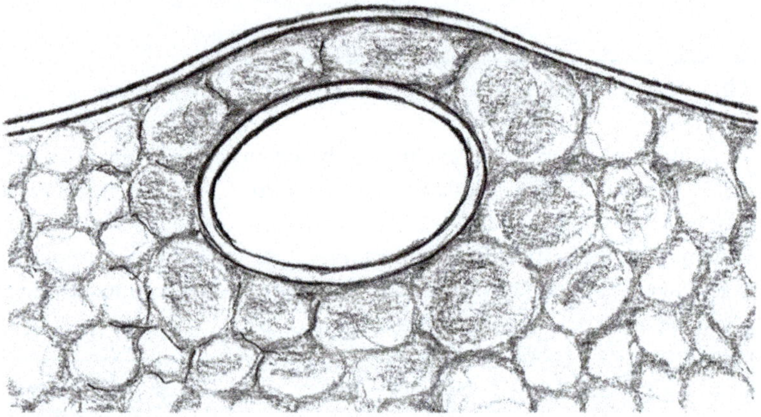

Fig. 10.2 Edema around the prosthesis

In this type, filtration persists for a longer time although the absorptive capacity seems to be sufficient. Differential diagnosis should include infections.

Frequency
10–15 %.

Therapy
- Conservative with cooling and immobilization of the raised extremity.
- No punctures as long as the edema persists.

Prognosis
After the edema subsides, complete healing can be expected. The time needed before we recommend the first puncture is significantly longer than usual.

10.2.3 Type III

Postoperative wound secretion (filtrate) or prolonged fluid drainage.

The volume of the filtrate exceeds the absorptive capacity. If the secretion persists after the third day or is profuse before that, redo surgery will be indicated.

Frequency
Rare after fibrin sealing.

Therapy
- Open the surgical wound and inspect the graft.
- If filtration is limited to the exposed segment of the graft near the arterial anastomosis, temporarily cross clamp the proximal and distal artery, and perform selective fibrin sealing of the exposed graft.
- If filtration involves the whole prosthesis, proceed as follows:
  1. With prior sequential fibrin sealing, repeated fibrin sealing does not seem to be a promising option. The graft must be removed.
  2. If there was no prior sequential fibrin sealing, the graft should be taken out, treated as above, and implanted again.

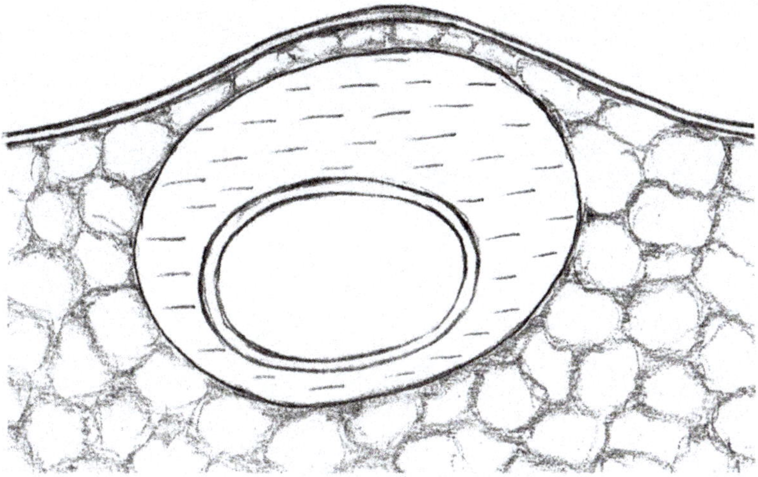

Fig. 10.3 Encapsulated fluid collection around the prosthesis

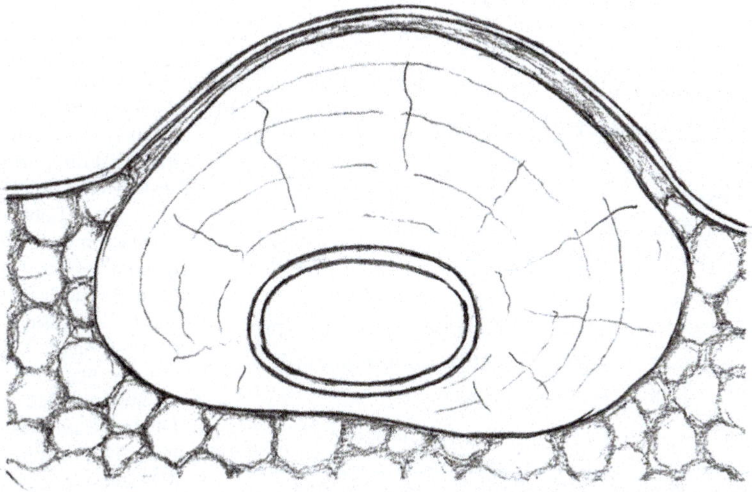

Fig. 10.4 Collection of hard protein coagula around the prosthesis

10.2.4 Type IV

After primary wound healing, a periprosthetic fluid collection leads to a prominence over the path of the prosthesis. Sonography can confirm the visual and palpatory findings.

Filtration exceeds the absorptive capacity. The graft is embedded in a fluid-filled capsula which develops over the course of mostly 3–4 weeks.

Frequency

Not observed after fibrin sealing.

Therapy

- Don't puncture the graft so as to avoid hematoma formation inside the capsula with the risk of secondary infection.
- Expose the graft at the anastomoses. The graft lies in a fluid-filled tunnel which sometimes also contains fibrin particles. The wall of this space consists of a shiny whitish capsula (Fig. 10.3).
- Further actions depend on whether fibrin sealant has been used previously (cf. Type III). In the case that the graft is reused, a new tunnel must be created.

10.2.5 Type V

Hard tumors possibly combined with cyst-like structures without inflammatory signs surround the whole graft or the arterial anastomosis. They appear weeks to months after the implantation. With persistent leakage they form a hard mass of fibrin-rich thrombi (Figs. 10.4 and 10.5).

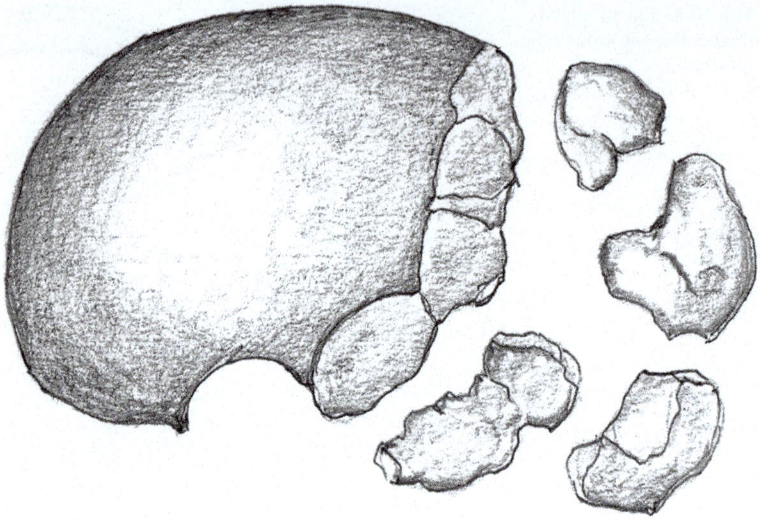

Fig. 10.5 Typical appearance of removed protein coagula

Frequency

Not observed after fibrin sealing.

Therapy

As for type IV.

If a fibrin-sealed prosthesis has to be removed because of a perigraft seroma, a special multilayer, primarily pressure watertight graft (produced by different manufacturers) should be placed into a separate tunnel.

Literature

Ahn SS, Williams DE, Thye DA, Cheng KQ, Lee DA (1994) The isolation of a fibroblast growth inhibitor associated with perigraft seroma. J Vasc Surg 20:202–208

Dauria DM, Dyk P, Garvin P (2006) Incidence and management of seroma after arteriovenous graft placement. J Am Coll Surg 203:506–511

Sobrinho G, Henriques SP (2001) Perigraft seromas complicating prosthetic bridge arteriovenous fistula-solution with autogenous vein interposition. Eur J Vasc Endovasc Surg 22:469–471

Tabata R, Mori A, Magara T, Watarida S, Nakamura Y, Onoe M, Okada Y, Kobayashi T (1989) Experimental study on the mechanism of serum leakage from expanded polytetrafluoroethylene (EPTFE) vascular prosthesis. Nihon Kyobu Geka Gakkai Zasshi 37:439–448

Tabata R, Kobayashi T, Mori A, Matsuno S, Watarida S, Onoe M, Sugita T, Shiraisi S, Nojima T (1993) A computer simulation of the plasma leakage through a vascular prosthesis made of expanded polytetrafluoroethylene. J Thorac Cardiovasc Surg 105:598–604

Tsuchida H, Kashyap A, Cameron BL, Peng SK, Wilson SE (1993) In vivo study of a high-porosity polytetrafluoroethylene graft: endothelialization, fluid leakage, and the effect of fibrin glue sealing. J Invest Surg 6:509–518

Zanow J, Kruger U, Settmacher U, Scholz H (2010) Treatment of perigraft seroma in expanded polytetrafluoroethlene grafts by sequential fibrin sealing of the outer graft surface. Ann Vasc Surg 24:1005–1014

Insufficient Peripheral Perfusion and Cardiac Strain After AV Access Creation

11

AV accesses may cause insufficient perfusion of the extremity distal to the AV anastomosis as well as excessive cardiac strain. The therapy for both follows the same principles and is therefore discussed together.

11.1 Insufficient Peripheral Perfusion

If there are clinically relevant symptoms distal to the AV anastomosis due to an inadequate blood supply, we call this state insufficient peripheral perfusion.

11.1.1 Pathophysiology and Stages of Insufficient Perfusion

In the literature the inadequate blood supply to the extremity distal to the AV anastomosis is mostly called steal syndrome. In a true steal syndrome, however, there is usually a retrograde flow in the distal artery, which actually is not obligatory for insufficient peripheral perfusion. Therefore we do not use this expression. Figure 11.1 shows a drawing of the peripheral circulation of an extremity with the corresponding flow resistances. The venous outflow resistance R_v is low unless there are hemodynamically relevant stenoses. Therefore it will be neglected in the following. Channeling flow portions from the proximal artery into the AV access leads to a decrease of pressure in the artery distal to the anastomosis (peripheral perfusion pressure p_p). This pressure drop depends on:

- Resistance of the feeding artery (R_{aprox})
- Resistance of the AV access (R_{av})
- Resistance of the distal artery (R_{adist}) and peripheral vasculature

Over the course of time these resistances may change.

- The inflow resistance R_{aprox} may decrease due to the dilation of the feeding artery.
- The outflow resistance of the distal artery (R_{adist}) may decrease due to the dilation of the peripheral vasculature.

Furthermore, collaterals, which can be quite pronounced between forearm and upper arm, must be taken into account. Anecdotal reports even mention cubital AV fistulas which are effectively fed by the distal stump of a proximally-occluded brachial artery without any signs of insufficient peripheral perfusion. Changing resistances may entail changes of the peripheral arterial perfusion pressure. After an initial pressure drop distal to the anastomosis, the following scenarios may develop (Fig. 11.2):

(a) The initial peripheral pressure drop may persist, if the resistance of the feeding artery (R_{aprox}) and the resistance of the AV access (R_{av}) remain constant (neither dilation of the proximal artery nor of the AV access) (Fig. 11.2a).
(b) The peripheral pressure increases due to the dilation of the proximal feeding artery (decrease of the inflow resistance R_{aprox}) (Fig. 11.2b).

H. Scholz, *Arteriovenous Access Surgery*,
DOI 10.1007/978-3-642-41139-7_11, © Springer-Verlag Berlin Heidelberg New York 2015

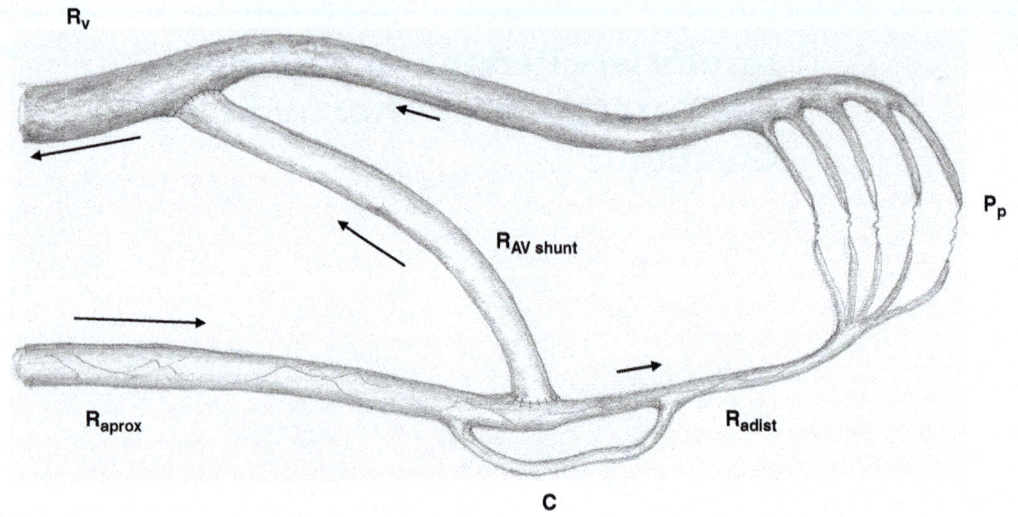

Fig. 11.1 Depiction of a peripheral circulatory segment with an AV shunt. R_{aprox} inflow resistance, R_{adist} peripheral resistance, R_{av} resistance inside the AV shunt, R_V central venous outflow resistance, P_p peripheral perfusion pressure, *C* collateral

(c) The peripheral resistance decreases continuously due to the dilation of the AV access (decrease of R_{av}) (Fig. 11.2c).

Depending on resistance and collaterals, three different flow patterns in the AV anastomosis can be observed (Fig. 11.3):

(a) Systolic and diastolic inflow both into the AV access as well as into the distal artery (Fig. 11.3a).
(b) Systolic inflow both into the AV access as well as into the distal artery, and diastolic inflow into the AV access both from the proximal and distal artery (Fig. 11.3b).
(c) Systolic and diastolic inflow into the AV access both from the proximal and distal artery (Fig. 11.3c).

The critical peripheral perfusion threshold – below which symptoms of insufficient perfusion occur – varies widely between individuals. Patients with high peripheral resistances such as diabetics suffering from small vessel disease are particularly prone to these complaints.

We distinguish between four stages of insufficient peripheral perfusion.

Stage I
Sensation of coldness and decrease in sensitivity in the affected extremity, particularly when exercising and during dialysis.
Stage II
Painful extremity particularly when exercising and during dialysis.
Stage III
Pain at rest.
Stage IV
Pain at rest and trophic disturbances possibly including tissue loss.

11.1.2 Vascular Investigations

The first step is to exclude a significant stenosis or occlusion of the feeding artery. Watch out for collateralized arterial occlusions. If there is a central stenosis or occlusion, it should be treated accordingly. Only with an unimpaired arterial inflow can the contribution of the AV access to the inadequate peripheral blood be evaluated.

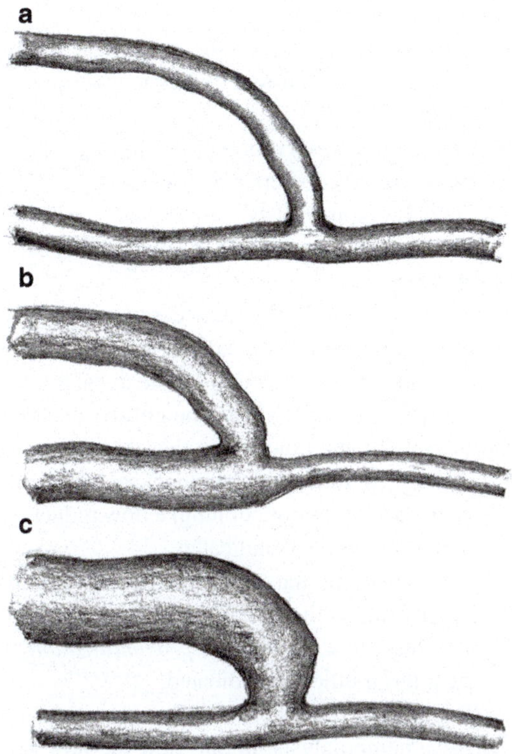

Fig. 11.2 Possible impact of an AV fistula on vascular morphology. (**a**) Absence of fistula dilation. (**b**) Dilation of the proximal artery. (**c**) Dilation of the vein

Apart from clinical examination, color duplex sonography is the primary diagnostic tool for measuring the flow in the AV access. As flow turbulence in the AV access may falsify the results, the flow should be determined in the proximal and distal feeding artery (Fig. 11.4). The flow direction of the distal artery should be noted (flow reversal with steal effect). The flow in the AV access (Q_{av}) is

$$Q_{av} = Q_{aprox} - Q_{adist}.$$

As the flow in the AV access is proportionately related to the blood pressure, the systolic blood pressure also has to be recorded simultaneously. In many patients who need hemodialysis, blood pressure varies widely. The flow rate in the AV access at the lowest blood pressure is important (frequently occurring directly after dialysis).

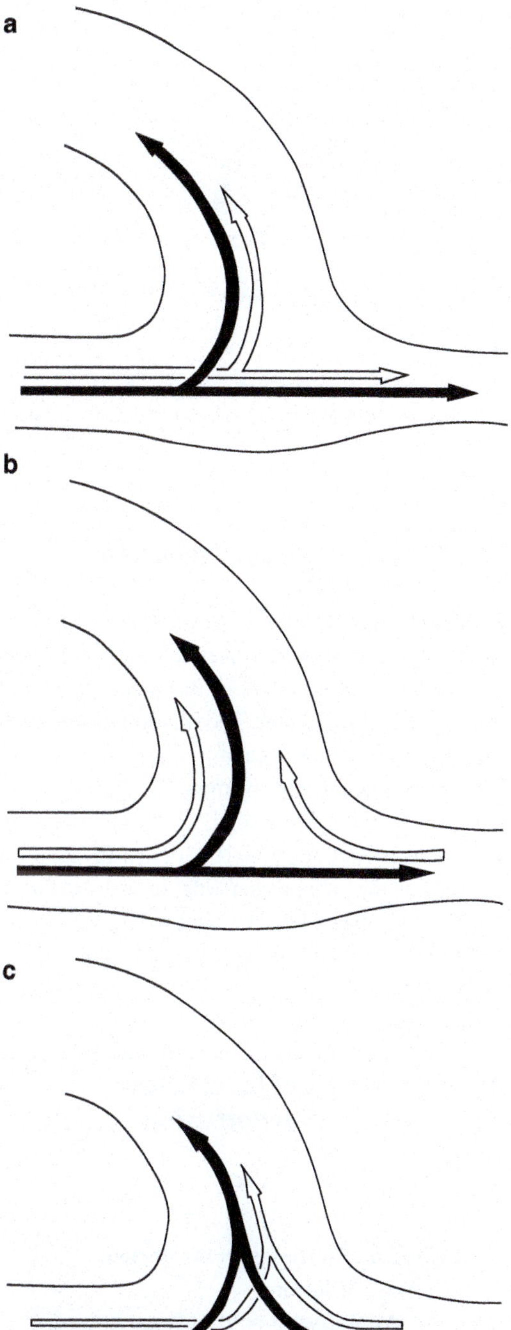

Fig. 11.3 Possible flow variants in the AV anastomosis (*black arrows*: systole, *white arrows*: diastole). (**a**) Systolic and diastolic inflow into the vein as well as into the distal artery. (**b**) Systolic inflow into the vein and the distal artery, diastolic (retrograde) inflow from the distal artery into the vein. (**c**) Systolic and diastolic inflow into the vein from the proximal as well as from the distal artery

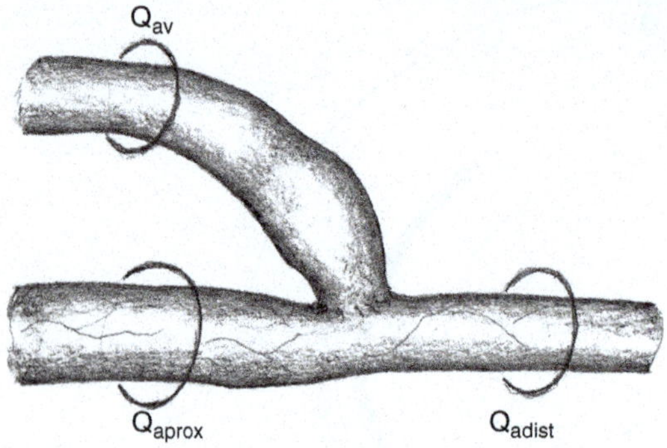

Fig. 11.4 Flow in the AV anastomosis. Q_{aprox} flow in the proximal artery, Q_{adist} flow in the distal artery, Q_{av} flow in the AV shunt

11.1.3 Indications for Treatment

Perioperative complaints corresponding to stages I and II should be treated conservatively. Symptoms may be relieved by keeping the hand warm and moving it in warm water. The dilation of the feeding artery and other regulatory processes mostly lead to significant improvement. If symptoms do not get better after 3–4 weeks, we see an indication for reconstruction in stage II patients. In stage I it depends on the patient's personal level of suffering and the complexity of potential procedures.

In stages III and IV we see principal indications for repair.

11.2 Therapy of Insufficient Peripheral Perfusion

Therapeutic Principles for Insufficient Peripheral Perfusion

1. An AV access should only be ligated if all other means to improve the inadequate peripheral perfusion have failed. As a measure of last resort this is hardly ever necessary.
2. It is highly likely that a new AV access in the same but contralateral position will lead to the same symptoms if all other conditions are equal.

Therapy aims at:

- Permanent increase of the peripheral perfusion pressure to correct insufficient peripheral perfusion
- Guaranteed preservation of the AV access
- Prevention of irreversible vascular damage

The literature lists numerous methods, which basically boil down to two therapeutic approaches:

- Flow reduction in the AV access
- Proximalization of the arterial inflow into the AV access or of the stump of the distal artery

The approach that should be chosen depends exclusively on the flow rate in the AV access:

- If the flow rate is higher than necessary for secure long term functioning, a flow reduction of the AV access is indicated.
- If the flow in the AV access is around or slightly higher than the rate required for secure long term functioning, the *proximalization* of the arterial inflow is indicated.

To guarantee a reliable long term function and effective hemodialysis, in our view the flow rate should be at least:

- Around 300 mL/min with AV fistulas
- 600–1,000 mL/min with ePTFE grafts (7 mm diameter)

In AV fistulas with extremely dilated veins, the necessary flow rate should be significantly higher.

The influence of flow reduction on peripheral perfusion cannot be exactly predicted. In some patients intraoperative flow and pressure readings distal to the anastomosis (in the cubital fossa) rise proportionally only above a certain systemic blood pressure threshold. In the rare cases when flow reduction does not suffice to raise peripheral perfusion pressure, proximalization should be carried out later. If even proximalization fails, the AV access should be abandoned possibly in favor of an arterioarterial graft. Figure 11.5 lists therapeutic options.

11.2.1 Flow Reduction

In the literature you can find numerous ways to reduce the flow with banding either involving circumscribed (ligature) or segmental (ribbon)

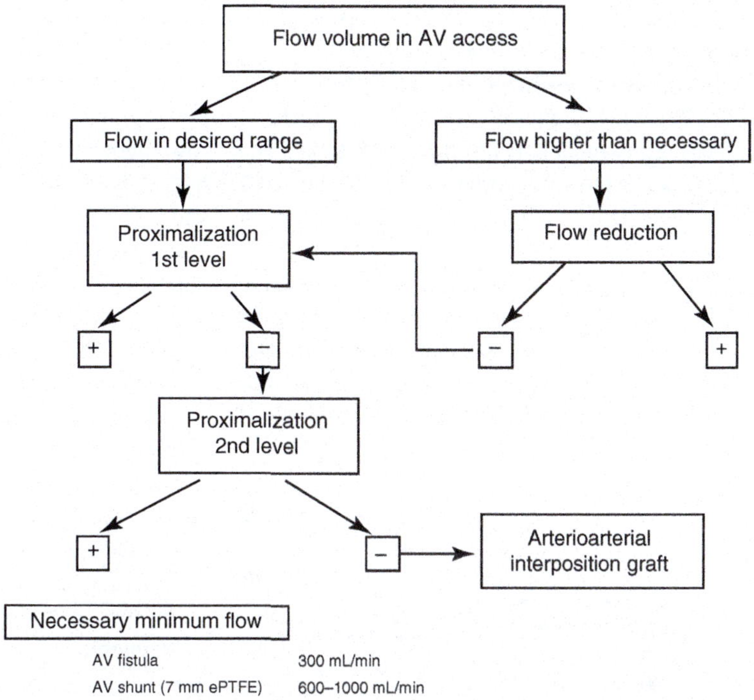

Fig. 11.5 Therapeutic strategy for insufficient peripheral perfusion

narrowing of the lumen. Basically two aims should be achieved:

- Precise reduction of the flow as desired
- Stable long term results

Physical Principles

The impact of a stenosis on blood flow depends on diameter and length. To achieve the same flow reduction, a wide stenosis has to be significantly longer than a narrow one. The longer a stenosis that was created on purpose is, the more precisely it can be adjusted. At the same time this stenotic segment is no longer available for puncture. The smaller the diameter of a stenosis that has been created on purpose is, the shorter it needs to be. Yet it is more difficult to realize exactly the diameter that is required.

We examined transparent silicone models in a pulsatile flow system to determine the effects of the length and diameter of a narrow segment on the extent of flow reduction. In this system the narrow segment was interspersed between a 6-mm artery and a 7-mm graft.

For better illustration, Fig. 11.6 shows narrow segments of different diameters (1.2, 3, and 4 mm, respectively) in scale as well as the different lengths that are required to reduce the flow by 40 %. The results were found in our pulsatile flow system (Chap. 21). The inflow through a 6-mm fake artery into the 7-mm fake AV graft (pipe) met the counter pressure of a 12-cm water column (venous outflow). For the 4-mm narrow segment we investigated lengths of up to 70 mm. This length resulted in a flow reduction of only 28 %. Its length (150 mm) required for the 40 % flow reduction shown in Fig. 11.6 was determined approximately by the Hagen–Poiseuille equation.

Already discrete variations in diameter of small caliber narrow segments lead to considerable flow changes. A different flow velocity in the stenotic segment has important implications in a biological system. The narrower the stenosis, the higher the flow velocity and the mechanical irritation at the vascular wall. Clinical experience shows that with very small diameters there is an elevated risk of tissue proliferation and occlusion of the lumen.

Therefore it is important to find a compromise between:

- The precise extent of the stenosis you want to create surgically.
- The partial loss of the segment that is suitable for puncturing because a narrow segment is not suited for needle placement.

Experiments on the Influence of Diameter and Length of a Narrow Segment on Shunt Flow in the Pulsatile Flow System

For these investigations we created precision acrylic glass models (Figs. 11.7 and 11.8). The diameters of the model arteries varied between 2 and 7 mm, and the lengths of the narrow segment between 0 and 70 mm.

Figure 11.9 shows the relative flow reduction with 4-mm narrow segments upstream from the prosthesis at an arterial pressure of 100 mmHg. Here the results are normalized to flow rates without a narrow segment (direct anastomosis of the graft).

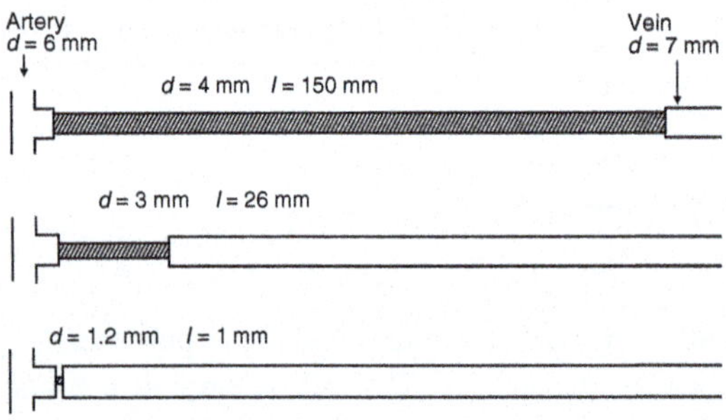

Fig. 11.6 Exemplary calculations to achieve a 40 % flow reduction via a narrow segment with diameters of 6 mm for the artery and 7 mm for the vein. Appropriate length/diameter combinations of the narrow segments would be 150/4, 26/3, and 1.2/1 mm

The relative flow rate decreases with an increasing diameter of the artery. Likewise, the same is true for an increasing length of the narrow segment. As an example the 70 mm long narrow segment (7 mm diameter) reduces the flow by 5 % if anastomosed to a 2 mm diameter artery and by 28 % if anastomosed to a 7 mm diameter artery (Krueger et al. 2001, 2004; Zanow et al. 2006a, b).

- If the diameter of the narrow segment is only 3 mm, the impact on flow reduction is much more pronounced (Fig. 11.10). Under these circumstances the flow reduction may be as high as 55 % (7 mm diameter artery, length of narrow segment 70 mm). The flow reduction after only 5 mm is already so pronounced that it would be difficult to achieve a flow reduction precisely as desired in a real life situation in the operating room with such a short segment.

The higher the inflow resistance is (narrow native artery), the less influence an intercalated narrow segment has on flow reduction. The lower the inflow resistance is (wide native artery), the more influence an intercalated narrow segment has on flow reduction.

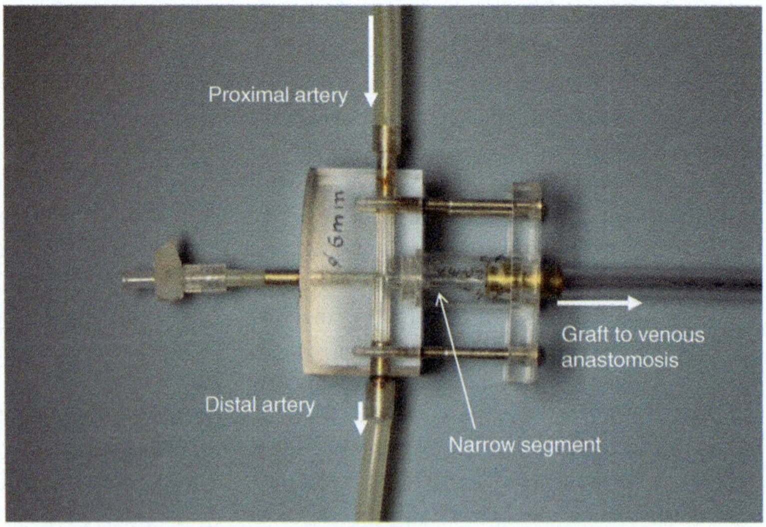

Fig. 11.7 Model of the arterial anastomosis with narrow segment. The other end of the prosthetic graft is connected to the venous model anastomosis (see Fig. 4.7)

Fig. 11.8 Model of a narrow segment. Cylinders with different diameters and lengths are mounted to the model's artery as narrow segments

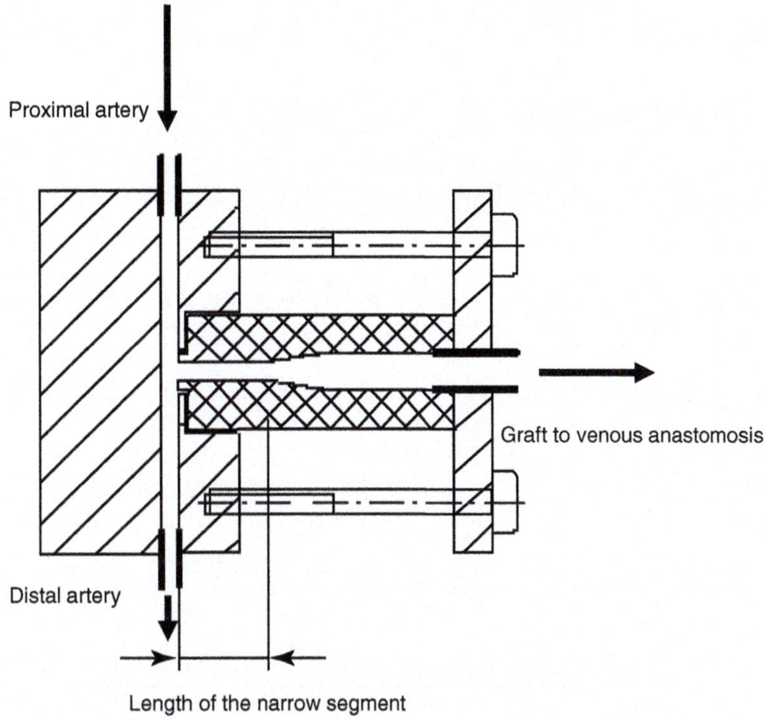

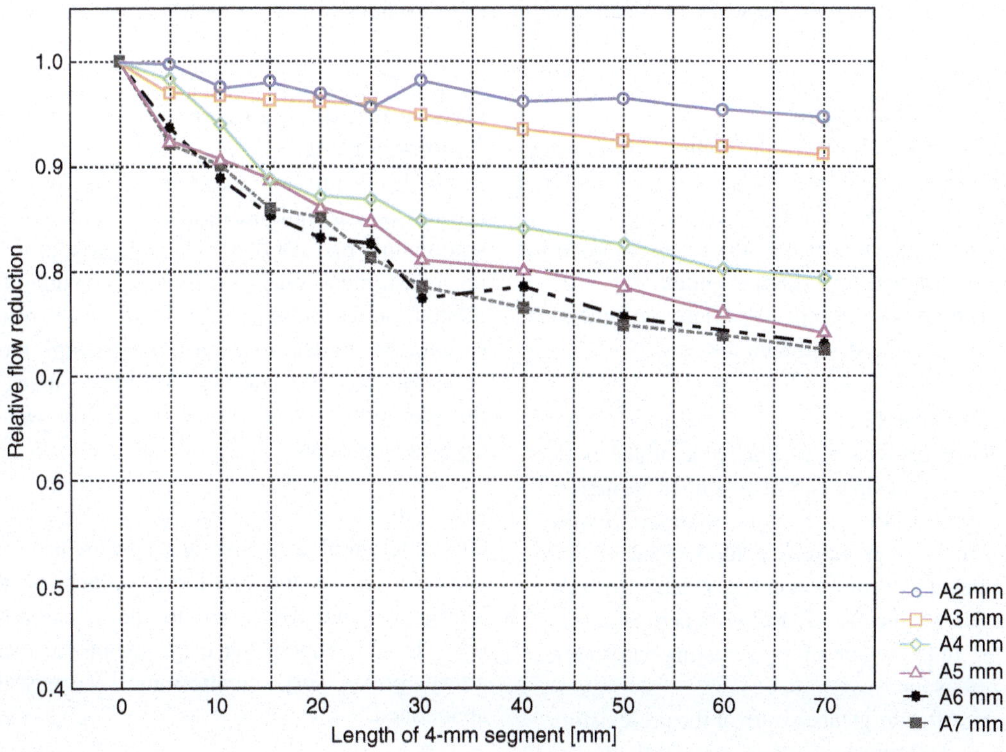

Fig. 11.9 Relative flow reduction by a 4 mm diameter narrow segment dependent on its length and the arterial diameter (2–7 mm)

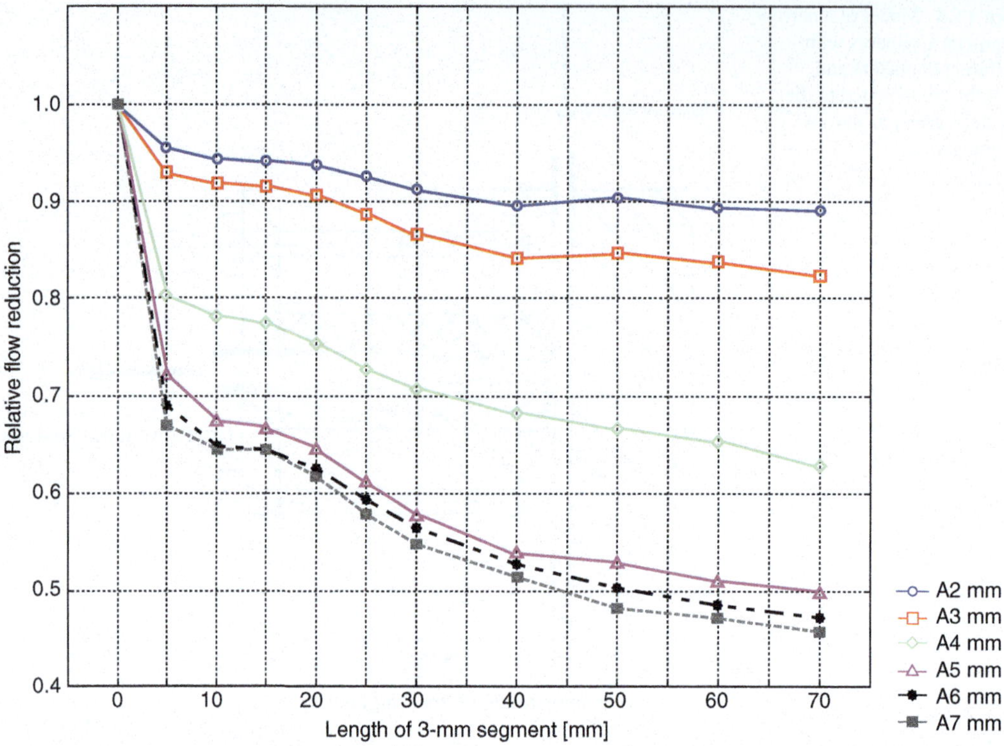

Fig. 11.10 Relative flow reduction by 3 mm diameter narrow segments of different lengths. Parameter: arterial diameter

Surgical Technique

Our technique involves the controlled, long segment narrowing of an AV access near the arterial anastomosis. We perform two variants:

- The narrowing of the AV access close to the anastomosis by a running suture.
- The interposition of a specially designed narrow prosthetic segment.

Technical Hint

If the anastomosis is close to the cubital fossa, there is a definite risk of kinking of the narrow segment when the elbow is flexed. Taking into account individual topographic conditions, preoperative planning includes the decision whether flow reduction is performed:

- In the region of a preexisting anastomosis, or
- After surgical closure of the pre-existing anastomosis further proximal to the cubital fossa with a then newly created anastomosis.

Flow Reduction by a Long Running Suture

From 1982 through February 2009 we performed this technique in around 450 patients who mainly had AV fistulas. Frequently, close to the anastomosis their veins were considerably dilated, and sometimes even to an extreme extent. Also, due to their lengthening, these veins followed meandering circuitous courses. If this morphology was present, surgery followed a six-step procedure.

Exposure

Circumferential exposure of the vein near the anastomosis, of the anastomoses, and of the artery proximal and distal to the anastomosis (Fig. 11.11). Should the exposure of the distal artery prove very cumbersome, it may be abandoned.

Shortening of the Vein

Separation of the vein from the anastomotic orifice for adequate shortening (Fig. 11.12).

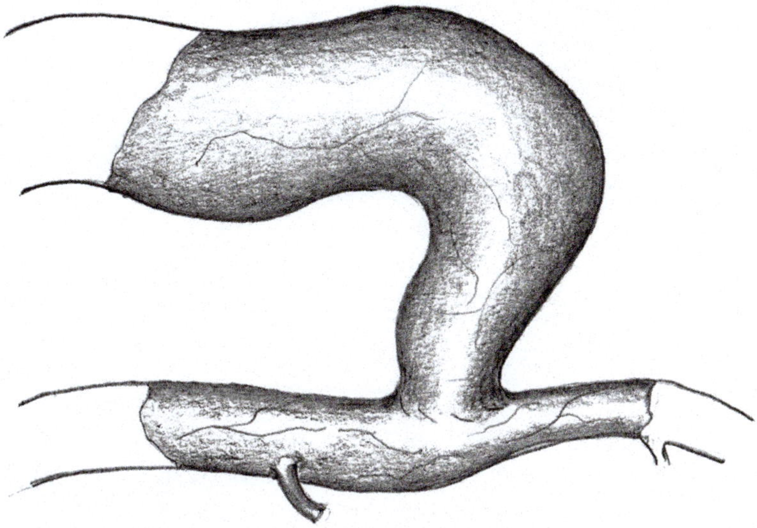

Fig. 11.11 Isolation of the artery and vein near the anastomosis

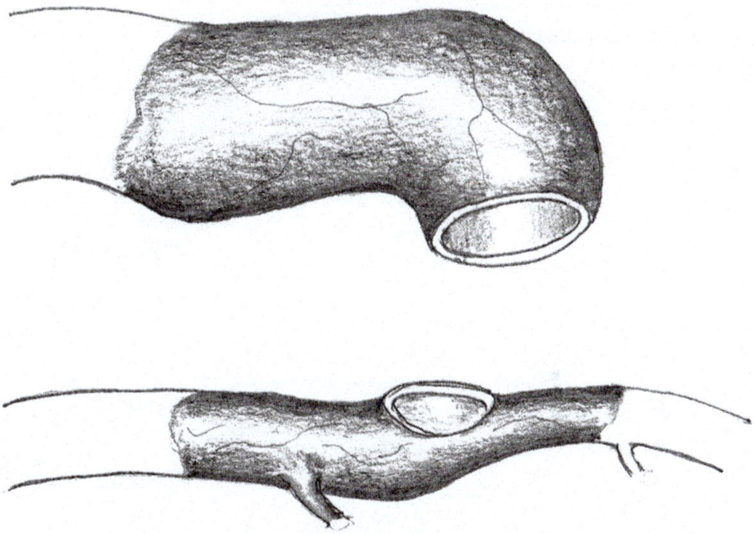

Fig. 11.12 Disconnection of the anastomosis

Plasty of the Vein Stump

The planned running suture for the defined narrowing of the vein may only be performed in a vein whose lumen has already been reduced to 5–6 mm. For this purpose it is necessary to excise a triangular portion of the venous wall over a distance of 3–5 cm (Fig. 11.13) so as to create a funnel-like narrower lumen by a running suture (Fig. 11.14).

Reanastomosis

The anastomotic orifice of the artery is frequently wider than the lumen of the prenarrowed vein. It is also easy to narrow the orifice using a running suture. After an adequate diameter has been created, the next step is to suture the lateroterminal anastomosis (Fig. 11.15).

Controlled Flow Reduction

The plasty of a vein to reduce its diameter to 5–6 mm most often does not lower the flow rate sufficiently by itself. Therefore we continue with a running (6-0) suture of the vascular wall over a 2–3-cm segment under constant monitoring of the blood flow. A stepwise approach with several rows of sutures upon each other yields the desired effect. The intended newly-created stenosis takes on a concave form (Fig. 11.16).

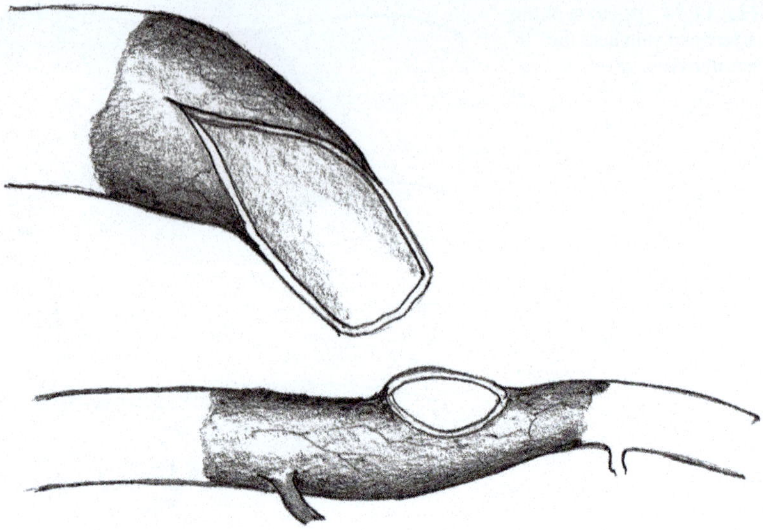

Fig. 11.13 Resection of a triangular wall portion to reduce the lumen

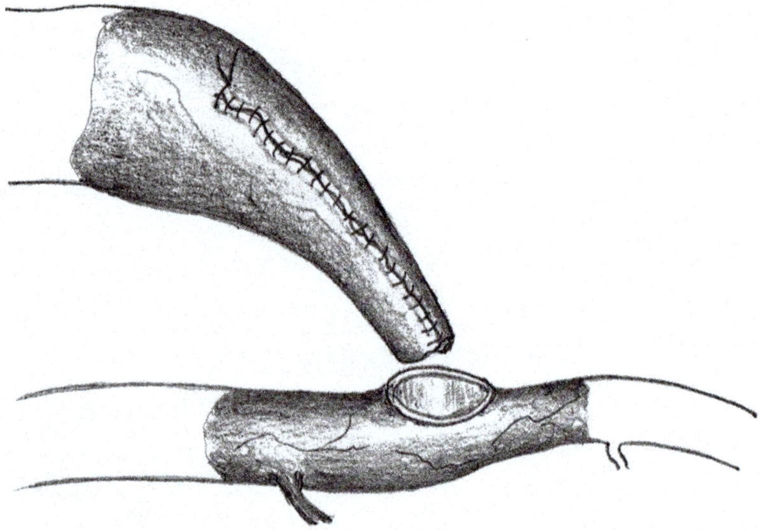

Fig. 11.14 Creation of a new lumen by suturing the wall margins

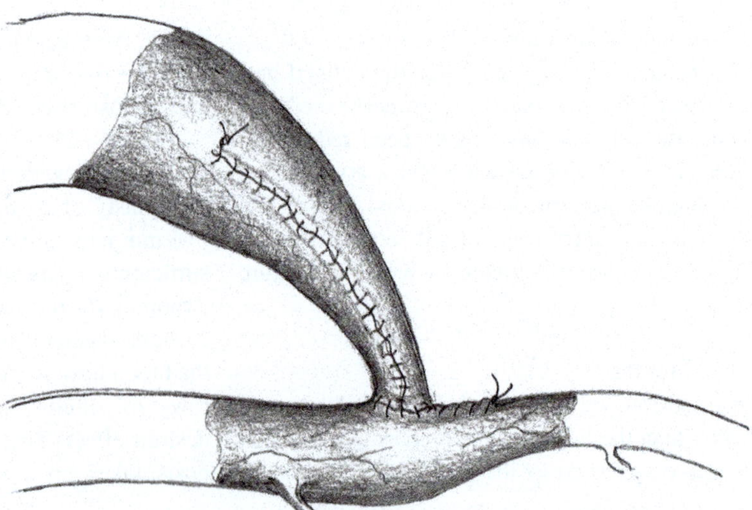

Fig. 11.15 Narrowing of the arteriotomy and reanastomosis with the venous stump

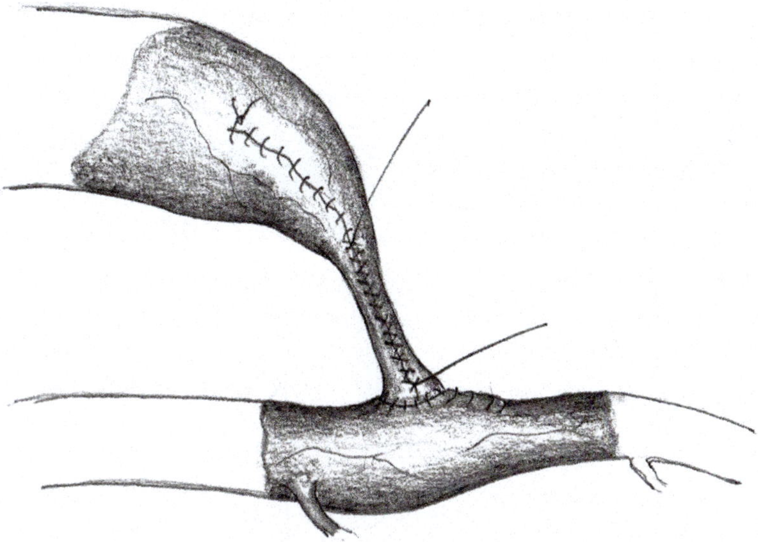

Fig. 11.16 Narrowing of the venous lumen using a running suture while measuring the flow

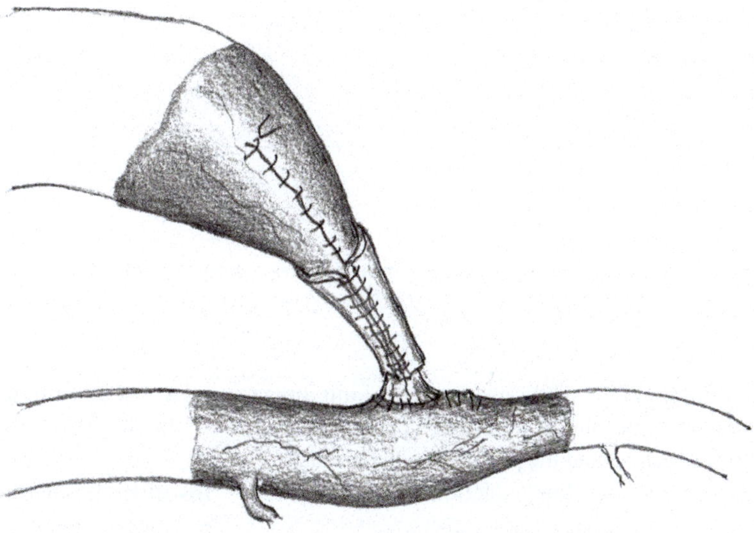

Fig. 11.17 Wrapping the narrow segment with an alloplastic cuff

When fine-tuning the flow rate, you should also watch the current arterial blood pressure so as to make adjustments for anesthesia-related differences from normal readings in each individual patient.

We measure the intraoperative flow by the sonographic transit-time method only. For best results use both the proximal and distal artery. Thus you can determine the flow rate in the AV access when taking into account the flow direction in the distal artery. According to our experience, the direct sonographic examination of the AV access is error-prone.

Wrapping of the Narrowed Segment

The vascular wall of the narrowed segment consists of a formerly (possibly extremely) dilated vein. We have seen secondary dilatations with subsequent increases in blood flow. To avoid this dilatation we wrap an ePTFE or polyurethane cuff around the narrowed segment and secure it with a running suture (Fig. 11.17). If this suture is too loose, dilation will occur anyway. If it is too tight, an additional unwanted flow reduction will arise. Therefore another control is necessary to verify the desired result. If the surgical field is in the cubital fossa, flow should also be checked during elbow flexion.

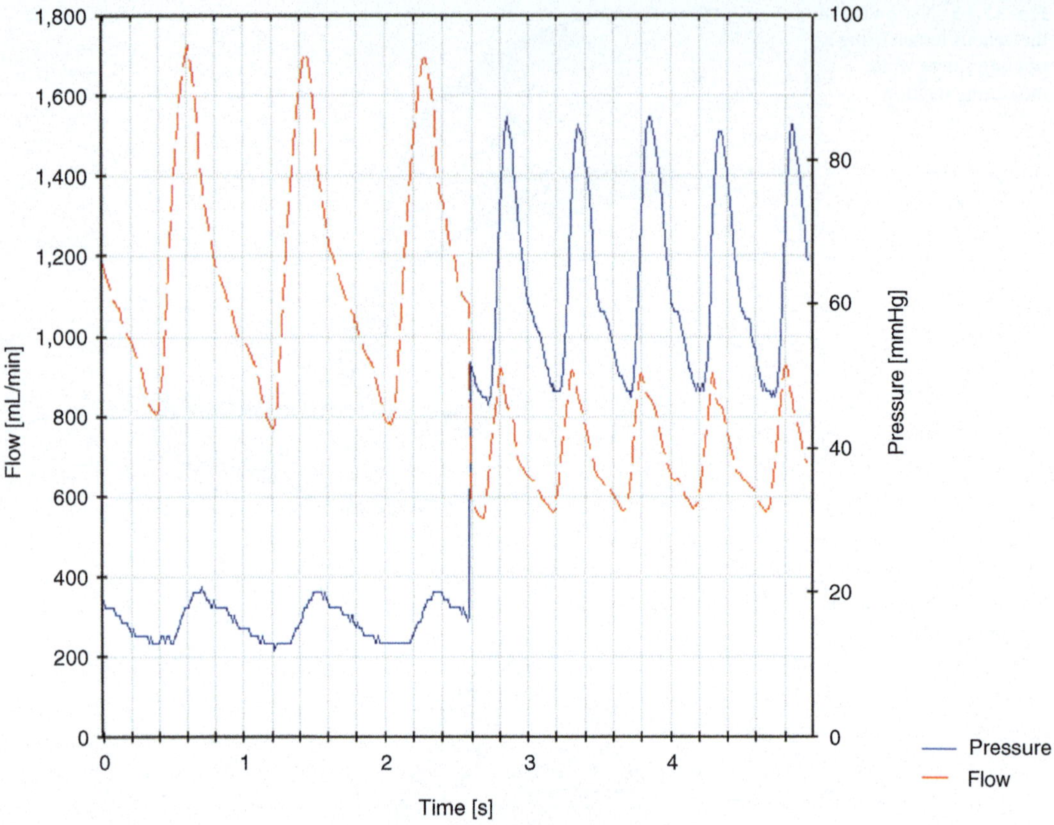

Fig. 11.18 Examples for pressure and flow curves before and after flow reductions. The mean pressure in the anastomosis rises from 16 to 63 mmHg. The mean flow drops from 1,170 to 700 mL/min

Figure 11.18 shows an example of intraoperative flow rates in the arterialized cephalic vein of the upper arm and the pressure in the distal artery before and after flow reduction.

Clinical Results

In 453 flow reductions (February 1981 through February 2009) we observed the results and complications detailed below within the first 12 months (no consistent follow up after the second postoperative week).

Thrombosis

- About 5 % early thrombosis
- About 10 % late thrombosis

Flow evolution

- About 10 % progressive decrease in flow (without late thrombosis)
- About 35 % significant increase in flow within the first year

Insufficient peripheral perfusion

- Normalization or significant improvement in 94.3 % (427 patients) directly after surgery.
- No significant improvement or again worsening symptoms within the first year in about 30 %. These patients either underwent another flow reduction or proximalization of the arterial inflow.

Critical evaluation

The *pros* of this method are:

- The exact intraoperative adjustment of the desired flow rate
- The high primary success rate

The *cons* of this method are:

- The time-consuming procedure.

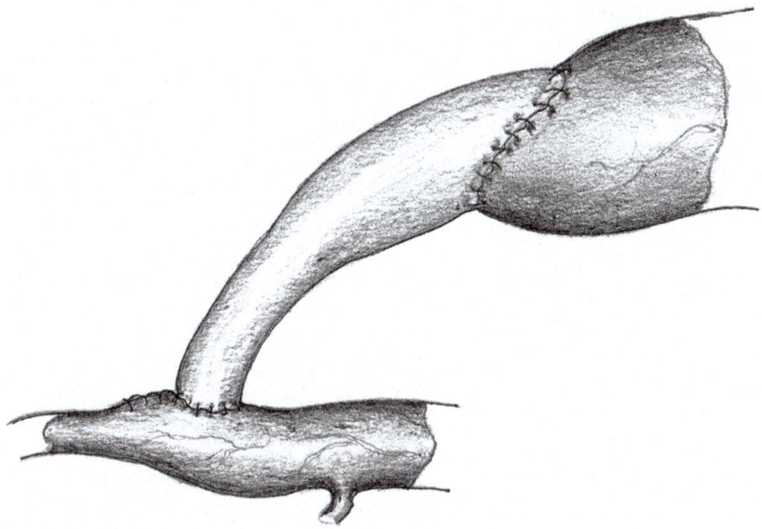

Fig. 11.19 Lateroterminal interposition of a conical graft segment between artery and vein

- The technical (flow measurement) and, to a lesser degree, material (cuff) effort.
- The possible future loss of the intended improvement by the narrowed segment either due to its dilation with an increased flow or due to its progressive stenosis caused by tissue proliferation with flow reduction possibly leading to thrombosis.

Flow Reduction Using a Narrow Graft Segment

We introduced the interposition of a narrow graft segment for flow reduction in March 2009. For this purpose we use the tapered segment of a 4–7-mm ePTFE graft. After its implantation, the 4-mm segment will be narrowed even further as necessary.

Approach/Technical Hints

We proceed as follows:

(a) Exposure

(b) Shortening of the vein
Separation of the vein from the anastomotic orifice and resection, so that a distance of 3–4 cm remains between the vein stump and the former anastomotic orifice.

(c) Interposition of the tapered graft segment
After the anastomotic orifice has been narrowed, a lateroterminal anastomosis between the 4-mm graft segment (at least 2-cm) and the artery is created. Then the 7-mm graft segment is sutured to the vein to form a terminoterminal anastomosis with the 7-mm end. Even large differences in diameter of vein and graft can be overcome by a beveled graft end (Fig. 11.19).

(d) Narrowing of the graft lumen
Longitudinal excision of a spindle-shaped (about 15-mm) wall segment from the 4-mm end of the graft (Fig. 11.20) and closure of the defect with a running suture (Fig. 11.21).

(e) Flow control and correction if necessary
After declamping, the flow in the proximal and distal artery is measured. Direct sonographic evaluation of the ePTFE graft may be impeded for a few days by gas inclusions in the graft wall. If the resulting flow reduction proves insufficient, further narrowing by additional running sutures is indicated.

Clinical Results

Since March 2009, narrow graft segments have been implanted in 41 patients for flow reduction (3 forearm cephalic fistulas, 6 superficialized basilic veins, and 32 cephalic fistulas in the cubital fossa and distal upper arm). During the first 8 weeks there was thrombosis in two cases when flow had been reduced too much (250–380 mL/min with venous diameter of up to 3.5 cm). During follow up (2–25 months) there was another thrombosis caused by a stenosis of the

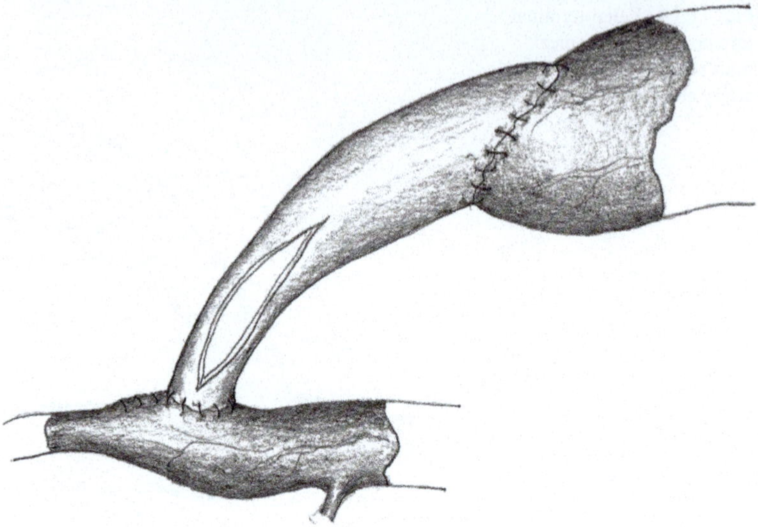

Fig. 11.20 Excision of an elliptic wall portion out of the narrow segment of the graft

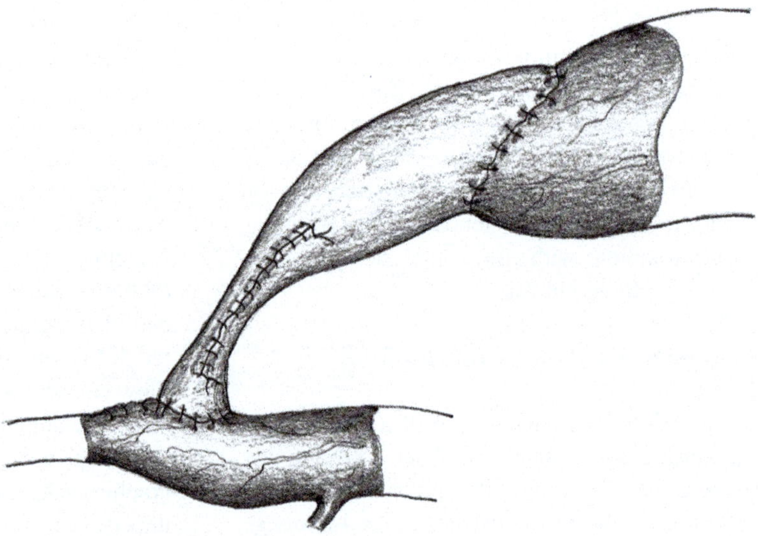

Fig. 11.21 Luminal narrowing by closure of the longitudinal graft defect with running suture

anastomosis to the vein. Color duplex sonography showed a constant flow in the other patients.

Evaluation

In our view, the advantages of this method are the low thrombosis rate and the stable results. The disadvantages include the necessary effort (exposure of the artery, flow measurements) and the difficulty to determine correctly the required extent of the intended stenosis.

Perspective

It would be desirable to have prefabricated graft segments with defined stenoses in stock. They should:

- Be short (3–4 cm) so as not to take up too much space that could otherwise be used for puncture.
- Have a wide lumen apart from the intended stenotic portion for creating an anastomosis with the vein.
- Have a hemodynamically optimized form.
- Be available in different standardized sizes.

If venous outflow of the AV access is uninhibited (no stenosis of the venous outflow) and the diameter of the feeding artery is known, a suitable graft with the right dimensions could also be selected preoperatively to achieve the desired effect. The relative flow reduction is independent of the arterial pressure if you neglect resistance changes of the distal artery.

We tested and optimized different designs and specifications of such narrow graft segments in our pulsatile flow system. Criteria for the best-suited stenosis of a prefabricated graft segment are only:

- The diameter of the feeding artery
- The flow in the AV access
- The desired proportional flow reduction

Diameter and flow volume can easily be determined preoperatively by duplex sonography. During surgery only a segment of the AV access of an adequate size is resected near the anastomosis, and the previously selected graft segment (with the correct predetermined stenosis) is implanted in its place.

Standardized graft segments for flow reductions offer the following advantages:

- Smaller operative field (no circumferential exposure of the proximal and distal artery, no flow measurements necessary).
- Less operative time and effort needed.

These prefabricated stenosed graft segments mentioned above are being developed.

11.2.2 Proximalization of the Arterial Inflow

If a shunt flow rate is so low that a further reduction is not possible, proximalization is indicated.

Basically there are two options for proximalization (Fig. 11.22) – the proximalization of the arterial feeding of:

- The AV access using a graft that takes off from an artery proximal to the previous anastomosis (PAI – proximalization of arterial inflow).
- The distal arterial stump using a graft that takes off from an artery proximal to the previous anastomosis (DRIL – distal revascularization and interval ligation).

Since 1984 we have exclusively used PAI if indicated (Scholz et al. 1988).

Proximalization of the Arterial Inflow (PAI)

The technique involves:

- Closure of the AV anastomosis.
- Separation of the puncturable vessel.
- Arterialization of the puncturable vessel via a graft that takes off from an artery which is more proximal.

Physiology

The principle of proximalization is based on:

- The closure of the AV anastomosis while maintaining the normal continuity of the artery.
- Feeding the AV access via a graft which is also anastomosed to a more proximal artery. In this proximal position, due to the larger arterial diameter and the shorter distance to the aorta, the arterial resistance is lower than in more peripheral arteries. Therefore the pressure drop in the distal artery of a proximal AV anastomosis is significantly less pronounced than with a distal AV anastomosis. Despite its branching, the design of the arterial tree of the arm lets the pressure remain constant almost up to the deep palmar arch. The mean diameters of the upper extremity arteries are listed in Table 11.1.

This data is based on the analysis of 17 (11 males, 6 females) upper extremity arteriographies at our institution. It corresponds to our intraoperative findings. For better visualization we depict the exemplary arteriography (from the aorta to the palmar arch) of a 58-year-old male without any obvious vascular pathology. We noted the lengths of equal-diameter segments with 1-mm steps (measuring inaccuracy less than 10 %) (Fig. 11.23a).

Flow resistance was determined according to the Hagen–Poiseuille equation:

$$R = \frac{8l\eta}{\pi r^4}$$

where η stands for viscosity, l for the length, and r for the radius of the vessel. Here we assumed that blood viscosity was 3.6 mPa × s. The unit for the resistance is PRU (peripheral resistance unit):

$$1\ \text{PRU} = 1\ \frac{\text{mmHg}}{\text{mL / min}}$$

For typical locations of AV anastomoses we calculated the inflow resistance by adding the upstream resistances (Table 11.2).

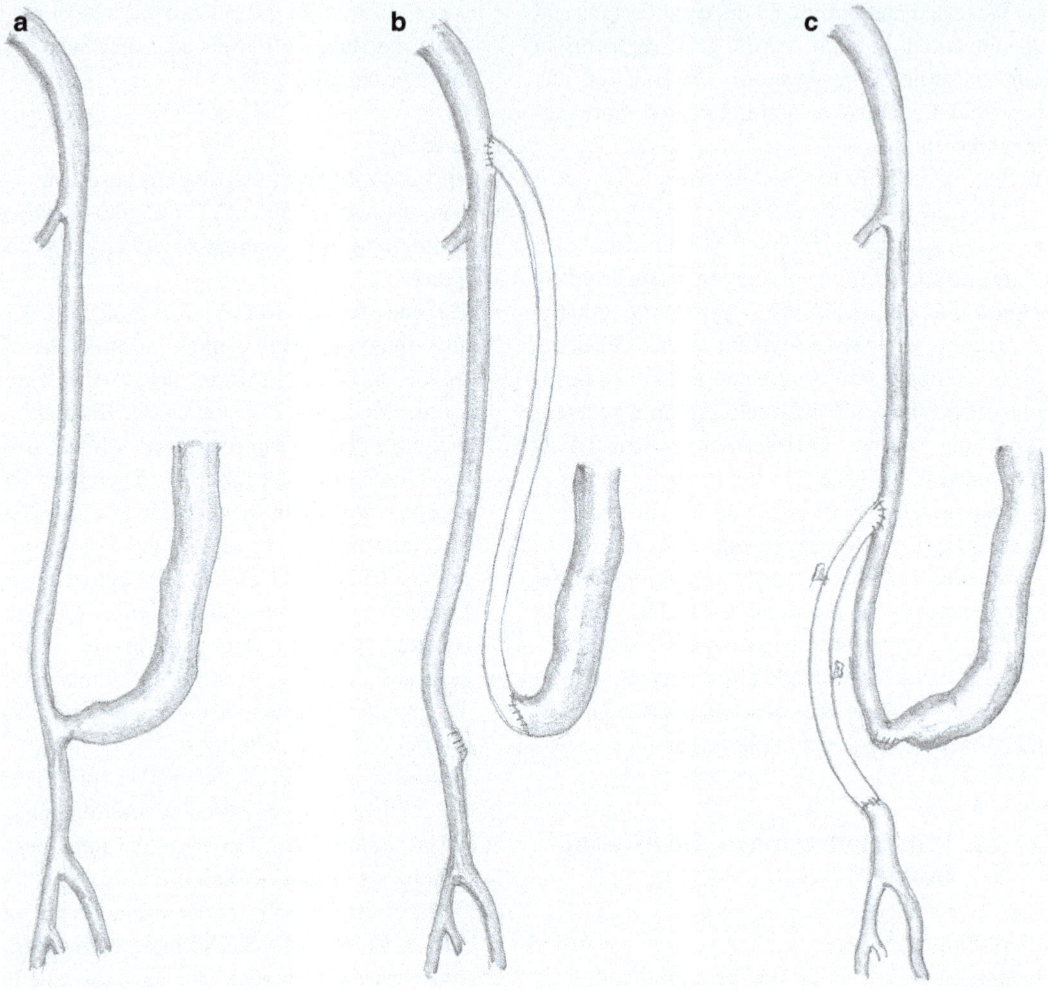

Fig. 11.22 Proximalization of an AV fistula. (**a**) AV fistula of the cephalic vein in the cubital fossa. (**b**) Proximalization of the arterial inflow via a graft originating from the axillary brachial artery. (**c**) Proximalization of the inflow to the distal arterial stump via a graft anastomosed to the brachial artery proximal to the cubital fossa

Table 11.1 Mean arterial diameters

Artery (region)	Diameter (mm)
Axillary (infraclavicular)	7
Brachial (axillary)	5
Brachial (cubital)	4
Radial/ulnar	2.5

The arterial inflow resistance of arteries increases from proximal to distal regions (Fig. 11.23b). The proximalization effect is based on this fact (see above). The true resistances in vivo differ from those shown above. Factors that have not been taken into account include:

- The presence of collaterals.
- The fact that the Hagen–Poiseuille equation is valid for Newtonian fluids and non-pulsatile flow only.

In vivo you would expect a significant increase of resistance proportionally to the flow, which is caused by the inertia of the blood column when it is accelerated during early systole (cf. Chap. 20).

Investigations on the Proximalization of the Arterial Inflow of the AV Access (PAI)

The influence of the location of the arterial anastomosis on distal perfusion was investigated in a silicone model of the arm (Figs. 11.24 and 11.25).

a

Segment	*D* (mm)	*L* (mm)	Σ*R* (mPRU)
1	10	35	0.06
2	9	35	0.16
3	8	20	0.25
4	7	40	0.55
5	6	10	0.70
6	5	45	2.02
7	4	150	12.77
8	2.5	290	68.34
9	2.5	200	

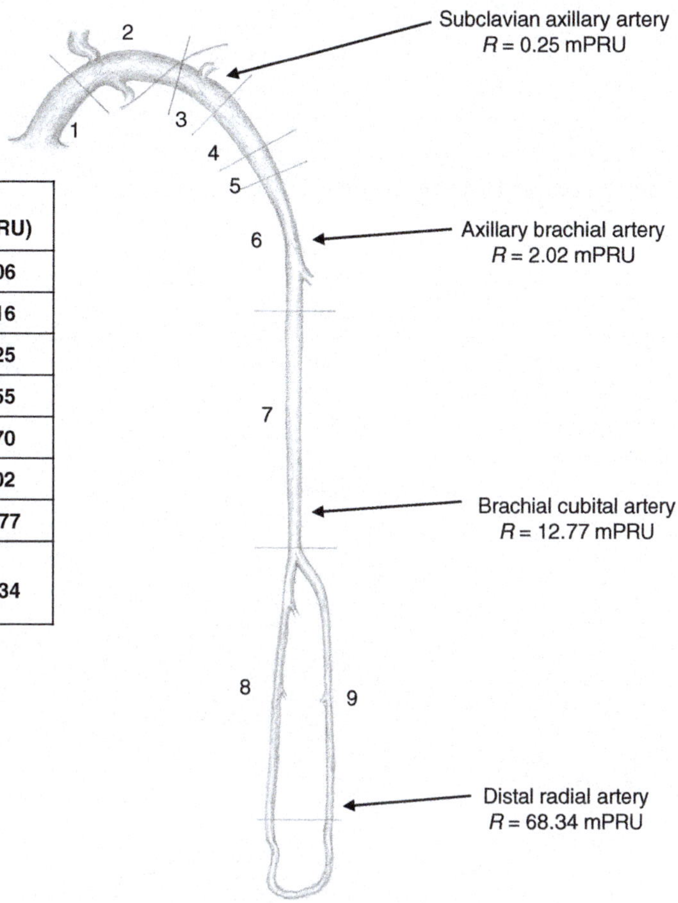

b

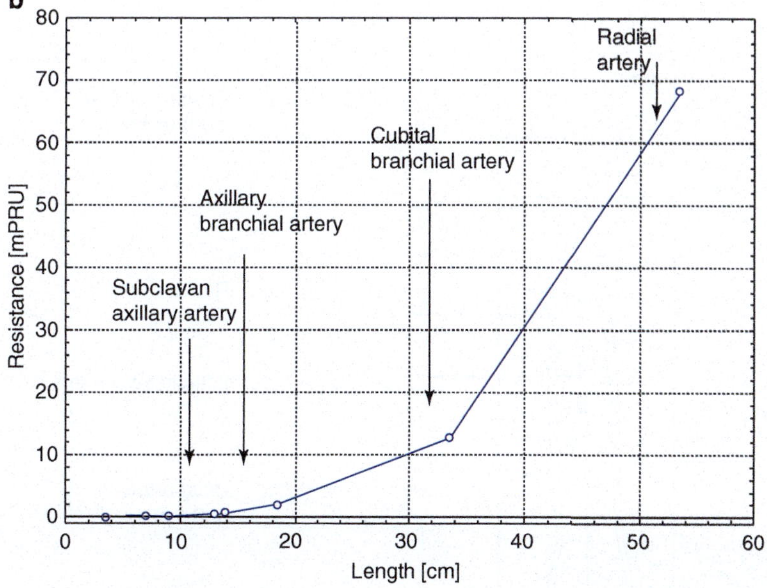

Fig. 11.23 (**a**) Imaging study of the arm arteries of a 58-year-old male with healthy vessels. The arteries were divided in segments of the same diameter with luminal differences (9) of 1 or 2.5 mm for the forearm (cf. table). (**b**) Increase of the inflow resistance of the arterial segments from the aorta to the radial artery

The model has several connectors. Three connectors are meant to simulate the venous drainage in the upper arm (V1), forearm (V2), and hand (V3). The outflow was set to 75 mL/min in the upper arm, 50 mL/min in the forearm, and 20 mL/min in the hand (based on intraoperative findings). A 7-mm pipe simulated the AV shunt that had five different connectors in the forearm and upper arm (A1–A5).

Positions

- A1: infraclavicular axillary artery
- A2: axillary brachial artery

Table 11.2 Inflow resistance at typical AV anastomosis sites

Location of the AV anastomosis, artery (region)	Inflow resistance (mPRU)	Relative increase of resistance as compared to infraclavicular position	Relative increase of resistance as compared to next proximal region
Axillary (infraclavicular)	0.25		
Brachial (axillary)	2.02	8.1	8.1
Brachial(cubital)	12.77	51	6.3
Radial (distal)	68.34	273	5.3

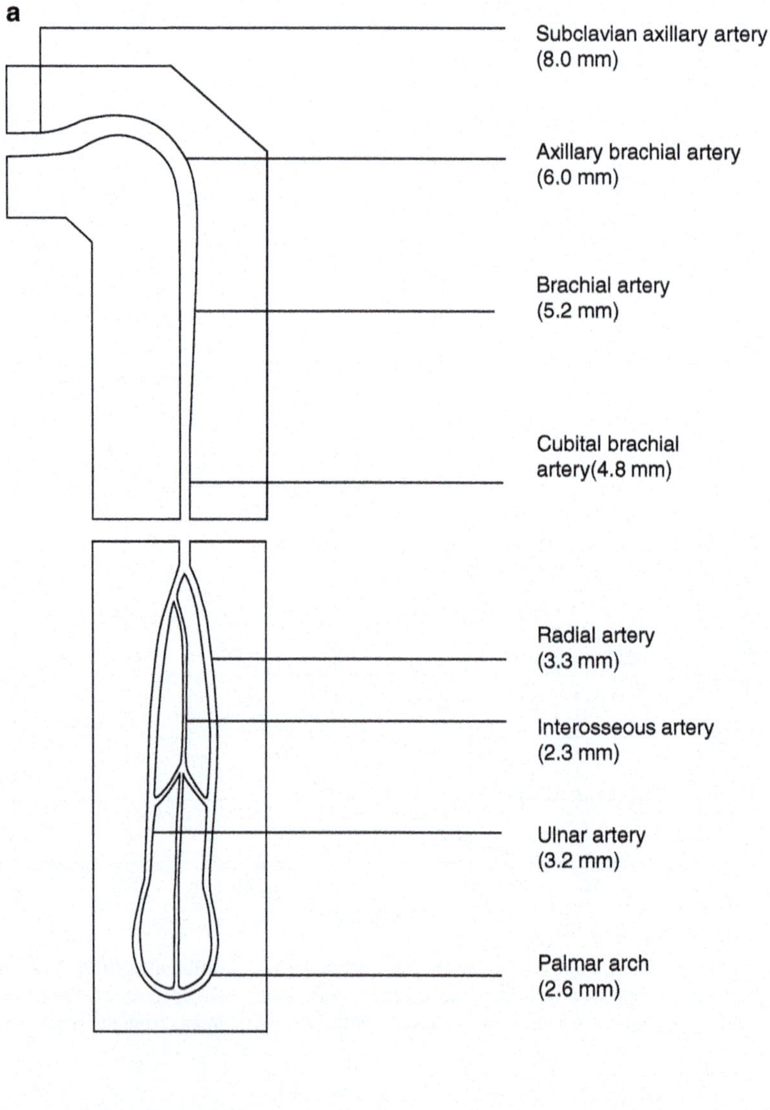

Fig. 11.24 (**a**) Sketch of the arm artery model. (**b**) Model of the arm arteries with options for connecting AV anastomoses, *K* collaterals, *P* measuring arterial pressure and *Y* flow volume, *S* simulation of stenoses, *V* venous outflow

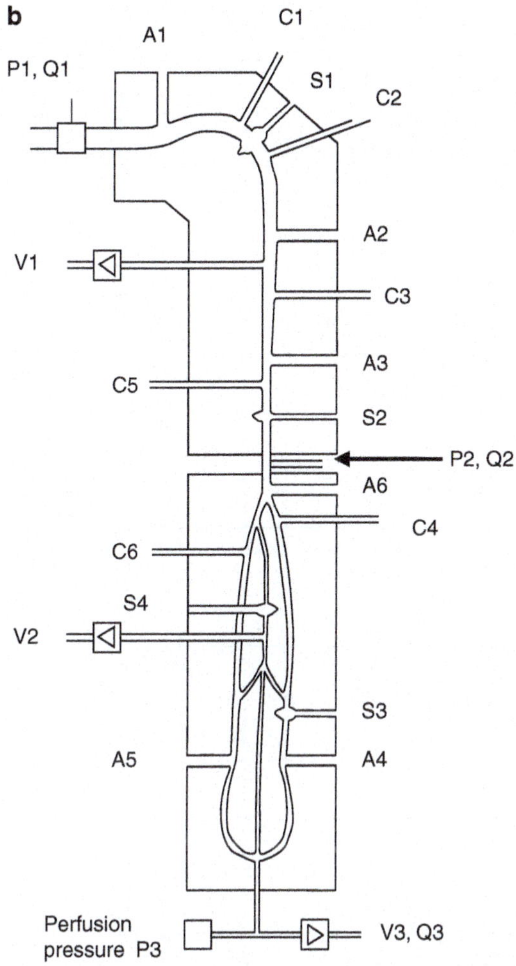

Fig. 11.24 (continued)

- A3: cubital brachial artery
- A4: radial artery
- A5: ulnar artery

Extra connectors were added to the model for collaterals (K1 to K6). The investigations were carried out at different shunt flow rates (300–900 mL/min) and three distinct arterial pressures (80, 100, and 120 mmHg). Flow rates could be reproducibly regulated by a variable outflow resistance (Zanow et al. 2008; Reddemann 2010).

The results are summarized in Figs. 11.26, 11.27, and 11.28. An increased pressure in the model palmar arch corresponds to a successful treatment in a real patient. Figure 11.26 shows the changes of pressure depending on the location and shunt flow rates from 300 to 900 mL/min at 80 mmHg, Fig. 11.27 at 100 mmHg, and Fig. 11.28 at 120 mmHg.

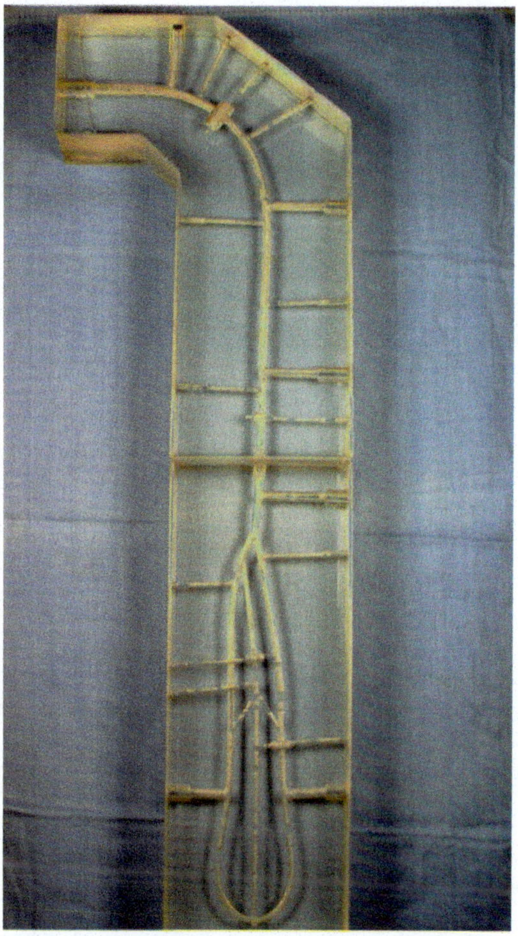

Fig. 11.25 Model of the arm arteries

As the data was collected in a model, there are no biological regulatory mechanisms. The lack of compliance of the vascular walls, the Newtonian property of the fluid, and the high internal resistance of the model cause systematic errors. A direct transfer of these results to patients is only permissible to a limited extent, but they are valuable approximations of clinical observations.

> At the same systemic arterial pressure and the same shunt flow, the peripheral perfusion pressure increases the more proximal the arterious anastomosis is situated.

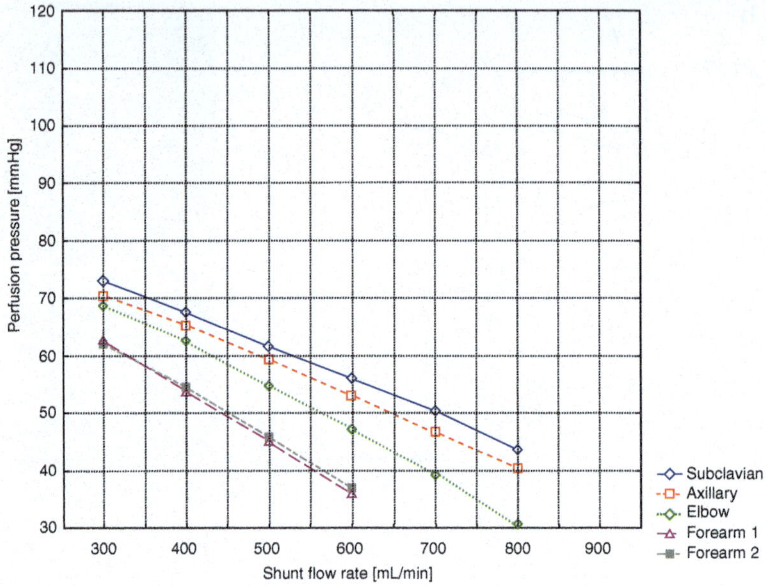

Fig. 11.26 Change of perfusion pressure dependent on site and flow at 80 mmHg

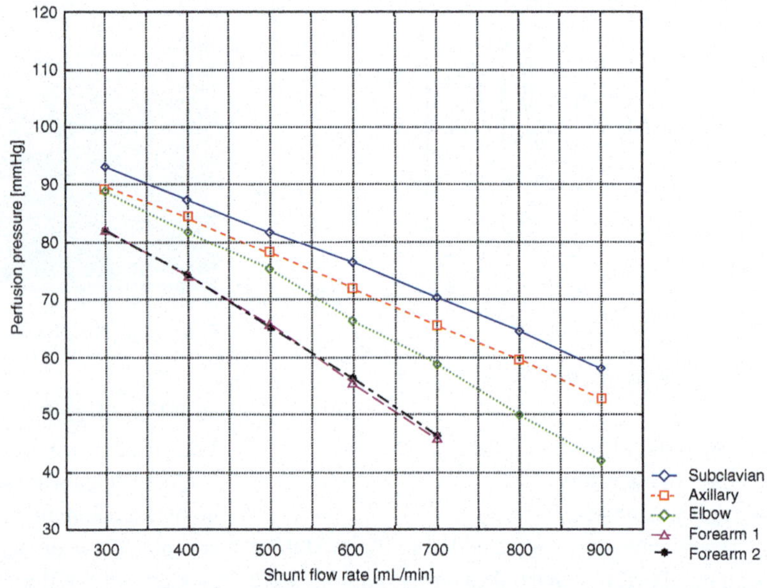

Fig. 11.27 Change of perfusion pressure dependent on site and flow at 100 mmHg

A change of the systemic arterial pressure (80, 100, 120 mmHg, see above) achieves corresponding changes of the peripheral pressure. Yet the influence of the location of the arterial anastomosis is still preserved.

Comparison of the Proximalization of Arterial Inflow of an AV Access (PAI) to That of the Distal Stump of the Artery (DRIL)

For the experiments comparing both techniques (PAI and DRIL) for the treatment of insufficient peripheral perfusion in a simulated elbow fistula (EBF), the model had to be changed (Figs. 11.29, 11.30, and 11.31).

The model setup mentioned above did not lead to a significant increase of the peripheral pressure with the DRIL method.

A changed setup taking this difficulty into account is shown in Fig. 11.30. The DRIL procedure is characterized by the ligation of the artery distal to the AV anastomosis. Bypassing of this occluded vessel with a 6-mm pipe (25 cm length, green in Fig. 11.30) did not noticeably change the

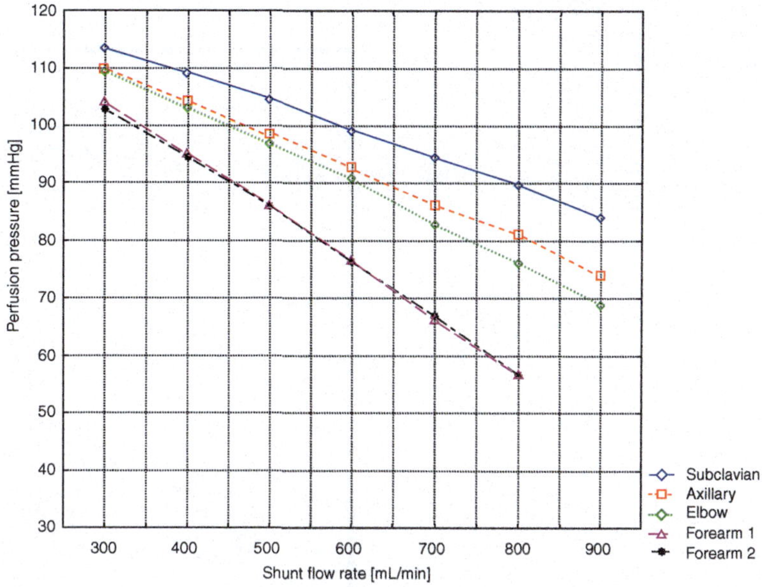

Fig. 11.28 Change of perfusion pressure dependent on site and flow at 120 mmHg

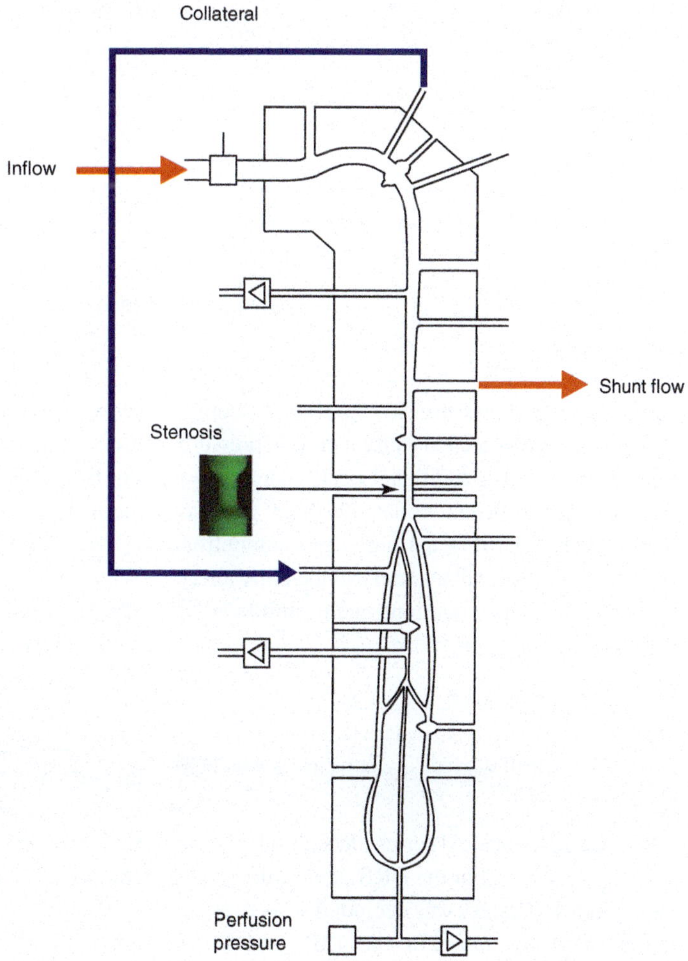

Fig. 11.29 Modified set up for the simulation of an elbow fistula

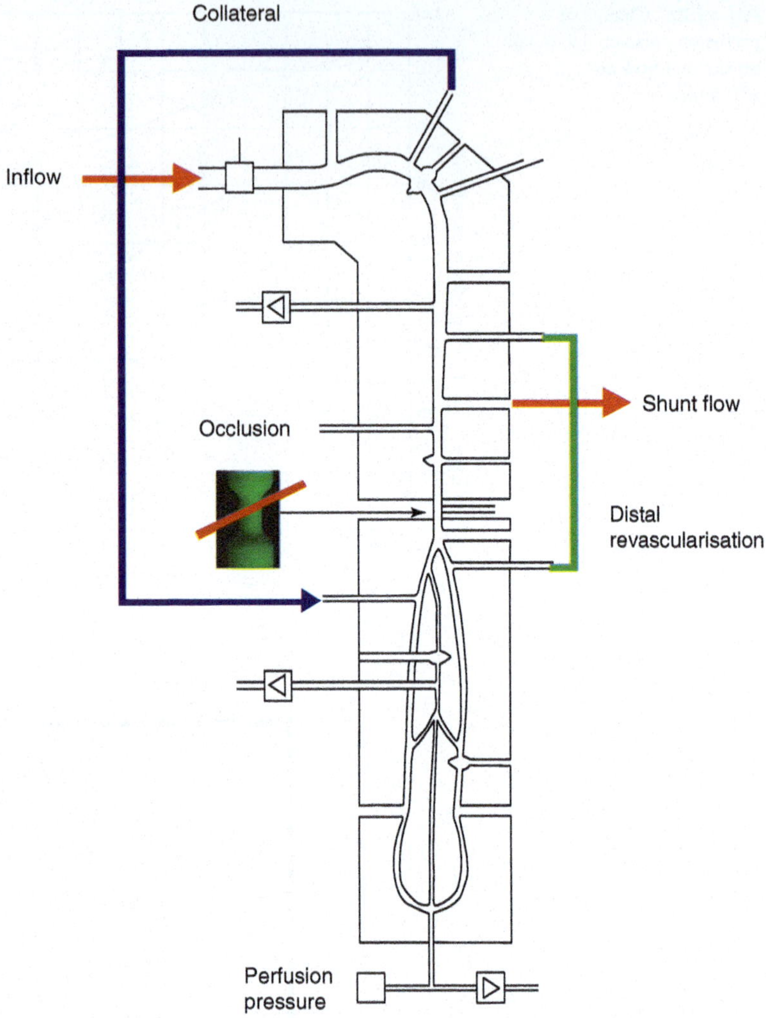

Fig. 11.30 Modified set up for the simulation of the DRIL method

peripheral arterial pressure. To gain results, a cubital stenosis was introduced to cause a drop in pressure. We also simulated an additional steal syndrome. For this purpose sufficient collaterals were needed. They were simulated by a 4-mm pipe running from the infraclavicular axillary artery to the ulnar artery.

Three different situations were simulated in the model:

1.	EBF	Elbow fistula, Fig. 11.29
2.	DRIL	DRIL procedure, Fig. 11.30
3.	PAI	Proximalization of arterial inflow, Fig. 11.31

For the EBF and PAI series, the cubital stenosis was kept constant. For the DRIL series, the model cubital brachial artery was occluded so as to simulate interval ligation. For the EBF and DRIL series, the shunt was connected to the elbow (position 3, red arrow (Q4) in Figs. 11.29 and 11.30). For the PAI series, the shunt was connected to the model axillary artery (position 1, Fig. 11.31).

Mean arterial feeding pressure was 100 mmHg. With open collaterals and a stenosed brachial artery, the initial perfusion pressure was 88 mmHg, when the shunt was closed in position 3 (elbow). This was the reference value to indicate relative changes of the perfusion pressure. The ligation of collateral had hardly any influence on the distal perfusion pressure (relative perfusion pressure 0.99), whereas the occlusion of the brachial artery with open collaterals reduced the perfusion pressure by 20 % (relative perfusion pressure 0.80).

The relative change of the perfusion pressure depending on shunt flow is shown in Fig. 11.32.

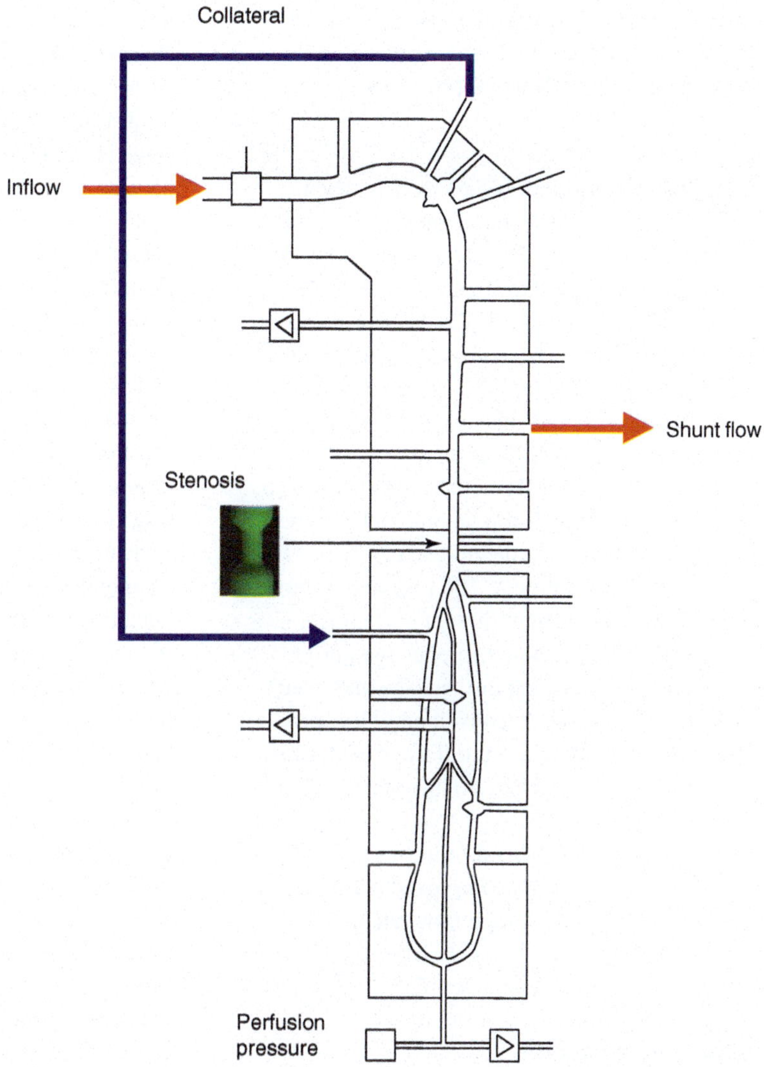

Fig. 11.31 Modified set up for the simulation of the PAI method

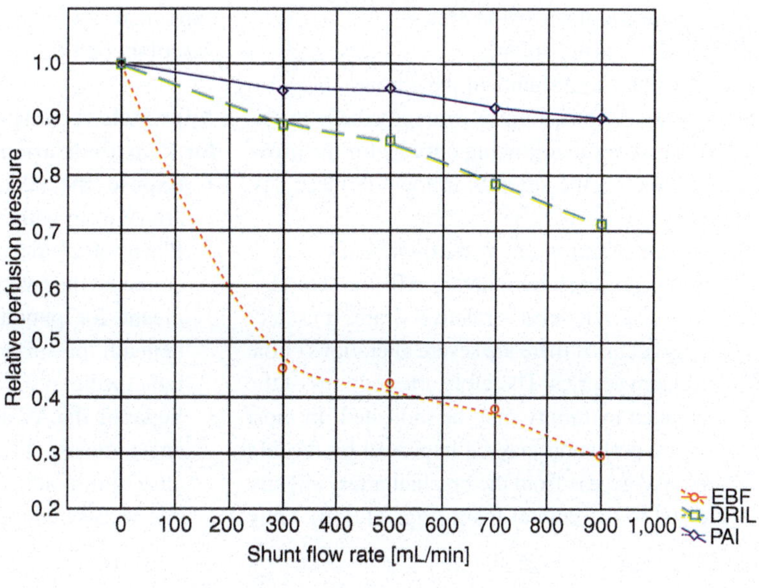

Fig. 11.32 Relative change of perfusion pressure dependent on shunt flow. The perfusion pressure we measured was related to the baseline pressure with a closed shunt (zero shunt flow)

Results of the Comparison Between PAI and DRIL for the Treatment of Insufficient Peripheral Perfusion

1. If the fistula/shunt of the model is attached to the elbow position, peripheral pressure decreases to 45 % with a shunt flow of 300 mL/min and to 30 % with a shunt flow of 900 mL/min as opposed to a closed fistula/shunt. The retrograde flow in the brachial artery increases with an increasing flow rate (–8 mL/min at 500 mL/min; –65 mL/min at 900 mL/min).
2. DRIL: The DRIL method improves the peripheral pressure significantly. The relative pressure decreases to only 91 % with a shunt flow of 300 mL/min and to 71 % with a shunt flow of 900 mL/min.
3. PAI: This method improves the peripheral pressure even further. The influence of the flow rate is considerably less pronounced. With a shunt flow of 300 mL/min, the relative perfusion pressure reached 95 %, and 90 % even with a flow rate of 900 mL/min. This means that PAI leads to an improved peripheral perfusion also at high flow rates.

Clinical Application

Variants of AV accesses that can typically show inadequate distal perfusion are:

- Distal forearm fistulas
- AV fistulas and shunts in the elbow
- Axillary AV anastomoses with prosthetic grafts

This leaves the following options for the proximalization of the arterial inflow of these AV accesses:

(a) *Proximalization of a forearm fistula*
The insufficient peripheral perfusion with distal forearm fistulas is relatively rare. It usually only occurs if there are severe alterations of the forearm arteries. Therefore arteriograms of the affected extremity may be indicated. In most cases, perfusion may be improved by feeding the AV access from the brachial artery slightly distal to the cubital fossa (Fig. 11.33b). Only under exceptional circumstances with severe changes of the upper arm brachial artery may it be necessary to feed the AV fistula from the infraaxillary brachial artery (second level) (Fig. 11.33c). Intraoperative measurements in patients showed an increase of 15–30 mmHg in the radial artery after proximalization to the cubital brachial artery, and of 30–50 mmHg to the infraaxillary brachial artery.

(b) *Proximalization of an elbow AV access*
Most peripheral perfusion disorders occur after both AV access creations in this position. This is true for AV fistulas as well as for AV shunts. The majority of patients benefit from proximalization to the infraaxillary brachial artery (Fig. 11.34b). If improvement is not sufficient – and in particular if the contralateral side shows signs of inadequate peripheral perfusion already without prior AV access surgery – we feed the AV access from the infraclavicular axillary artery (second level) (Fig. 11.34c). At the level of the then ligated old anastomosis, intraoperative measurements in patients showed increases of 15–30 mmHg after proximalization to the infraaxillary brachial artery and of 25–30 mmHg to the infraclavicular axillary artery.

(c) *Proximalization of an infraaxillary AV graft*
It is possible to feed the access from the infraclavicular axillary artery (Fig. 11.35b). Intraoperative measurements showed that pressure increased by 20–40 mmHg.

Figure 11.36 shows the expected pressure increase after proximalization. The wide range is explained by interindividually inhomogeneous vascular conditions.

Approach/Technical Hints for Proximalization

- Expose the AV anastomosis and proximal artery from which to feed the AV access.
- Place a graft in a new subcutaneous tunnel that connects the two incisions. As this graft is not meant for puncturing, it should run deeper beneath the surface so as to avoid inadvertent puncturing.
- Separate the AV access form its former arterial anastomosis, close the arterial defect, and create a terminoterminal anastomosis between the AV access and the newly-placed prosthesis.

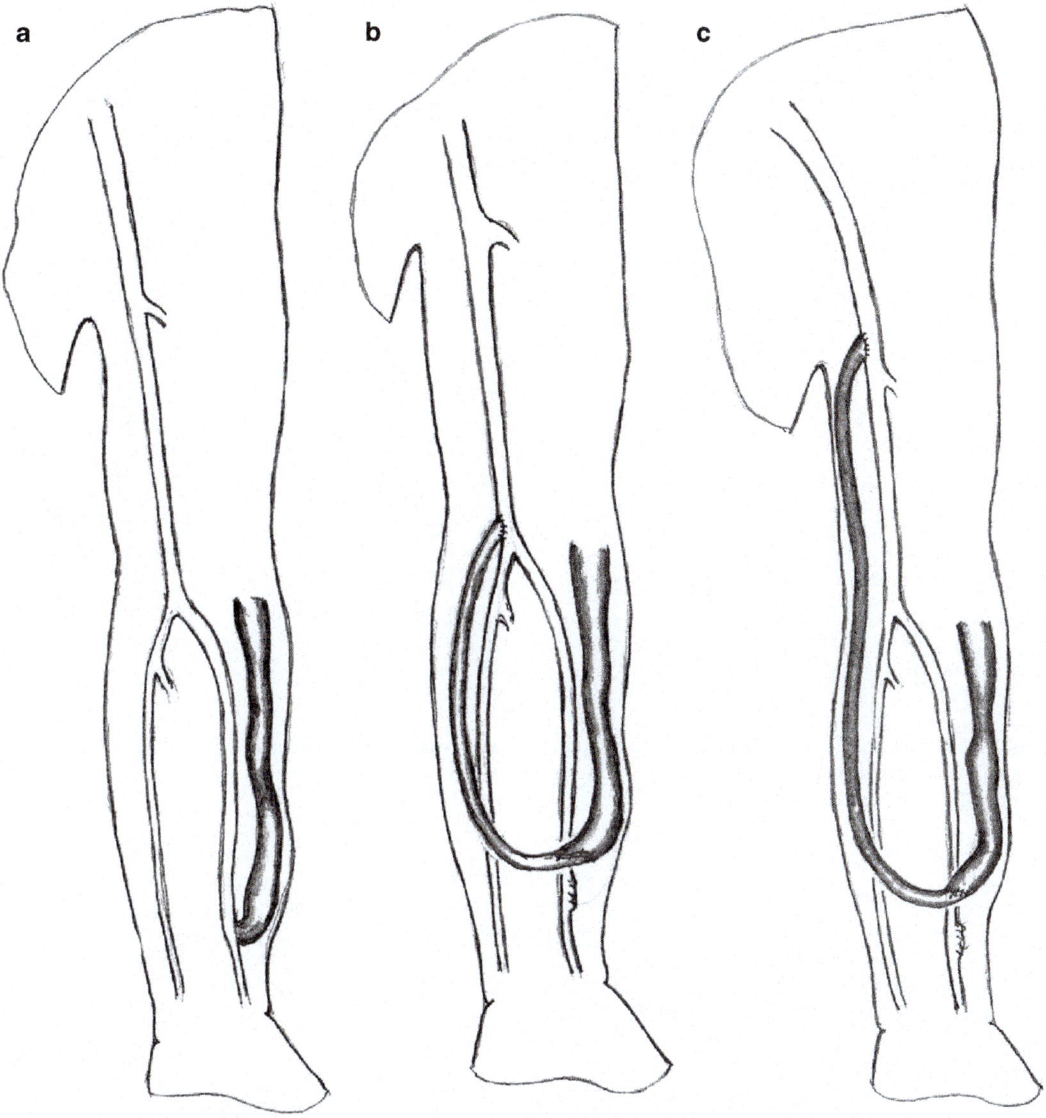

Fig. 11.33 (**a**) Cephalic forearm fistula before proximalization of the arterial inflow. (**b**) Feeding the vein via a graft originating from the brachial artery distal to the cubital fossa. (**c**) Feeding the vein via a graft originating from the infraaxillary brachial artery (second level)

- Create the lateroterminal anastomosis of the proximal artery to the graft.

From 1983 to 1991 we used preserved allogeneic veins and preserved allogeneic bovine sacral arteries (Scholz et al. 1988). Since 1991we have been using ePTFE grafts with 4 or 5 mm diameters, the latter mostly for the proximalization of the axillary artery.

Clinical Results

We performed proximalizations of the arterial inflow of AV accesses in more than 100 patients. There was only one patient with an elbow fistula fed from the axillary artery, in whom we had to ligate the AV access because of severe alterations of the arm arteries. This patient received an arterioarterial graft. With almost all other patients, the proximalization to the next proximal level could relieve their symptoms. Just in a few cases the second next level had to be tapped. Figure 11.37 shows the pressure curves of a brachial artery in the elbow before and after proximalization of an elbow fistula to the infraaxillary brachial artery.

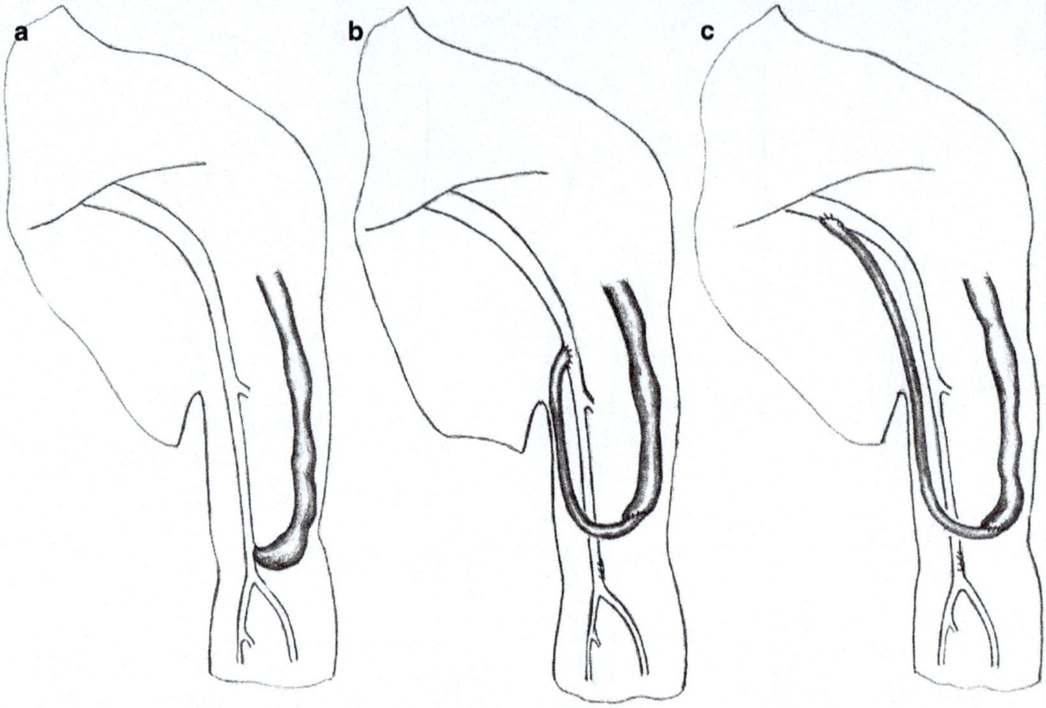

Fig. 11.34 (**a**) Cephalic elbow fistula before proximalization of the arterial inflow. (**b**) Feeding the vein via a graft originating from the brachial artery. (**c**) Feeding the vein via a graft originating from the infraclavicular axillary artery (second level)

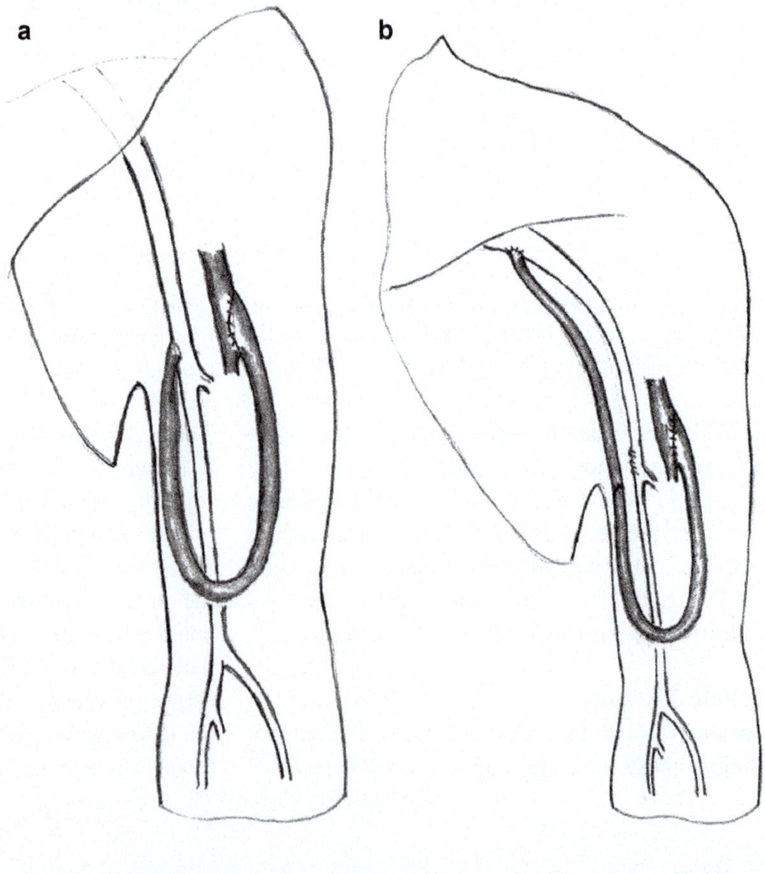

Fig. 11.35 (**a**) Infraaxillary AV loop. (**b**) Feeding the AV loop via a graft originating from the infraclavicular axillary artery

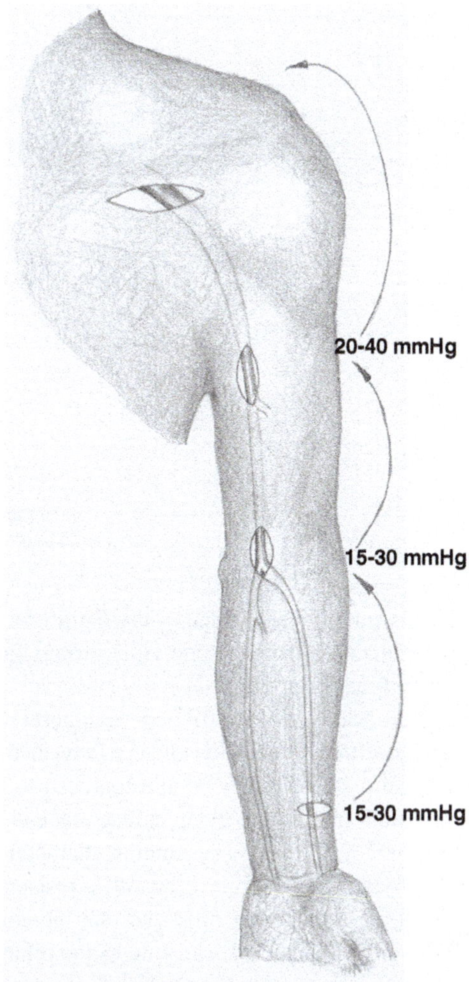

Fig. 11.36 Sketch showing by how much the peripheral perfusion pressure rises if the arterial inflow is proximalized to the next central level

Unless there were contraindications, all patients with ePTFE grafts received oral anticoagulants. The most frequent complications included thrombosis due to stenosed anastomoses between vein and graft. These could be repaired surgically also using a new graft if indicated.

11.2.3 Proximalization of the Arterial Inflow into the Distal Arterial Stump

This procedure called DRIL (distal revascularization and interval ligation) is often reported in the literature. Directly distal to the AV anastomosis, the artery is ligated, and the distal arterial stump is fed via a venous graft that (according to the literature) is anastomosed 5–8 cm proximal to the old anastomosis. Figure 11.22 compares both methods for an elbow fistula. With DRIL the distal arterial stump is proximalized, whereas with PAI the arterial inflow of the AV fistula is proximalized. We do not use DRIL.

11.2.4 Comparison of Both Methods for Proximalization

Both methods are based on the same principle of reducing the inflow resistance by proximalizing the arterial inflow. With PAI the arteries remain intact apart from the obligatory anastomosis. The peripheral drop in pressure caused by the flow in the AV access is diminished by feeding it from a proximal artery with a lower inflow resistance. With DRIL the intended increase in peripheral pressure is brought about by feeding the distal stump of the peripheral artery via a (venous) graft that is anastomosed to a proximal artery. There the inflow resistance is also lower.

In our view there are *disadvantages of DRIL*:

- The transection of the healthy artery (distal to the new AV anastomosis) should be taboo.
- The proximalization over only a short distance (5–8 cm as often reported in the literature) can possibly only lead to a slight increase of peripheral perfusion pressure.
- Harvesting a vein significantly prolongs the time needed for surgery.

11.3 Cardiac Strain Caused by AV Accesses

Even in young patients, high shunt flow rates (1.5–2.5 L/min) lead to reduced physical fitness. This effect is more pronounced in patients with previous cardiac disease. Furthermore, cardiac complications are among the leading causes of death among hemodialysis patients. It seems necessary to monitor AV access flow continuously. Frequently a physical examination can

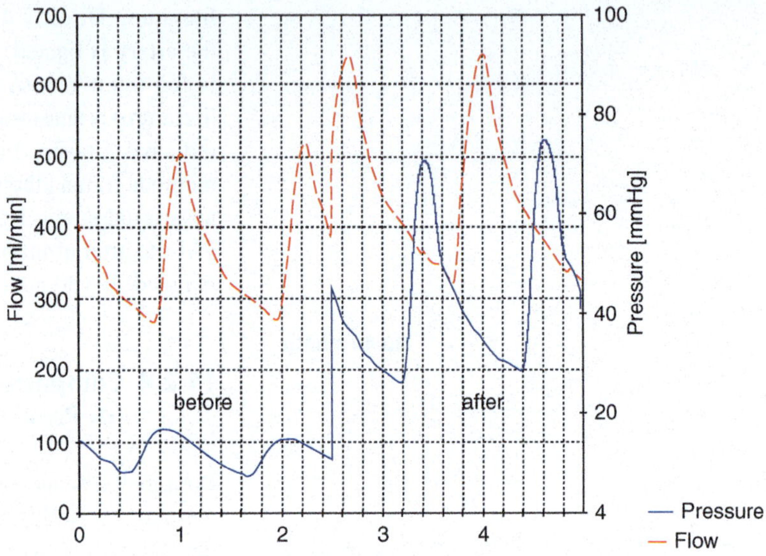

Fig. 11.37 Example for pressure and flow curves before and after a proximalization. The mean pressure in the anastomosis here rises from 12 to 43 mmHg. The mean flow rises from 360 to 450 mL/min

help detect an unnecessarily high flow, which duplex sonography can confirm. The indication for flow reduction should be discussed in an interdisciplinary team including a cardiologist. If a clinically significant cardiac strain caused by high shunt flow has been shown, we proceed as follows:

- If the shunt flow is considerably higher than required for a stable long term functioning (about 300 mL/min for an AV fistula, about 600–1,000 mL/min for a 7-mm ePTFE graft), flow reduction is indicated.
- If the shunt flow is so low that a flow reduction would probably lead to thrombosis, but still causes cardiac failure refractory to therapy, we create an arterioarterial graft and ligate the AV access (very rare).

11.4 Prevention of Insufficient Peripheral Perfusion

When creating an AV fistula, the most distal suitable vein should always be chosen. Therefore perfusion disorders seem inevitable and not entirely predictable. In the following situations preventive measures seem possible:

- If peripheral perfusion is already impaired preoperatively (e.g., in diabetics) and the cephalic vein in the forearm or upper arm seems suitable, we primarily use a graft for its arterialization from the cubital or infraaxillary (rare) brachial artery.
- If there is a risk of insufficient peripheral perfusion after the creation of an elbow fistula, the vein should either be anastomosed to the proximal radial or ulnar artery instead of the brachial artery. The smaller diameter of the forearm arteries raises the inflow resistance and leads to a lower flow rate. An increased flow can be expected later due to the dilation of the feeding arterial segment.
- AV accesses with prosthetic grafts may also be created with arterial anastomoses as proximal as possible (e.g., axillary loop instead of a straight upper arm graft).

Literature

Berman SS, Gentile AT, Glickman MH, Mills JL, Hurwitz RL, Westerband A, Marek JM, Hunter GC, McEnroe CS, Fogle MA, Stokes GK (1997) Distal revascularization-interval ligation for limb salvage and maintenance of dialysis access in ischemic steal syndrome. J Vasc Surg 26:393–402

Callaghan CJ, Mallik M, Sivaprakasam R, Iype S, Pettigrew GJ (2011) Treatment of dialysis access-associated steal syndrome with the "revision using distal inflow" technique. J Vasc Access 12:52–56

Chemla ES, Morsy M, Anderson L, Whitemore A (2007) Inflow reduction by distalization of anastomosis treats efficiently high-inflow high-cardiac output vascular access for hemodialysis. Semin Dial 20:68–72

DeCaprio JD, Valentine RJ, Kakish HB, Awad R, Hagino RT, Clagett GP (1997) Steal syndrome complicating hemodialysis access. Cardiovasc Surg 5:648–653

De Lima JJ, Vieira ML, Molnar LJ, Medeiros CJ, Ianhez LE, Krieger EM (1999) Cardiac effects of persistent hemodialysis arteriovenous access in recipients of renal allograft. Cardiology 92:236–239

Duijm LE, Liem YS, van der Rijt RH, Nobrega FJ, van den Bosch HC, Douwes-Draaijer P, Cuypers PW, Tielbeek AV (2006) Inflow stenoses in dysfunctional hemodialysis access fistulae and grafts. Am J Kidney Dis 48:98–105

Illig KA, Surowiec S, Shortell CK, Davies MG, Rhodes JM, Green RM (2005) Hemodynamics of distal revascularization-interval ligation. Ann Vasc Surg 9:199–207

Gradman WS, Pozrikidis C (2004) Analysis of options for mitigating hemodialysis access-related ischemic steal phenomena. Ann Vasc Surg 18:59–65

Guerra A, Raynaud A, Beyssen B, Pagny JY, Sapoval M, Angel C (2002) Arterial percutaneous angioplasty in upper limbs with vascular access devices for hemodialysis. Nephrol Dial Transplant 17:843–851

Gupta N, Yuo TH, Konig G 4th, Dillavou E, Leers SA, Chaer RA, Cho JS, Makaroun MS (2011) Treatment strategies of arterial steal after arteriovenous access. J Vasc Surg 54:162–167

Haimov M, Schanzer H, Skladani M (1996) Pathogenesis and management of upper-extremity ischemia following angioaccess surgery. Blood Purif 14:350–354

Knox RC, Berman SS, Hughes JD, Gentile AT, Mills JL (2002) Distal revascularization-interval ligation: a durable and effective treatment for ischemic steal syndrome after hemodialysis access. J Vasc Surg 36:250–255

Krisper P, Martinelli E, Zierler E, Schilcher G, Tiesenhausen K, Schneditz D (2011) More may be less: increasing extracorporeal blood flow in an axillary arterio-arterial access decreases effective clearance. Nephrol Dial Transplant 26:2401–2403

Krueger U, Heise M, Huhle A, Krys K, Zanow J, Scholz H (2001) Effects of arterial and venous anastomotic design on hemodynamics in arteriovenous prosthetic grafts. In: Henry ML (ed) Vascular access for hemodialysis VII. W.L. Gore & Associates, Inc./Precept Press, Chicago, pp 177–191

Krueger U, Huhle A, Krys K, Scholz H (2004) Effect of tapered grafts on hemodynamics and flow rate in dialysis access grafts. Artif Organs 28:623–628

Lazarides MK, Staramos DN, Panagopoulos GN, Tzilalis VD, Eleftheriou GJ, Dayantas JN (1998) Indications for surgical treatment of angioaccessinduced arterial "steal". J Am Coll Surg 187:422–426

Mickley V (2008) Steal syndrome–strategies to preserve vascular access and extremity. Nephrol Dial Transplant 23:19–24

Ori Y, Korzets A, Katz M, Perek Y, Zahavi I, Gafter U (1996) Haemodialysis arteriovenous access–a prospective haemodynamic evaluation. Nephrol Dial Transplant 11:94–97

Parmar CD, Chieng G, Abraham KA, Kumar S, Torella F (2009) Revision using distal inflow for treatment of heart failure secondary to arteriovenous fistula for hemodialysis. J Vasc Access 10:62–63

Plumb TJ, Lynch TG, Adelson AB (2008) Treatment of steal syndrome in a distal radiocephalic arteriovenous fistula using intravascular coil embolization. J Vasc Surg 47:457–459

Reddemann P (2010) Der Einfluss der Lokalisation der arteriellen Anastomose und des Flussminutenvolumens von arterio-venösen Gefäßzugängen auf den peripheren Perfusionsdruck bei in vitro Untersuchungen am Kreislaufmodell. Dissertation, Medizinische Fakultät Charité – Universitätsmedizin Berlin

Saratzis N, Saratzis A, Sarafidis PA, Melas N, Ktenidis K, Kiskinis D (2008) Quantitiave evaluation of the systemic effects of transposed basilic vein to brachial artery arteriovenous fistula: a prospective study. J Vasc Access 9:285–290

Schanzer H, Schwartz M, Harrington E, Haimov M (1988) Treatment of ischemia due to "steal" by arteriovenous fistula with distal artery ligation and revascularization. J Vasc Surg 7:770–773

Scholz H, Nauendorf M, Precht K, Schulze BD, Rössler E, Buder HW, Matthes G, Schoepke W (1988) Gerade arterio-venöse Interponater am Oberarm aus allogenem Gefößersaztmaterial unter verschiedenen hämodynamischen Bedingungen. Zent.bl.Chir 113:249–253

Scholz H, Nauendorf M, Matthes G, Precht K, Rössler E, Schulze BD, Reinke P, Schoepke WD (1988) Untersuchungen zum Einsatz formaldehydkonservierter, innenflächensilikonierter und formfixierter boviner Gefäße als Gefäßtransplantate. Zentr bl Chir 113:441

Thermann F, Wollert U (2009) Proximalization of the arterial inflow: new treatment of choice in patients with advanced dialysis shunt-associated steal syndrome? Ann Vasc Surg 23:485–490

Thermann F, Wollert U, Ukkat J, Dralle H (2010) Proximalization of the arterial inflow (PAI) in patients with dialysis access-induced ischemic syndrome: first report on long-term clinical results. J Vasc Access 11:143–149

Tordoir JH, Dammers R, van der Sande FM (2004) Upper extremity ischemia and hemodialysis vascular access. Eur J Vasc Endovasc Surg 27:1–5

van der Meer S, Zeebregts C, Tielliu I, Verhoeven E, van den Dungen J (2007) Modified distal revascularization with interval ligation procedure for steal syndrome after arteriovenous fistula creation for hemodialysis access. Vascular 15:226–230

van Duijnhoven EC, Cheriex EC, Tordoir JH, Kooman JP, van Hooff JP (2001) Effect of closure of the arteriovenous fistula on left ventricular dimensions in renal transplant patients. Nephrol Dial Transplant 16:368–372

van Tricht I, De Wachter D, Tordoir J, Verdonck P (2004) Hemodynamics in a compliant hydraulic in vitro model of straight versus tapered PTFE arteriovenous graft. J Surg Res 116:297–304

Wixon CL, Mills JL Sr, Berman SS (2000a) Distal revascularization-interval ligation for maintenance of dialysis access and restoration of distal perfusion in ischemic steal syndrome. Semin Vasc Surg 13:77–82

Wixon CL, Hughes JD, Mills JL (2000b) Understanding strategies for the treatment of ischemic steal syndrome after hemodialysis access. J Am Coll Surg 191: 301–310

Yee-Moon Wang A, Lai KN (2008) Use of cardiac biomarkers in end-stage renal disease. J Am Soc Nephrol 19:1643–1652

Zanow J, Petzold K, Petzold M, Krueger U, Scholz H (2006a) Flow reduction in high-flow arteriovenous access using intraoperative flow monitoring. J Vasc Surg 44:1273–1278

Zanow J, Kruger U, Scholz H (2006b) Proximalization of the arterial inflow: a new technique to treat access-related ischemia. J Vasc Surg 43:1216–1221

Zanow J, Krueger U, Reddemann P, Scholz H (2008) Experimental study of hemodynamics in procedures to treat access-related ischemia. J Vasc Surg 48: 1559–1565

12 Arterial Reconstructions of AV Accesses

With only 0.3 % of all AV access cases, arterial reconstructions related to AV accesses are rare events in our patients. Arterial stenoses and occlusions of the large vessels (subclavian, axillary, and femoral arteries) are almost exclusively caused by atherosclerotic changes, whereas in peripheral arteries secondary changes after AV surgery are predominant.

12.1 Clinical Presentation and Investigations

12.1.1 Reduced Arterial Inflow into the AV Access

A reduced thrill and a slowed refilling after emptying the vessel are signs of an arterial inflow that is too low (cf. Chap. 18). Then the pressure in the AV access is also reduced. During dialysis, pathologic recirculation may be present. There are different causes (Fig. 12.1):

- Stenosis of the AV anastomosis (Fig. 12.1a)
- Stenosis or occlusion of the feeding artery (Fig. 12.1b)
- Small lumen of the feeding artery (Fig. 12.1c)
- Relative narrowing of the lumen of the feeding artery in combination with arterial hypotension (Fig. 12.1d)

Often sonography is sufficient to find the correct diagnosis. If there is a suspicion or proof that the feeding artery is occluded, we also rely on arteriograms.

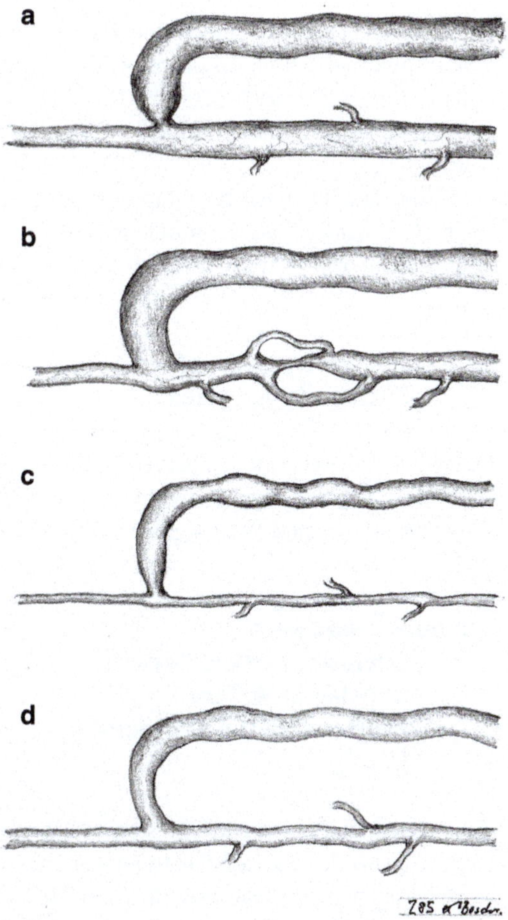

Fig. 12.1 Potential causes of a low arterial inflow. (**a**) Stenosis of the anastomosis. (**b**) Stenosis of the feeding artery. (**c**) Narrow artery. (**d**) Hypotension with sufficient artery

H. Scholz, *Arteriovenous Access Surgery*,
DOI 10.1007/978-3-642-41139-7_12, © Springer-Verlag Berlin Heidelberg New York 2015

12.1.2 Insufficient Peripheral Perfusion

Mainly in patients with repeated previous AV access surgery or surgery dating back some time, multiple arterial occlusions or stenoses may lead to clinically relevant insufficient perfusion with symptoms ranging from pain to tissue loss (Chap. 11). Duplex sonography may prove helpful, but before surgery we also order arteriograms if indicated.

12.1.3 Indications for Arterial Reconstructions

An occlusion or stenosis should only be treated if it causes relevant symptoms or loss of function.

Indications for arterial reconstructions are:

- Indadequately low arterial feeding of the AV access
- Indadequately low peripheral perfusion

The following is based on our experience in 59 documented cases from 1982 through 2011.

12.2 Reconstruction of Upper Extremity Arteries

Taking into account anatomy, occurrence of stenoses, and therapy, we suggest dividing the arteries of the arm into seven (I–VII) segments (Fig. 12.2).

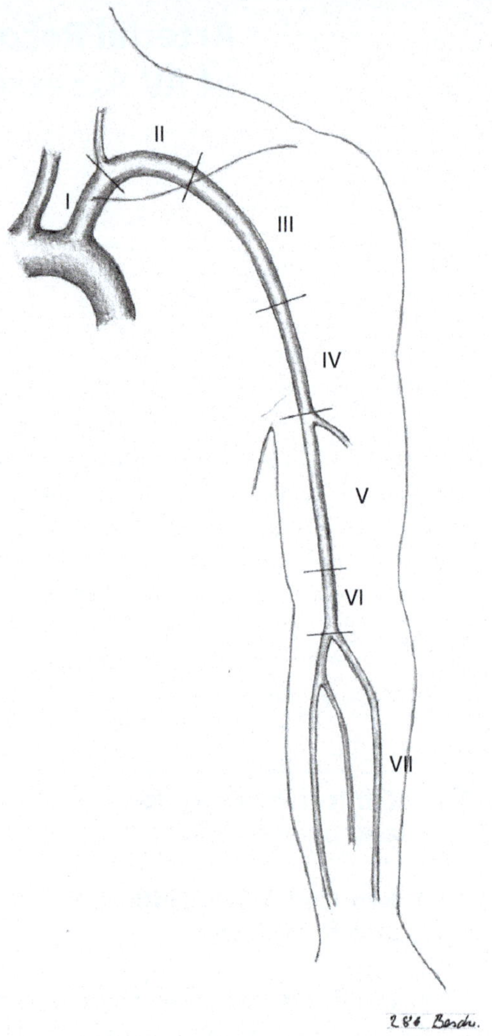

Fig. 12.2 Division of the arm arteries into seven segments according to surgical aspects

Segment I: Stenoses/Occlusions of the Central Subclavian Artery (Aortovertebral Segment) (*n* = 5)

If the vertebral artery is patent, a steal effect may arise. In general, endovascular treatment should be tried first, which is successful in about 75 % of these cases. Only if it fails will surgery be indicated. There are three local options. Vascular morphology and topography dictate the choice.

Transposition of the Subclavian to the Common Carotid Artery (Fig. 12.3)

Prerequisite and indication

- The subclavian artery is accessible via a supraclavicular approach, and
- The distance between the subclavian and common carotid arteries is not too long for the transposition.

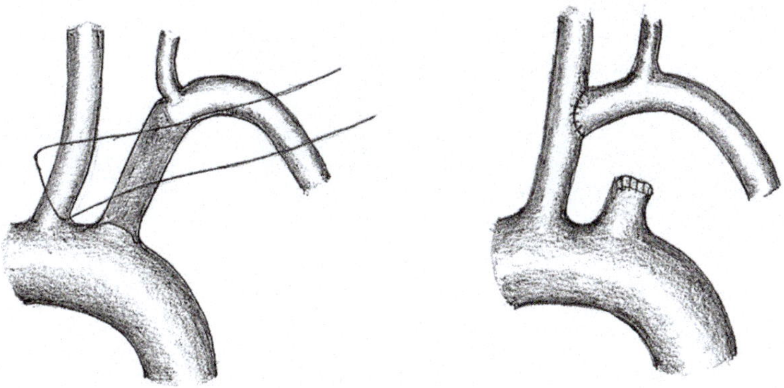

Fig. 12.3 Transposition of the subclavian artery to the common carotid artery

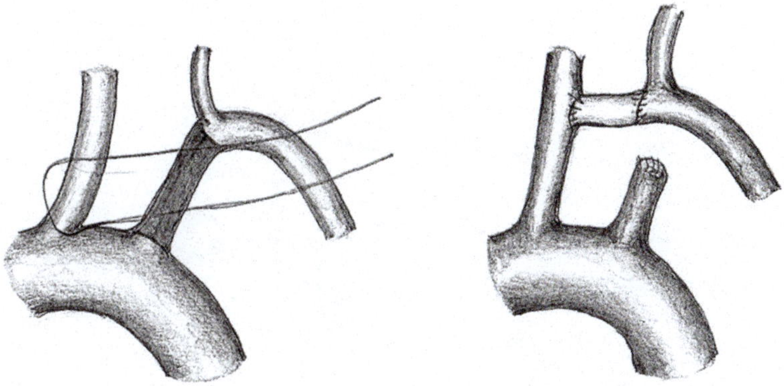

Fig. 12.4 Carotidsubclavian bypass

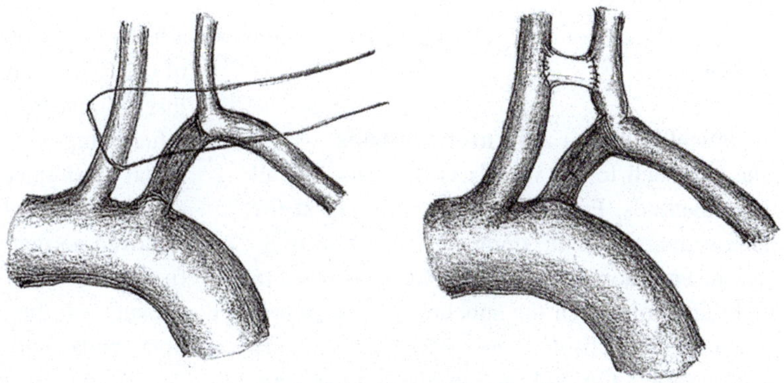

Fig. 12.5 Carotidvertebral bypass

Carotidsubclavian Bypass (Fig. 12.4)

Prerequisite and indication

- The subclavian artery is accessible via a supraclavicular approach.
- Due to the long distance between the vessels a bypass graft is needed.

Carotidvertebral Bypass (Fig. 12.5)

Prerequisite and indication

- The subclavian artery is not accessible via a supraclavicular approach as a result of its deep path.
- The lumen of the vertebral artery is large enough (>3 mm).

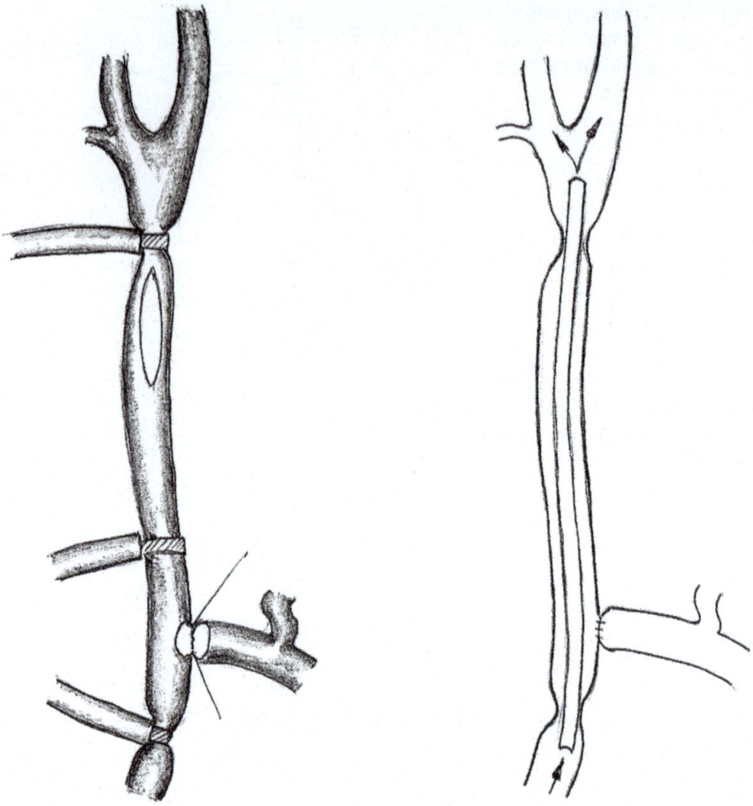

Fig. 12.6 Intraluminal shunt for creating an anastomosis of the common carotid and subclavian arteries

- The take off of the vertebral artery is not stenosed.

Technical Hints for All Three Methods

The approach to the vessels is the same for all three methods. From an oblique incision at the anterior margin of the sternocleidomastoid muscle, the common carotic artery (CCA) is freed to its bifurcation. Then the subclavian or vertebral arteries, respectively, are exposed dorsally between the CCA and the internal jugular vein. To avoid ischemic brain damage, we almost always use an intraluminal shunt for the CCA. We proceed as follows:

- After systemic heparinization and a longitudinal arteriotomy of the CCA approximately 3 cm caudad to its bifurcation, we insert a shunt which is secured and sealed by proximal and distal tourniquets (Fig. 12.6). The cranial end of the shunt is placed caudal to the carotid bifurcation. For the anastomosis, a further arteriotomy of the excluded segment of the CCA (caudal to the arteriotomy for the insertion of the intraluminal shunt) is made.
- After completion of the anastomosis, an additional tourniquet is placed cranial to this new anastomosis, and the most caudal tourniquet is removed so that the anastomosis will be perfused (Fig. 12.7).
- Closure of the arteriotomy is started from both ends with continuous sutures (6-0). Before this is completed, the intraluminal shunt is severed after bilateral clamping and removed through the remaining small arterial defect without further trauma to the vessel (Fig. 12.8).
- After flushing the suture is completed, clamps or tourniquets are removed, and the heparin effect is antagonized by the systemic administration of protamine (Fig. 12.9).
- We use 7-mm ePTFE prostheses for both carotidsubclavian and carotidvertebral bypasses.

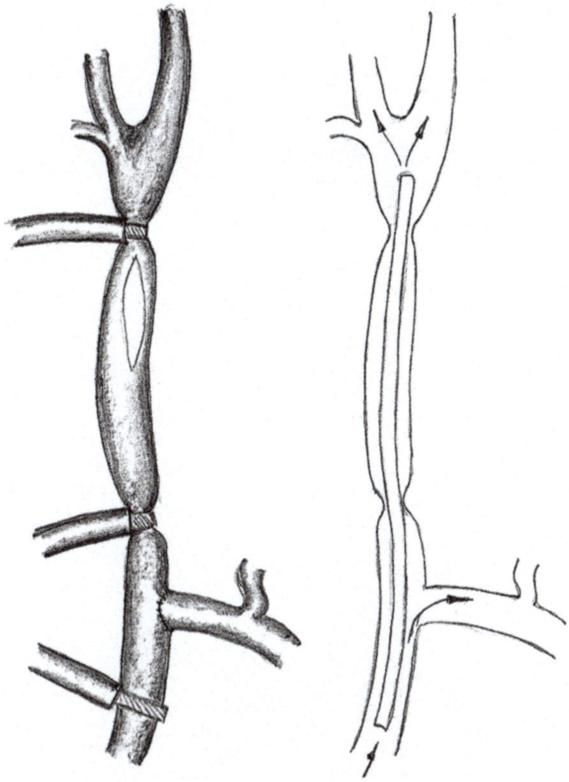

Fig. 12.7 After creating the anastomosis, let blood flow into the subclavian artery with an intraluminal shunt inside the common carotid artery

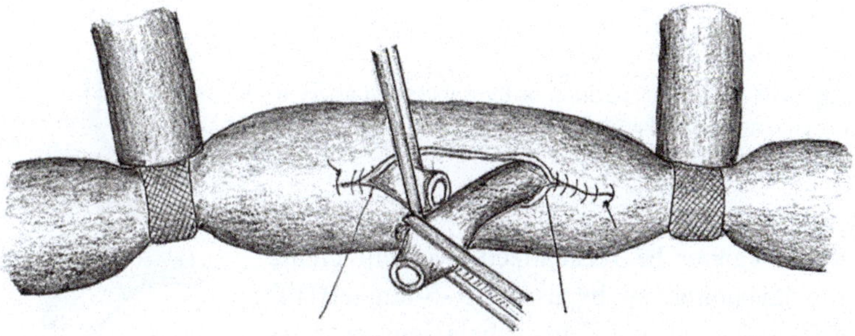

Fig. 12.8 Cutting and removal of the intraluminal shunt

12.2.1 Segment II: Peripheral Subclavian Artery (Vertebroaxillary Segment) (*n* = 2)

An occlusion of the peripheral subclavian artery should be recanalized by endovascular means if possible. Should this fail, a carotidaxillary bypass (Fig. 12.10) is indicated. We proceed as described above. For the axillary artery, an additional infraclavicular transverse skin incision is made.

12.2.2 Segment III: Axillary Artery (*n* = 9)

With stenoses or short occlusions of the axillary artery, endovascular therapy should also be tried first. If this fails or if there are long occlusions

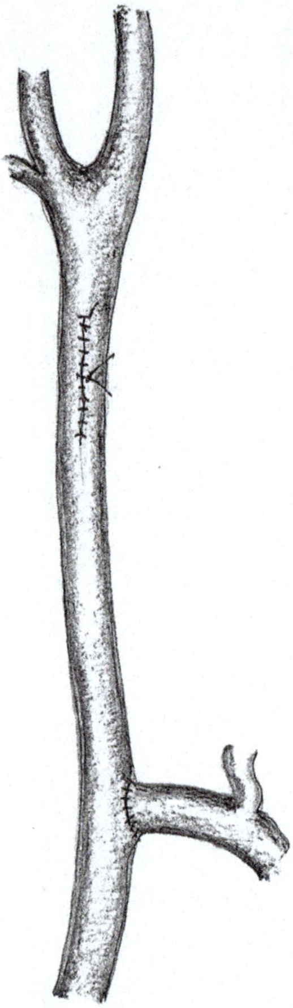

Fig. 12.9 After transposition of the subclavian artery to the common carotid artery (with intraluminal shunt)

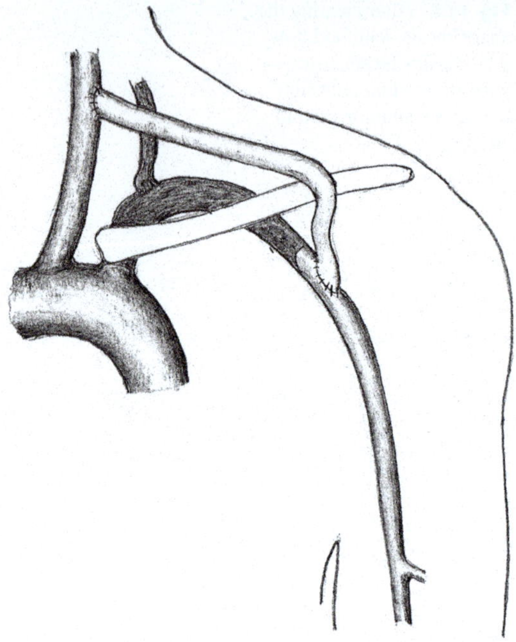

Fig. 12.10 Carotidaxillary bypass

which cannot be recanalized, we will create subclavianbrachial bypasses (5–6-mm ePTFE graft) (Fig. 12.11). The subclavian artery is exposed via a supraclavicular transverse incision, and the proximal brachial artery via an infraaxillary longitudinal incision. The extraanatomic subcutaneous tunnel runs anterior to the clavicula.

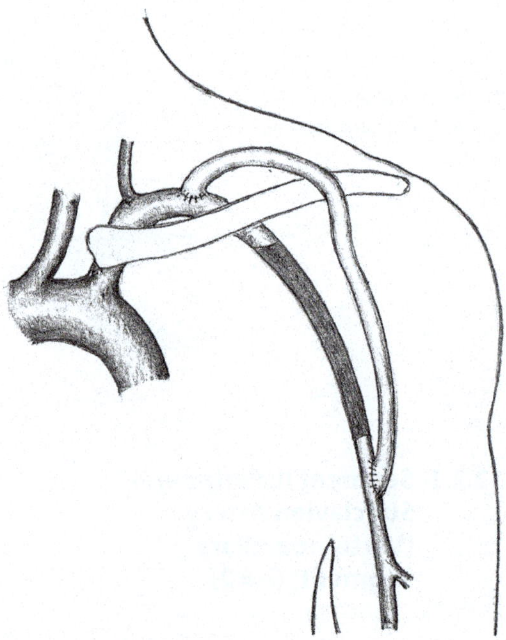

Fig. 12.11 Subclavianbrachial bypass

12.2.3 Segment IV: Proximal (Infraaxillary) Brachial Artery (*n* = 7)

The most important causes of occlusions are complications after shunt surgery. Frequently heavy scarring after previous surgery involves the nerves. Therefore we do not expose the occluded segments in these cases. We rather expose the artery proximal and distal to an occlusion for bypass implantation, usually with a 4- or 5-mm PTFE graft.

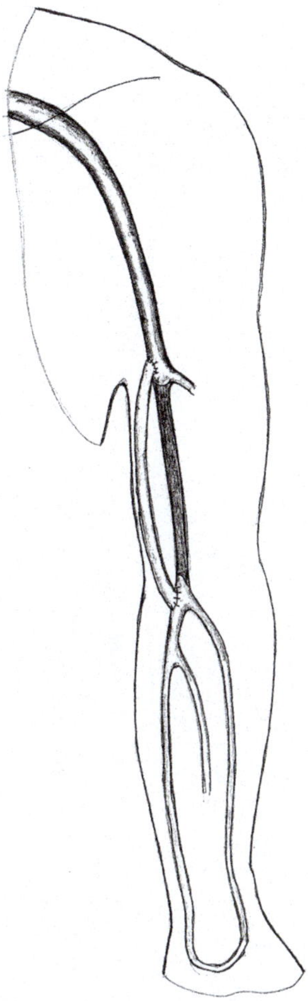

Fig. 12.12 Brachiocubital bypass

12.2.4 Segment V: Middle Brachial Artery (*n*=11)

Should it not be possible to recanalize the artery by endovascular means, we see an indication for a brachiobrachial bypass (Fig. 12.12). For this purpose a 4-mm ePTFE graft, which is placed in a subcutaneous tunnel, seems suited. For an anastomosis distal to the elbow, the graft should pass near the center of rotation in order to prevent kinking with elbow flexion.

12.2.5 Segment VI: Peripheral Brachial Artery (*n*=13)

Occlusions mainly arise after previous AV access surgery. Near the elbow primary surgical reconstruction is indicated. As the occluded segments tend to be relatively short, autologous vein grafts or 4-mm ePTFE prostheses may be chosen.

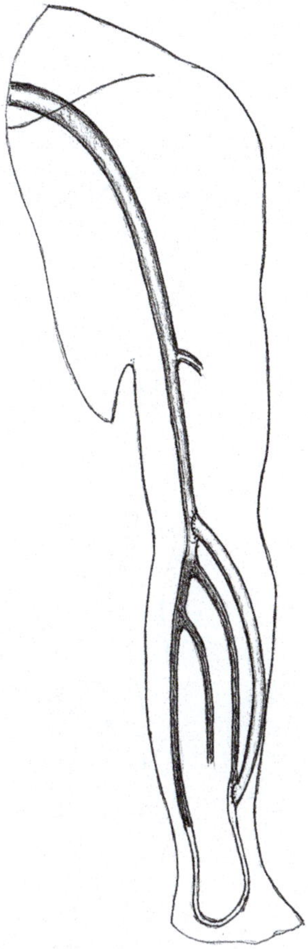

Fig. 12.13 Cubitoradial bypass

12.2.6 Segment VII: Forearm Arteries (*n*=5)

These occlusions are likewise mostly due to previous AV access surgery (possibly combined with diabetic angiopathy). If there is no autologous vein available for grafting, we choose a 4-mm ePTFE prosthesis (Fig. 12.13). The distal anastomosis close to the wrist is either sutured to the radial artery or ulnar artery.

12.2.7 Long Occlusions (*n*=7)

With extended long stenoses it has been possible to preserve the arm through long bypasses from

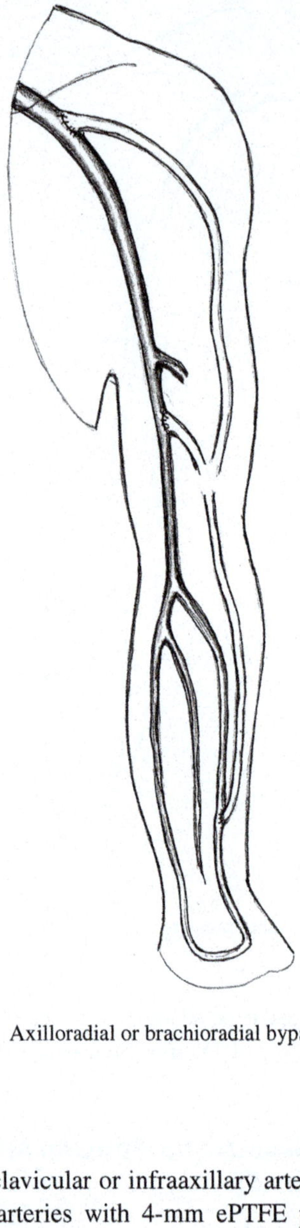

Fig. 12.14 Axilloradial or brachioradial bypass

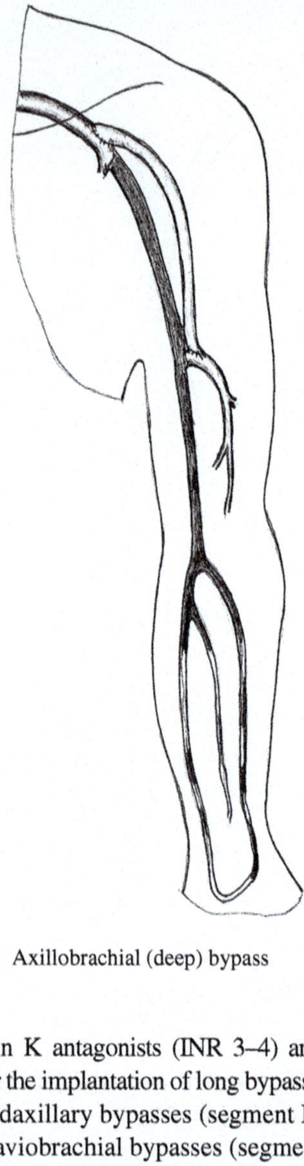

Fig. 12.15 Axillobrachial (deep) bypass

the infraclavicular or infraaxillary arteries to the forearm arteries with 4-mm ePTFE prostheses ($n = 6$) (Fig. 12.14) or to the deep brachial artery ($n = 1$) (Fig. 12.15).

Drug Regime After Reconstructions of the Arm Arteries

Acetylsalicylic acid only is administered after:

- Reconstructions for occlusions of the subclavian artery
- Short infraaxillary grafts (segment IV)
- Short cubital grafts (segment VI)

Vitamin K antagonists (INR 3–4) are administered after the implantation of long bypasses such as:

- Carotidaxillary bypasses (segment II)
- Subclaviobrachial bypasses (segment III)
- Brachiobrachial bypasses (segment V)
- All bypasses to the forearm arteries and bypasses with long occlusions (segments VII and VIII)

12.3 Extreme Dilatation of the Feeding Artery

After years the feeding artery of an AV fistula may dilate excessively often in the forearm and elbow regions. Most cases develop under long term steroid treatment (e.g., after organ transplants). With an elbow fistula it is usually only the feeding artery that dilates. With forearm fistulas to either the ulnar or radial artery, the other artery frequently also dilates via the palmar arch provided that there is a high flow. In case of a low venous outflow resistance with dilated veins and a strong inflow (i.e., arterial hypertension), the flow may well exceed 3 L/min. The dilation of the artery is always associated with:

- *Decrease in wall thickness.* (Through a gossamer arterial wall you can detect the whirls with the naked eye. Sometimes it may be difficult to distinguish the artery from the vein during surgery in particular in the elbow region.)
- *Lengthening.*

There may be bizarre formations of extremely meandering and loopy vessels (Fig. 12.16). The diameter of the brachial artery can reach 25 mm, and that of the radial artery 12 mm. We advocate:

- Preservation of a puncturable vessel for potential future use (even with a well-functioning renal graft).
- Flow reduction in case of cardiac strain.

Technical Hints

If flow reduction is overdone, the ensuing slowing of the flow might lead to thrombosis. Even in widely dilated high flow arteries there may be wall-adherent thrombi. We then proceed as follows:

1. Preservation of an AV fistula which is not needed presently.

   In this case we reduce the flow to 200–300 mL/min. With extreme dilatation or preexisting mural thrombi we recommend long term oral anticoagulants.
2. With cardiac strain we reduce to 500–800 mL/ min.

   In our experience there will only be a slight regression of the dilatation.

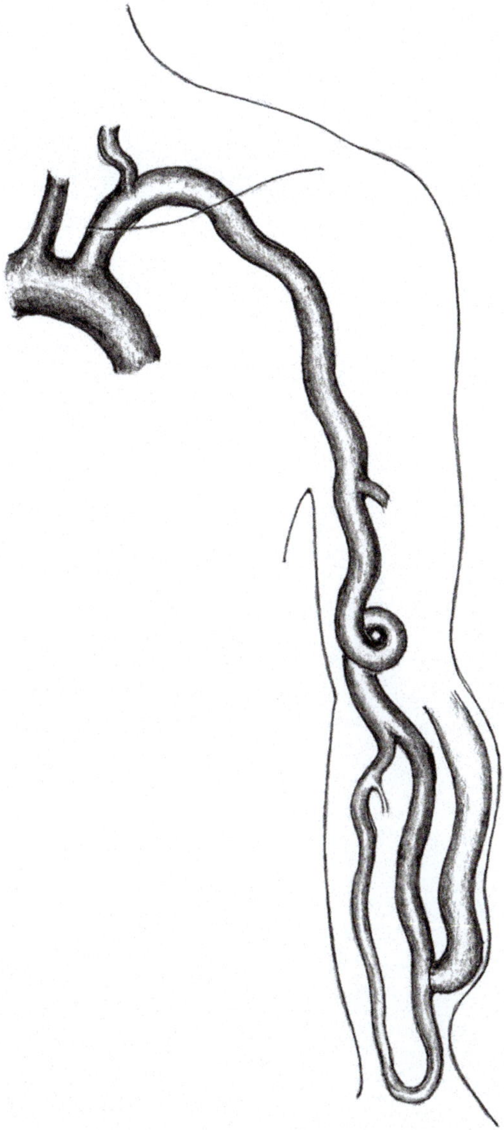

Fig. 12.16 Extreme dilation of the arm arteries with distal AV fistula

Literature

Scholz H, Rükert R, Settmacher U (1997) The proximal carotid-vertebral bypass. Eur J Vasc Endovasc Surg 13:214–216

13 Lymph Edema of the Arm After AV Access Surgery

Secondary lymph edema of the arm after AV access surgery is rare, but it seriously compromises a patient's well-being.

13.1 Pathophysiology

Starting in the periphery, lymphatic capillaries, precollectors, and collectors converge into trunks. Beginning with precollectors, lymphatic vessels have valves, which determine the flow direction. Lymphatic fluid is propelled by contractions of the vessel walls, which follow a complex regulation as required. The lymphatic system of the arm resembles the venous system. It consists of a deep (subfascial) as well as a superficial system, which is interconnected by perforators. In the arm, the collectors of the deep lymphatic system follow the arteries. Those of the superficial system form three bundles (median, radial, and ulnar). In the upper arm there are three bundles (median, dorsolateral, and dorsomedial) as well. Collaterals interconnect collectors. A lymph edema occurs if the lymphatic load surpasses the transport capacity.

Lymph edema after AV accesses is caused by:

- Transection of lymphatic vessels
- Compression of lymphatic vessels (e.g., hematoma, lymphocele, or seroma)
- Inflammatory changes of the lymphatic vessels
- Decompensation of the lymphatic system (with venous congestion)

Postoperative lymph edemas are either temporary or chronic.

13.2 Postoperative Lymph Edemas

13.2.1 Local Lymph Edema

Local lymph edemas can often be found on the inside of a looped graft. They mostly appear in the volar forearm and ventral thigh, more rarely in the upper arm. They almost always recede within days or weeks, not requiring further treatment.

13.2.2 Lymph Edema Distal to Operated Site

With a lymph edema distal to the surgical incision, which concern the whole periphery (e.g., forearm edema with elbow fistulas, arm edemas with axillary or infraclavicular AV access) a venous congestion and/or inflammation should be excluded. Other possible causes include the transection or compression of lymphatic vessels (e.g., by a fluid collection). The latter may be diagnosed by ultrasound and treated accordingly including surgery. If important lymphatic vessels have been transected during AV access surgery, therapy directly after surgery should include the elevation of the extremity and optional antibiotic prophylaxis. In the majority of these cases, an almost complete resolution of the lymph edema can likewise be expected within days to weeks.

H. Scholz, *Arteriovenous Access Surgery*,
DOI 10.1007/978-3-642-41139-7_13, © Springer-Verlag Berlin Heidelberg New York 2015

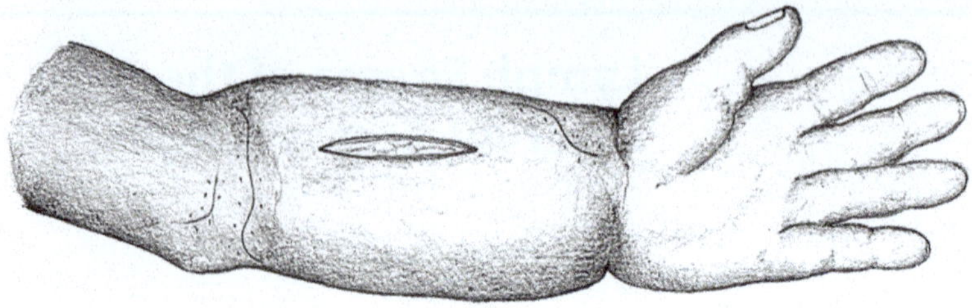

Fig. 13.1 Chronic lymph edema of the forearm after multiple operations

13.3 Chronic Postoperative Lymph Edema

13.3.1 Lymph Edema with Venous Congestion

Stenoses or occlusions of the venous outflow of AV accesses with insufficient venous collateralization lead to a venous backlog with raised capillary pressure and increased lymphatic load. If it exceeds the transport capacity, lymph edema will occur. The clinical presentation includes:

- Venous congestion
- Lymph edema
- A typical water-hammer pulse of the AV access may be palpated

The cause of the venous backlog should be repaired. Timely treatment may lead to the resolution of the edema within days. It rarely takes longer than that. If it takes weeks, most likely the valves of the lymphatic vessels are impaired. After months or years of venous congestion, connective tissue fibrosis develops. Even if the venous congestion is no longer prevalent, residual swelling will remain.

13.3.2 Lymph Edema Without Venous Congestion

Patients with chronic lymphedemas without venous congestion of the affected extremity mostly had a history of:

- Mulitple operations of the same arm with
- Long transverse skin incisions

These transverse incisions with the transection of lymphatic vessels and a lack of collaterals are, fortunately, rare causes of lymph edema. In three patients on hemodialysis, who could not close their fists due to pronounced edema, we performed forearm fasciectomies (Fig. 13.1). Starting from a 12-cm radiovolar longitudinal incision of the proximal forearm, the fascia was exposed, and a 2-cm band resected (Fig. 13.2). In all cases the fascia was thicker than usual (up to 5 mm). Postoperatively the edemas receded, and the patients could close their hands again.

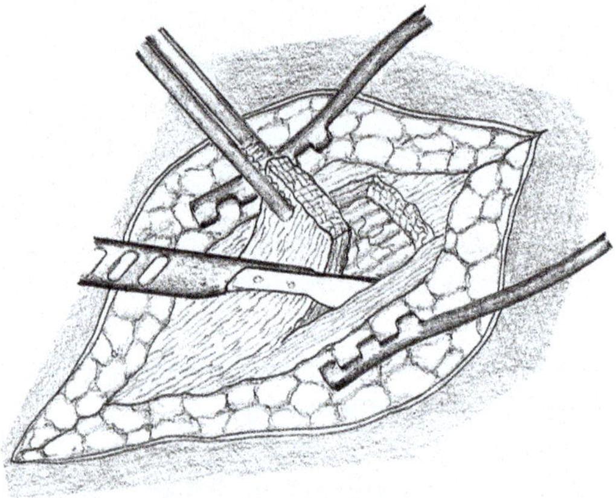

Fig. 13.2 Fasciectomy site

13.4 Prevention of Lymph Edema After AV Access Surgery

Lymphatic vessels should be left intact during AV access surgery by choosing:

- Longitudinal incisions
- Short approaches to the vessels
- Not to create cavities (don't force the tissue apart in a transverse sense)

Apart for distal forearm fistulas with arteries and veins which run close to each other, transverse incisions in general are not necessary and should be avoided.

Literature

Földi M (2010) Lehrbuch Lymphologie 7. Auflage, Urban & Fischer

14 Nerve Lesions After AV Access Surgery

Fortunately, despite the close proximity of nerves and vessels, nerve lesions are rare.

14.1 Concerned Nerves

Surgery determines the site of lesions. The following list is based on clinical observations without exact statistics.

14.1.1 Distal Cephalic Fistula

The superficial branch of the radial nerve, which innervates dorsal parts of the thumb and the back of the hand, is in or close to the field. The 1–2-mm nerve has to be preserved.

Clinical deficits: Loss of sensitivity and pain in the territory. Altogether a rare occurrence in spite of the frequent choice of this site.

14.1.2 Distal Basilic Fistula

The 3–4-mm ulnar nerve is situated laterally and deeply in the operative field and can hardly be overlooked. We have not encountered ulnar nerve lesions in this rare approach.

14.1.3 Elbow Fistula

Distal to the elbow, the median nerve almost always runs separately from the brachial artery. Unlike in our patients with longitudinal incisions over or close to the brachial artery, we have seen lesions in patients who had surgery elsewhere with long transverse incisions in the cubital fossa (which are not indicated).

14.1.4 Superficialization of the Basilic Vein in the Upper Arm

With the superficialization of the basilic vein in the upper arm, the ulnar and the ulnar cutaneous brachial nerves (and their branches), which run close to the vein, are involved. There are interconnections between the nerve trunks. The special care that this surgery requires to preserve the nerves makes it challenging.

14.1.5 Anastomosis Central to the Elbow

With straight AV grafts in the upper arm, the anastomosis to the brachial artery is sutured proximal to the cubital fossa. The median nerve often runs close to the artery on its ulnar side, but may also form a partially U-shaped sheath around it. The latter situation calls for an extended longitudinal exposure of the artery.

H. Scholz, *Arteriovenous Access Surgery*,
DOI 10.1007/978-3-642-41139-7_14, © Springer-Verlag Berlin Heidelberg New York 2015

14.1.6 Axillary Anastomosis

With an anastomosis close to the axilla, the median and ulnar nerves (and also the radial nerve) are involved. The brachial artery and the lateral brachial vein are situated between and behind the nerves. We always prefer the shortest approach to the vessels and take special care to preserve the nerves. During primary surgery, nerve lesions can almost always be avoided. There were median nerve lesions in two of our patients after redo surgery.

14.1.7 Infraclavicular Anastomosis

Here we always come across all three major arm nerves with numerous anatomical variants.

14.1.8 Jugular Anastomosis (Internal Jugular Vein)

The vein is close to the vagus nerve, which can hardly be missed. Although it is not really at risk for this reason, we have seen two lesions of the recurrent laryngeal nerve after surgical implantations of central venous catheters.

14.1.9 Supraclavicular Approach to the Subclavian Artery

In the supraclavicular approaches for the revascularization of the subclavian artery or transposition of the vertebral artery, we have only encountered lesions of sympathetic fibers (Horner's syndrome in 50 %). About half of these subside completely within the next few days or weeks following surgery. Chronic Horner's syndrome will persist in around 25 % of the patients whom we inform accordingly before obtaining consent.

14.2 Prevention of Nerve Lesions

The risk of nerve lesions is drastically reduced if the following principles are observed:

(a) Incisions that do not cross the nerves.
(b) No infiltration of the nerve itself, but only of the perineurium if need be.
(c) Take care not to squeeze the nerve with surgical instruments.
(d) Don't use diathermy on the vessels of the perineurium.

You should place tissue between a graft and a nerve. Seromas and hematomas should be evacuated in time to prevent compression damage.

Special Patient Groups 15

15.1 Renal Transplant Recipients

When creating a new AV access or before closing an access which is no longer required, special aspects need to be considered.

15.1.1 Creation of a New Vascular Access

- Patients who are under long term glucocorticoid treatment may require an additional perioperative stress dose due to the suppression of the hypothalamic-pituitary-adrenal axis.
- Transplanted patients have a higher risk for impaired wound healing and infections, and also sometimes increased propensity to bleed. The skin and blood vessels may be extremely friable, so that atraumatic surgical techniques, careful hemostasis, and extra cautious draping and placement of incise film if applicable are particularly important.

15.1.2 Request for the Closure of an AV Access

Many patients with a reliably stable transplant function inquire whether it is possible to ligate the AV access. Crucial aspects include:

- Kidney graft function
- Time passed since transplant surgery,
- Biological age and general condition of the patient
- Remaining options for future AV access surgery

Closure of the Vascular Access

We only close the vascular access if:

- The kidney transplant function is good.
- There are further possibilities for the creation of potential future accesses.

Frequency

Very rare.

Technical Hint

The continuity of the vein should be preserved if possible, so as to be able to use it for a potential future new vascular access. Illustrated examples are Fig. 15.1 which shows the closure of a cephalic fistula, and Fig. 15.2 that of an elbow fistula. Under certain circumstances the vein may remain patent due to the inflow from side branches.

Preservation of the Vascular Access with Flow Reduction

We try to preserve the vascular access if:

- Options for future access surgery are limited
- The patient is young

The procedure is different for AV fistulas and AV shunts.

AV Shunt

Flow reduction to the necessary minimum flow (cf. Chap. 11).

H. Scholz, *Arteriovenous Access Surgery*,
DOI 10.1007/978-3-642-41139-7_15, © Springer-Verlag Berlin Heidelberg New York 2015

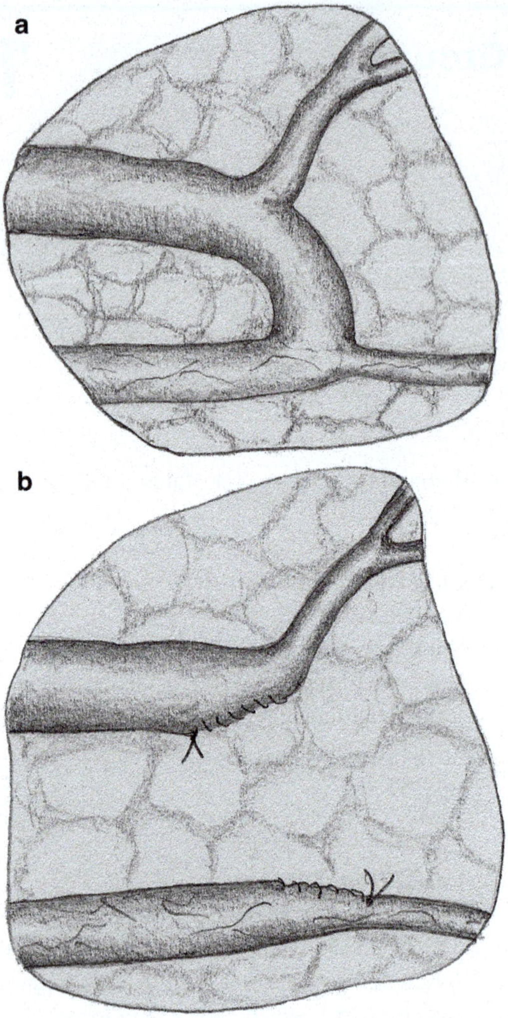

Fig. 15.1 Surgical occlusion of a cephalic forearm fistula while preserving the venous continuity. (**a**) Before. (**b**) After

AV Fistulas

Depending on the local situation there are the following options:

- Perform flow reduction if there is an only slightly dilated vein (cf. Chap. 11).
- With extreme dilatation of the vein and possibly additional dilatation of the artery, extensive surgical correction seems necessary. The interposition of a narrow graft segment

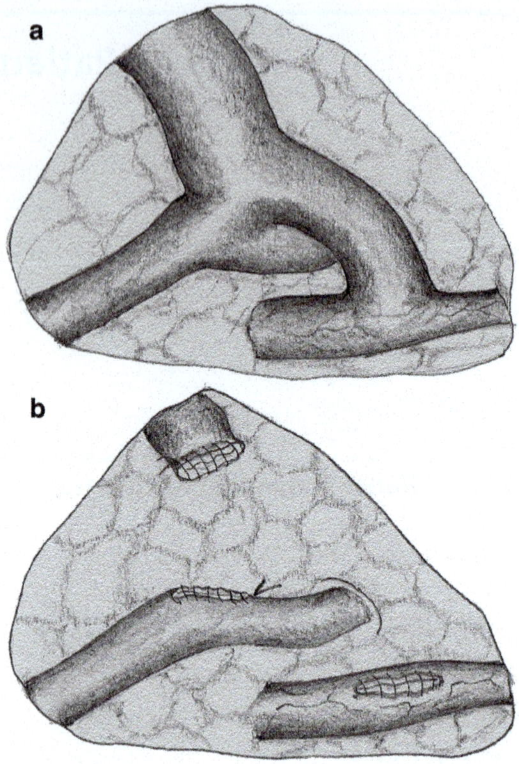

Fig. 15.2 Surgical occlusion of an elbow AV fistula while preserving the continuity of the basilic vein. (**a**) Before. (**b**) After

for flow reduction is an appropriate solution (Fig. 15.3).

Preservation of the AV Access Without Further Action

With an impaired renal graft function and difficult conditions for the creation of a new AV access, we would not close an AV access unless there are other compulsive reasons.

15.2 Patients Who Require Extra Attention

Comorbidity may have a crucial influence on the selection of an adequate vascular access and require additional therapy. Details have already

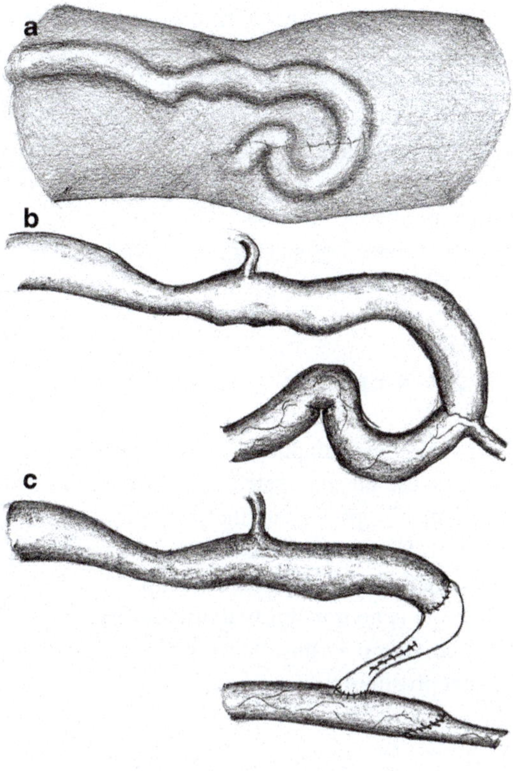

Fig. 15.3 (**a**, **b**) Elbow cephalic fistula with pronounced dilatation and elongation of the afferent brachial artery and vein. (**c**) Shortening of the artery, re-establishment of its continuity and anastomosis to the vein via a flow-reduced prosthetic graft

been mentioned elsewhere. Here we discuss the specific considerations for some frequent diagnoses.

15.2.1 Diabetics

Macro- and microangiopathy frequently cause difficulties.

Macroangiopathy

The lower arm arteries in chronic diabetics can resemble rigid calcified pipes. Then an AV anastomosis of such an artery does not lead to its dilation. The arterial inflow that is determined during surgery does not increase. Preoperatively the wall texture and the luminal diameter of the selected artery should be examined by ultrasound. The respective artery is not suited if the arterial inflow is insufficient.

Microangiopathy

The increased peripheral resistance due to microangiopathy calls for increased perfusion pressure. If as a result of an AV shunt the peripheral arterial pressure decreases, it may fall below a critical threshold. Therefore there is a higher risk for peripheral perfusion disorders after AV access surgery in diabetics. Resulting consequences are:

- With a history of an already previously low peripheral perfusion, this fact has to be taken into account when choosing the hemodynamically correct AV access.

Even without this history, the risk for insufficient peripheral perfusion is higher than in non-diabetic patients. The patient should be informed accordingly, and also about possible future surgery (e.g., proximalization of the arterial inflow).

15.2.2 Obesity

- The deep position of the vessels buried in adipose tissue necessitates preoperative imaging studies. Frequently veins can only be punctured after their superficialization.
- Near folds (mostly upper arm), subcutaneous prosthetic grafts may kink.
- In extremely obese patients, the risk of thrombosis caused by compression is elevated with axillary anastomoses.
- Obesity is the most frequent reason to place a loop graft in the forearm position.

15.2.3 Heart Failure

The flow of a vascular access causes extra strain on the already impaired heart. This aspect has to be taken into account, especially in young patients. There are two conclusions:

- The flow rate of an AV access should be as low as possible.
- A patient with heart failure refractory to therapy does not tolerate the additional strain of an AV access. Then an arterioarterial interposition graft may be indicated.

15.2.4 Hypotension

The decrease of access flow with hypotension may entail an insufficient dialysis and an increased risk for thrombosis. This is especially true for prosthetic grafts. To maintain the necessary flow rate, a vascular access with a centrally placed anastomosis should be chosen (e.g., an elbow fistula instead of a distal cephalic fistula, despite a suitable cephalic vein in the forearm). In spite of the central position of the vascular access, the flow rate may be so low that additional oral anticoagulants may be required to prevent thrombosis.

15.2.5 Malignancy

Malignancy-related coagulation disorders (paraneoplastic syndrome) may lead to hypercoagulopathy. This is particularly true for plasmocytomas with paraproteinemia. Two therapeutic strategies to prevent thrombosis are:

- The choice of a high flow access (AV anastomosis to a central artery)
- Anticoagulation

It is an individual decision to find the right solution for each patient.

15.2.6 Hypercoagulability

Unexplained thrombosis (deep vein thrombosis) in a patient's history can be a sign of hypercoagulability, just like:

- Thrombosis of an AV-fistula despite optimal hemodynamic conditions
- White or mixed thrombi in the AV access

If there is a suspicion of hypercoagulability, extensive coagulation tests should be performed, and anticoagulant therapy initiated if indicated. In some cases all tests were normal despite repeated thrombosis. Then we also administered anticoagulants.

15.2.7 Amputees

With unilateral amputees of the upper extremities, we use the amputated side (axillary or infraclavicular loop) to spare the sound arm.

With lower extremity amputees we create an AV access of the amputated side, if:

- There is no possibility to use the arms
- The stump is unsuited for a weight-bearing exoprosthesis

15.2.8 Pareses

We try to place the vascular access in the paretic upper extremity.

15.2.9 Dermatologic Diseases

Areas which are afflicted by (inflammatory) dermatologic disorders should not be used for vascular access surgery if possible. If we can't spare them (e.g., generalized psoriasis), we create a subcutaneous tunnel farther from the surface than usual (5–8 mm). We act likewise with extremely thin and friable skin such as after long term steroids usage or in sclerodermia.

15.2.10 Septic Disease

Septic disease should ideally be over prior to surgery. With chronic disease such as osteomyelitis, a vascular access should resort to the patient's own veins. Alloplastic grafts should only be used if there are no suitable autologous veins.

15.2.11 IV Drug Abuse

- Even primarily well-developed peripheral veins tend to show spasms and long stenoses with sclerosis after their arterialization.
- It is quite possible that patients will use their vascular accesses for drug injections. A lack of hygiene may lead to infections, particularly with alloplastic grafts.

  The two consequences are:
- Even after prior futile attempts with native veins, you should still prefer them.
- If there is no alternative to alloplastic grafts, you should place them as deep as possible to offer at least some protection from autopuncture-related complications resulting from doubtful hygienic conditions.

16 Anticoagulation with AV Accesses

In our experience, the following course of action has proved useful:

(a) With physiological circulatory conditions and normal coagulation, neither AV fistulas nor AV shunts require drugs that influence coagulation.

(b) We start primary anticoagulation (INR around 3) only in patients with:
- Confirmed hypercoagulability
- Arterioarterial grafts
- Hypotension (systolic RR < 80 mmHg) with prosthetic grafts

(c) After thrombosis we proceed according to intraoperative findings at thrombectomy. Criteria comprise:
- Arterial inflow and venous outflow resistance
- Vascular morphology as shown by intraoperative angiography (which we recommend)
- Kind of thrombus material (white, mixed, or red)
- Anamnestic suspicion of possible expressed temporary hypotension (e.g., severe diarrhea with pre-existing hypotension, shock, general anesthesia)
- Long-lasting compression of the vascular access (bandage, joint position)

Typical aspects of a coagulation disorder are white or mixed thrombi.

Without suspicion of a persistent
- Hemodynamic,
- Morphological, or
- Coagulation-related

cause, we do not order extra tests or introduce additional drug therapy after thrombectomy, but observe the clinical course.

With suspicion of
- A morphological cause (arterial or venous stenoses or occlusions)

we complete imaging studies and repair pathologic findings if possible.

With suspicion of
- Hypercoagulability

we initiate further coagulation tests.
- If they prove positive, we start with (oral) anticoagulants.
- If they prove negative, we observe the clinical course. Should there be repeat thrombosis in the absence of other evident causes, we start with anticoagulants despite negative standard test results.

(d) An increased hematocrite also means a higher blood viscosity. Nonetheless if erythropoietin therapy or transfusions are indicated, they should not be cancelled for fear of AV access occlusion. Their effect should only be risky as to access occlusion under already unstable conditions.

(e) We have not observed a definite effect of platelet inhibitors on rates of thrombosis of hemodynamically stable AV fistulas and ePTFE AV shunts. Therefore we do not administer antiplatelet drugs.

H. Scholz, *Arteriovenous Access Surgery*,
DOI 10.1007/978-3-642-41139-7_16, © Springer-Verlag Berlin Heidelberg New York 2015

Literature

Chan KE, Lazarus JM, Thadhani R, Hakim R (2009) Anticoagulant and antiplatelet usage associates with mortality among hemodialysis patients. J Am Soc Nephrol 20:872–881

Crowther MA, Clase CM, Margetts PJ, Julian J, Lambert K, Sneath D, Nagai R, Wilson S, Ingrom AJ (2002) Low-intensity warfarin is ineffective for the prevention of PTFE graft failure in patients on hemodialysis: a randomized controlled trial. J Am Soc Nephrol 13: 2331–2337

Dember LM, Beck GJ, Allon M, Delmez JA, Dixon BS, Greenberg A, Himmelfarb J, Vazquez MA, Gassman JJ, Greene T, Raeva MK, Braden GL, Ikizler TA, Rocco MV, Davidson IJ, Kaufman JS, Meyers CM, Kusek JQ, Feldman HI (2008) Effect of clopidogrel on early failure of arteriovenous fistulas for hemodialysis: a randomized controlled trial. JAMA 299: 2164–2171

Dixon BS, Beck GJ, Dember LM, Vazquez MA, Greenberg A, Delmez JA, Allon M, Himmelfarb J, Hu B, Greene T, Radeva MK, Davidson IJ, Ikizler TA, Braden GL, Lawson JH, Cotton JR, Kusek JQ, Felman HI (2011) Use of aspirin associates with longer primary patency of hemodialysis grafts. J Am Soc Nephrol 22:773–781

Elliott MJ, Zimmerman D, Holden RM (2007) Warfarin anticoagulation in hemodialysis patients: a systematic review of bleeding rates. Am J Kidney Dis 50: 433–440

Kaufmann JA, O'Connor TZ, Zhang JH, Cronin RE, Fiore LD, Ganz MV, Goldfarb DS, Peduzzi PN (2003) Randomized controlled trial of clopidogrel plus aspirin to prevent hemodialysis access graft thrombosis. J Am Soc Nephrol 14:2313–2321

O'shea SI, Lawson JH, Reddan D, Murphy M, Ortel TL (2003) Hypercoagulable states and antithrombotic strategies in recurrent vascular access site thrombosis. J Vasc Surg 38:541–548

Osborn G, Escofet X, Da Silva A (2008) Medical adjuvant treatment to increase patency of arteriovenous fistulae and grafts. Cochrane Database Syst Rev (8):CD002786

Sreedhara R, Himmelfarb J, Lazarus JM, Hakim RM (1994) Anti-platelet therapy in graft thrombosis: results of a prospective, randomized, double-blind study. Kidney Int 45:1477–1483

Yevzlin AS, Conley EL, Sssanchez RJ, Young HN, Becker BN (2006) Vascular access outcomes and medication use: a USRDS study. Semin Dial 19:535–539

17 Puncture Techniques

In this chapter we discuss puncture sites, puncture techniques, how to remove cannulas, and the hemodynamic results of single-needle and double-needle dialysis. For a start we will look at morphological changes of the vessel wall after puncture.

17.1 Pathophysiology of the Punctured Vessel Wall

The walls of a vein and of a prosthesis are quite different.

17.1.1 Vein

From a biomechanical point of view, the essential structure of the venous wall is the tunica media, which mainly consists of elastic and muscle fibers. The fibers follow a spiral course with only a slight rise. They cross in a grid pattern. A puncture severs this pattern. At the puncture site, a circumscribed dilation of the wall occurs (Fig. 17.1). Thus narrow venous segments can be dilated intentionally by selective puncturing (Krönung 1984a, b). Apart from the severance of the fibers, the mechanically less resistant connective tissue, which fills the defect, is responsible for the dilation. Frequent punctures of a vein at a specific site will almost always lead to its aneurysmatic dilatation (Fig. 17.2).

17.1.2 ePTFE Prosthesis

The wall of an ePTFE prosthesis shows a nodulous fibrillary structure. Each puncture leaves a wall defect through which connective tissue proliferates into the lumen (Fig. 17.3). Frequent punctures close to each other may then cause stenoses of the prosthesis. Only extensive destruction of the wall structure may lead to aneurysms due to the reduced resistance of the scar tissue.

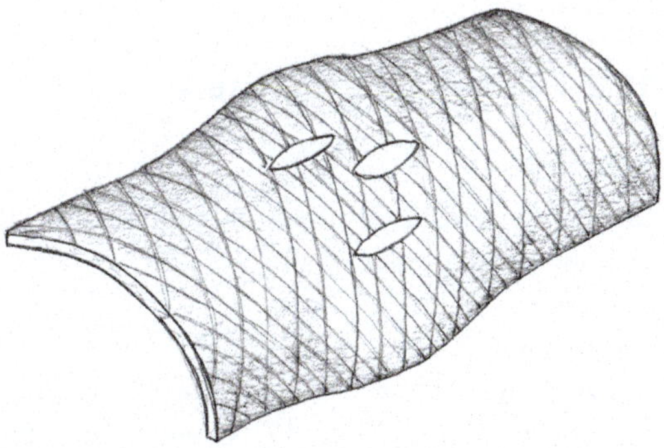

Fig. 17.1 Dilation of the venous wall caused by destruction of the wall structure

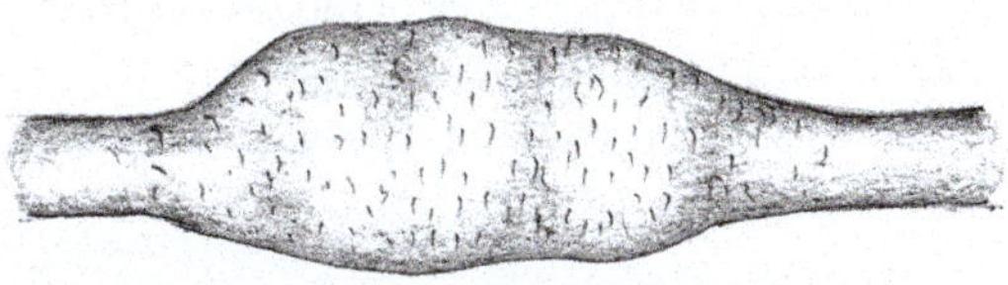

Fig. 17.2 Venous aneurysm of a frequently punctured venous segment

H. Scholz, *Arteriovenous Access Surgery*,
DOI 10.1007/978-3-642-41139-7_17, © Springer-Verlag Berlin Heidelberg New York 2015

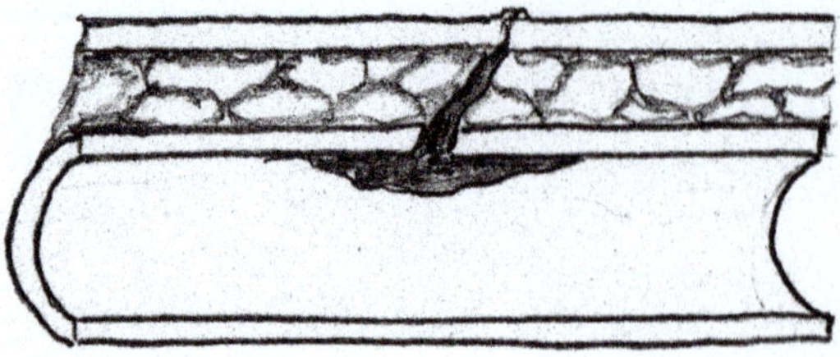

Fig. 17.3 Sprouting of connective tissue through a puncture site into the lumen of an ePTFE prosthesis

17.2 Puncture Site Selection

Basically there are three patterns of how puncture sites are distributed:

- Rope ladder puncture
- Area puncture
- Buttonhole puncture

The choice of puncture sites and their distribution should avoid unfavorable damage to the vessel.

The available puncturable surface of the vessel wall decisively determines the puncture pattern.

17.2.1 Rope Ladder Puncture

Principle
Regular systematic distribution of punctures all over the suitable vessel wall.

Indication
Long(ish) puncturable stretch. For the reasons mentioned above (Fig. 17.1) puncture sites should vary as much as possible as far as topography and time intervals are concerned. Thus the area used for punctures should include large portions of the total surface area of the AV vessel that may be used for punctures (Fig. 17.4).

These punctures should follow an individual pattern (e.g., Fig. 17.5).

17.2.2 Area Puncture

Principle
Even distribution of punctures across a limited area.

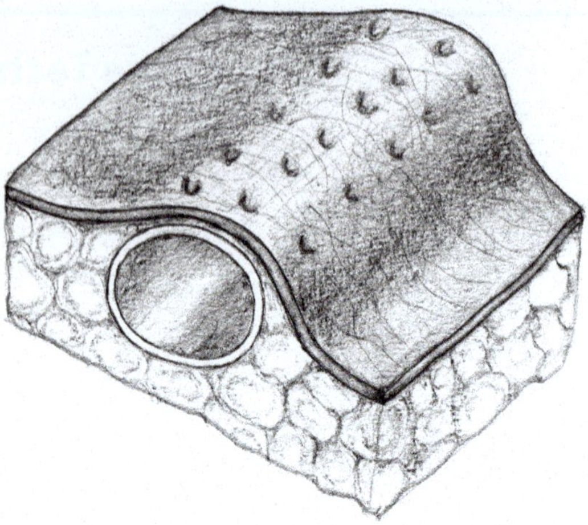

Fig. 17.4 Recommended puncture sites using the whole suited surface

Indication
Exclusive indications are:

- Only short puncturable segment
- Stenosed segment of an AV fistula

Intentional repetitive punctures of a stenosed segment may cause its dilation to allow for its future easier use. Area punctures very often lead to the dilation of the punctured segment.

17.2.3 Buttonhole Puncture

Principle
Punctures of always the exact same site. There are two distinct forms of buttonhole punctures.

Punctures of the Same Site Not Using a Long Subcutaneous Tunnel

We disapprove of this technique for theoretical and practical reasons.

Repetitive punctures of the exact same puncture canal without a long subcutaneous tunnel:

- Preclude the occlusion of the canal by connective tissue
- Widen the puncture canal (filled with thrombi and closed with slough) with each following puncture
- Eventually often lead to a localized inflammation and its possible progression up to a spontaneous perforation (Fig. 17.6a)

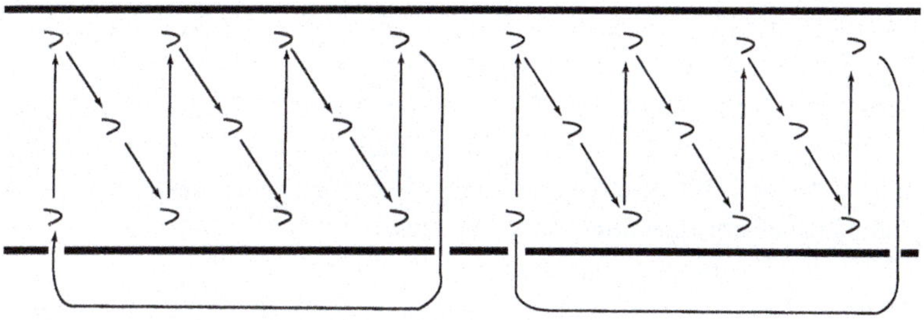

Fig. 17.5 Example for a puncture pattern

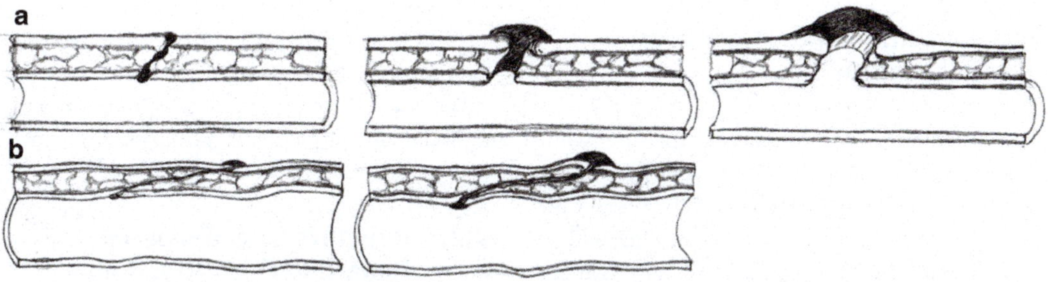

Fig. 17.6 (a) Increasing damage to the puncture site after multiple puncturing. (b) Buttonhole punctures. Creation of a long subcutaneous tunnel by repeated puncturing

Indication
In our opinion this technique is only justified under exceptional circumstances. Instead we recommend the speedy creation of a new vascular access if need be.

Punctures of the Same Site Using a Long Subcutaneous Tunnel

Under special circumstances the conscious systematic puncturing of the exact same site with a long subcutaneous tunnel is chosen.

Principle
- Creation of a single subcutaneous tunnel by repeated punctures with sharp cannulas over a 3–4-week period (Fig. 17.6b).
- Following a routine with:
  (a) Sufficiently long time for disinfection of the puncture site (several minutes).
  (b) Removal of scab with sterile instruments and repeat long disinfection.
  (c) Puncture vessel via the formed track using a (less sharp) blunt cannula.

Indication
Only limited cannulation sites of an AV fistula with sufficient subcutaneous cover.

Contraindication
Alloplastic material (prosthetic AV shunts).

Requirement
Specially trained and motivated staff.

Evaluation
No personal experience. Plausible good results in specialized centers.

17.3 Puncture Technique

Four factors characterize puncture techniques:
- The angle of insertion, which also determines the length of the subcutaneous tunnel
- The position of the cannula's aperture
- The way a cannula is inserted into the vessel
- The direction of puncture in relation to the flow direction

17.3.1 Angle of Insertion

In order to prevent infections, and for better hemostasis, we recommend a subcutaneous tunnel which is as long as possible. Therefore the angle of insertion should be as acute as possible. For this purpose the cannula needs to be sufficiently long (usual available lengths 5–25 mm with 5-mm intervals). The sketch in Fig. 17.7, which was drawn to scale, shows that only an adequately long cannula can create a long subcutaneous tunnel. The internal resistance of a long cannula is higher, though.

17.3.2 Position of the Cannula's Aperture

The orientation of the cannula aperture while puncturing (either to or from the lumen of the vessel) determines the V-shaped incision of the vessel wall. If the aperture faces the lumen, the flap will be pushed into the lumen and will later seal the defect from the inside after the cannula's removal (Fig. 17.8b). Conversely, with the aperture looking away from the lumen, the V-shaped incision is pushed out (Fig. 17.8a). Clinical experience confirms these theoretical considerations.

Fig. 17.7 Scale drawing of 5–25 mm cannulas (5 mm steps). Angle necessary for puncture dependent on cannula length

17.3.3 Vascular Puncture

The puncture of a vessel should involve these steps:

- Pierce the skin (Fig. 17.9a).
- Advance the cannula through the subcutaneous tissue to the vessel at a small angle thus forming a subcutaneous tunnel (Fig. 17.9b).
- Insert the cannula into the vessel at a larger angle.
- Complete placement of the cannula in the vessel at a small angle, and then secure the cannula needle (Fig. 17.9c).

The choice of an angle which is too large might damage or pierce the posterior vessel wall.

17.3.4 Puncture Direction with Regard to Flow Direction

The puncture direction should follow the flow direction.

17.4 Removal of the Cannula

Frequently we observe lengthwise lesions of the posterior access wall.

They may be caused by:

- Compression of the puncture site while the cannula is still in place

Fig. 17.8 (**a**, **b**) Shape of the punch defect depending on cannula orientation

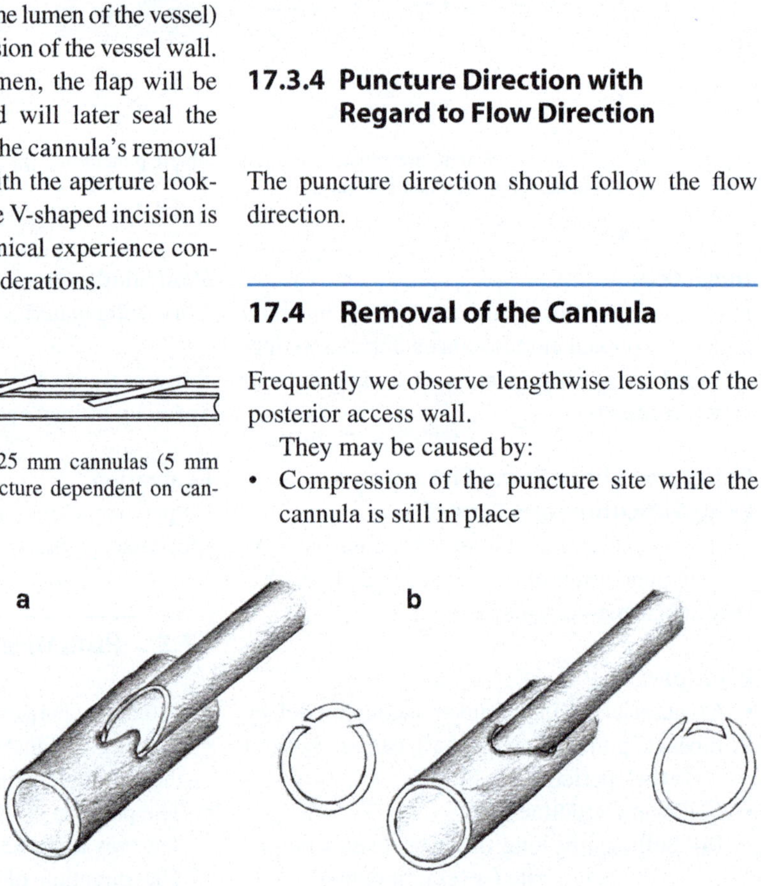

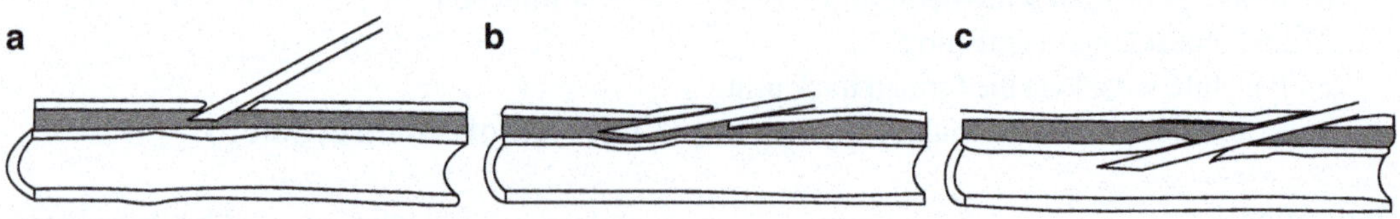

Fig. 17.9 (**a**–**c**) Steps of vascular puncture

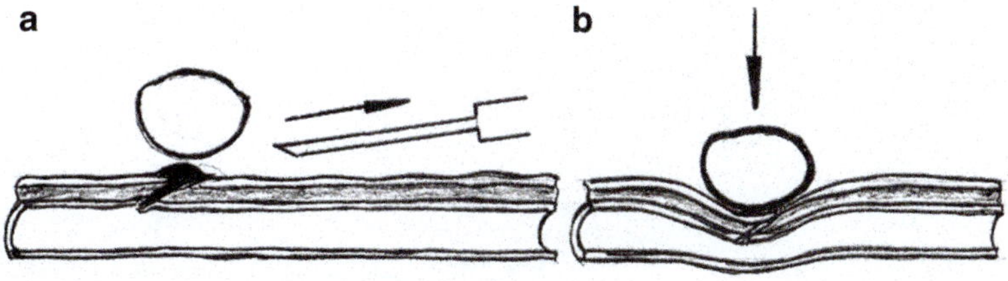

Fig. 17.10 Removal of the cannula. (**a**) Small angle for withdrawal of the needle. (**b**) Compression of the puncture site only after removal of the cannula

- Removal of the cannula at an angle which is too large

  They can safely be avoided by:
- Using a flat angle to withdraw the cannula (Fig. 17.10a)
- Compression of the puncture site only after the cannula has been removed (Fig. 17.10b)

  Compression should not be stronger than necessary to stop bleeding so that the thrill is still palpable.

17.5 Influence of Single-Needle Dialysis on the Hemodynamics of the Venous Anastomosis

With single-needle (SN)-dialysis, only one needle is inserted into the vascular access. A Y-shaped adaptor connects both the arterial and the venous sides to the cannula, which serves for blood removal as well as for blood return. There are two dialysis phases: during the *arterial* phase blood from the patient will be pumped into the dialyzer, which is subsequently returned during the *venous* phase.

Some dialysis units use this technique not only if an access is unsuitable for double needle puncture but also as a routine alternative concept (Trakarnvanich et al. 2007; Wilson et al. 2009; Rostoker et al. 2009; Breuch et König 2008). We discuss the influence on hemodynamics in the vascular anastomosis below.

A drop in blood flow in the venous anastomosis of an AV shunt during the arterial phase and its rise during the venous phase are typical for SN dialysis (Fig. 17.11).

If, for example, the flow of the dialyzer were set to a usual mean rate of 200 mL/min and both phases each continued for 30 s (assumed settings for easier illustration), the flow in the venous anastomosis would drop by 400 mL/min during the arterial phase and would rise by 400 mL/min during the venous phase.

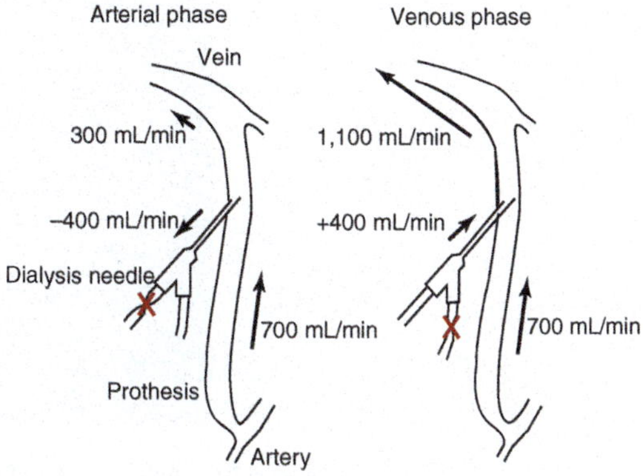

Fig. 17.11 Phases of SN-dialysis. *Arterial phase*: in this example, the flow in the anastomosis is reduced by 400 mL/min. *Venous phase*: the flow in the anastomosis is increased by 400 L/min

If 200 mL have to pass through the dialyzer and there is only 30 s available, during this time the flow needs to rise to 400 mL/min. The same fluid volume then needs to be returned during the second 30 s.

In the literature you can find recommendations to increase venous blood flow settings for up to 20 %, and for up to 50 % with poor shunt flow so as to shorten blood return in favor of the arterial phase (Breuch and König 2008). The differences of the anastomotic flow rates in both phases would thus be enhanced.

17.5.1 Investigations in the Circular Flow System

We compared SN dialysis with double-needle (DN) dialysis in a circular flow model. For this purpose we created the silicone perfusion model of an AV shunt (Fig. 17.12a) with a simulated arterial anastomosis, an interposition graft,

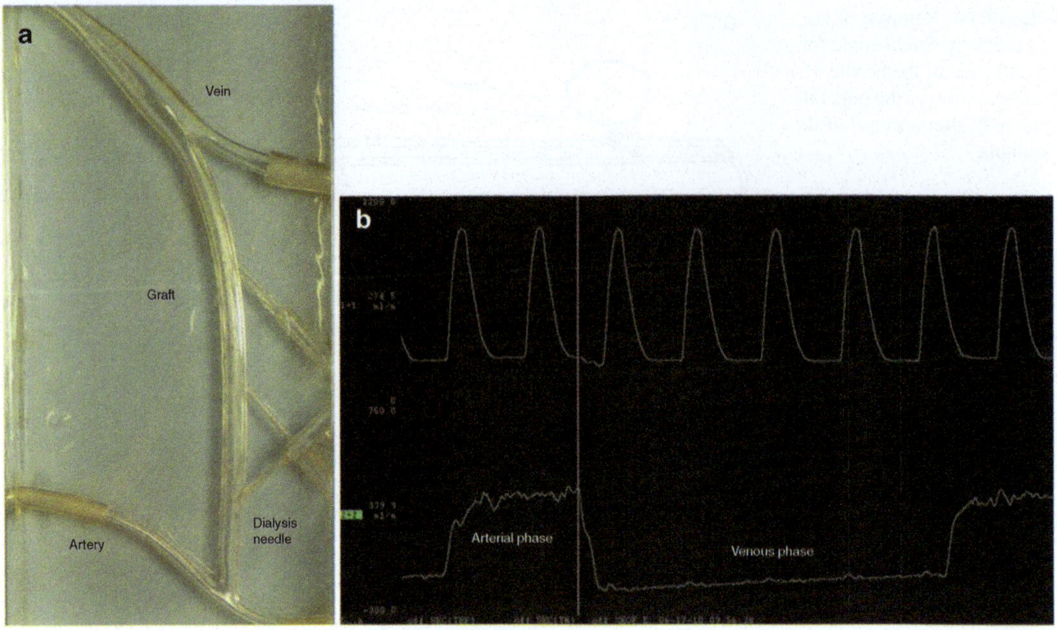

Fig. 17.12 (**a**) Model of a shunt with arterial anastomosis, graft, and venous patch anastomosis. The graft has openings for placing dialysis needles. (**b**) Screenshot from the SN-simulation in the pulsatile flow system. The *upper curve* shows the pulsatile flow in the shunt. The *lower curve* shows the flow in the dialysis needle during the arterial and venous phases

and a patchless venous anastomosis. We left three canals for the insertion of dialysis cannulas. Dye injections made the flow in the venous anastomosis visible.

Single Needle-Dialysis

During the arterial phase there was a backflow from the venous anastomosis into the dialysis needle. The two curves in Fig. 17.12b were gained from the flow system in SN mode. The upper curve depicts flow pulsations in the shunt, whereas the lower curve depicts the flow in the dialysis needle. During diastole the shunt flow falls below the needle flow (275 mL/min vs 340 mL/min, vertical line). This proves the *retrograde* flow in the venous anastomosis. The venous phase is markedly prolonged in our experimental setting, as the dialyzer had no pump on the venous side. Therefore the venous flow rate was also lower than in real life, when both pump-controlled phases are of around equal length (Breuch and König 2008).

Double Needle-Dialysis

With normal flow rates, the flow patterns in the venous anastomosis correspond to those observed without dialysis (Figs. 4.9 and 4.10).

17.5.2 Numerical Simulation

For the numerical simulations the following inflow boundary conditions were chosen:

- Entry of prosthesis: pulsatile flow rate, systolic 1,500 mL/min (*Re* 1,389), mean 700 mL/min (*Re* 648).
- Entry of needle: constant flow rates of −400 mL/min during the arterial phase, and +400 mL/min during the venous phase, respectively.

For these calculations a conventional terminolateral venous model anastomosis without patch was chosen in order to stress the differences between the two phases. Results are summarized in Figs. 17.13, 17.14, 17.15, and 17.16.

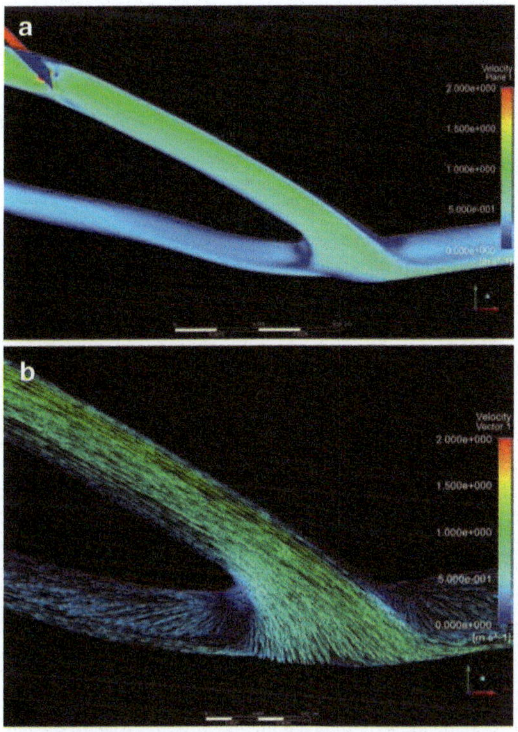

Fig. 17.13 Arterial phase of SN-dialysis. (**a**) Velocity distribution at systolic flow maximum. (**b**) Velocity vectors at systolic flow maximum

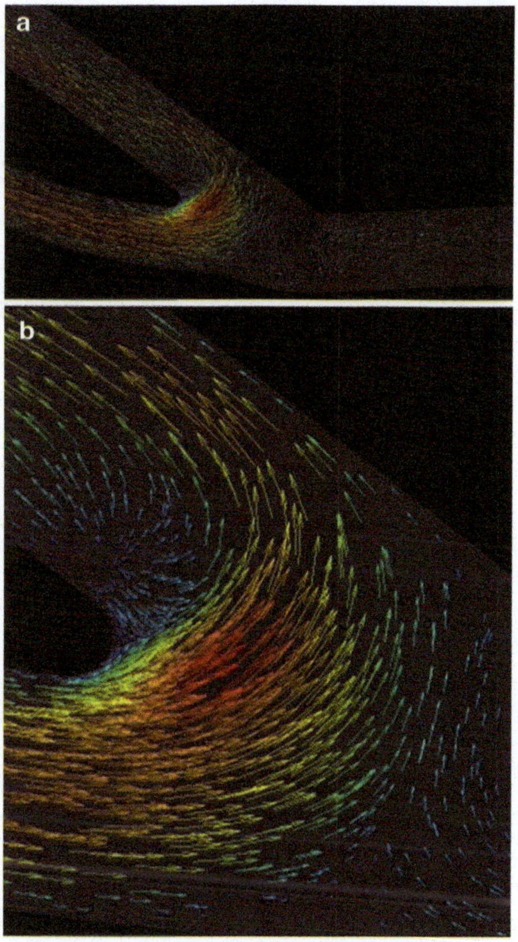

Fig. 17.15 Arterial phase of SN-dialysis. (**a**) Velocity vectors during late diastole. Almost all over the anastomosis, flow is retrograde. (**b**) Detail of (**a**)

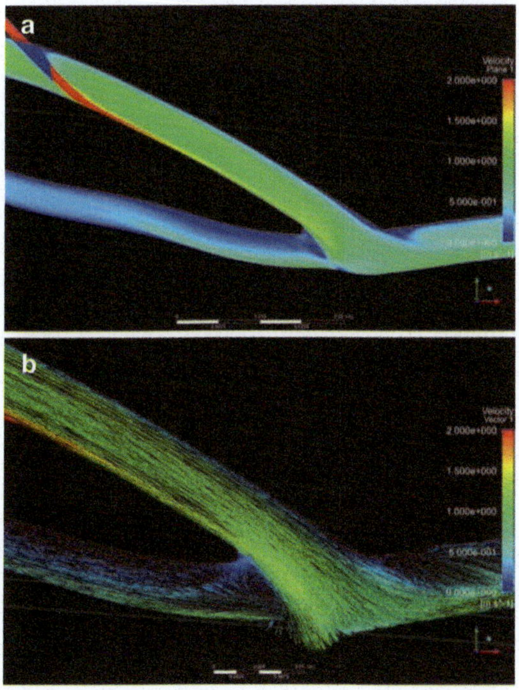

Fig. 17.14 Venous phase of SN-dialysis. (**a**) Velocity distribution at systolic flow maximum. (**b**) Velocity vectors at systolic flow maximum

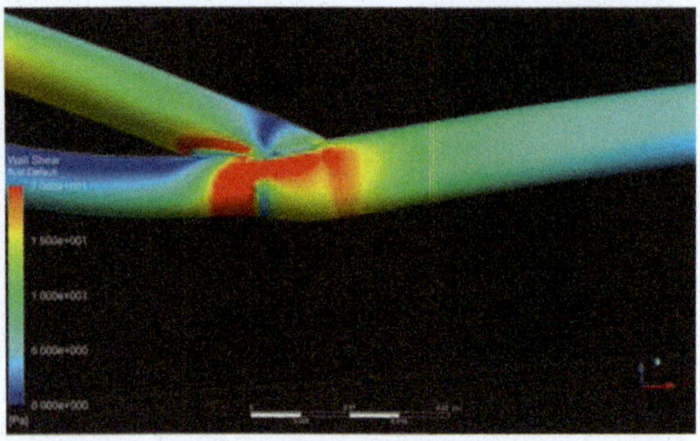

Fig. 17.16 Venous phase of SN-dialysis: wall shear stress at systolic flow maximum

Velocity Distribution and Vectors

Arterial phase, systolic maximum (Fig. 17.13a, b):

- High velocities at the outer wall of the prosthesis
- Flow separation in the proximal vein
- Small vortex in the distal vein

Venous phase, systolic maximum (Fig. 17.14a,b):

- High velocities at the inner side of the prosthesis
- Pronounced impact of the flow on the venous wall
- Large vortex in the distal vein during the entire cardiac cycle

Arterial phase, late diastole (Fig. 17.15):

- Retrograde flow almost over the whole anastomosis. The stationary flow in the needle is higher than the late diastolic inflow into the prosthesis.

Wall Shear Stress

Venous phase, systolic maximum (Fig. 17.16):

- The mean of the wall shear stress is twice as high as during the arterial phase.

17.5.3 Results and Conclusions

SN dialysis reinforces flow disturbances in the venous anastomosis due to:

- Marked differences of the flow rates in the venous anastomosis during the arterial and venous phase of the dialyzer
- Flow reversal (recirculation) during the arterial phase

This increase of already unphysiological flow patterns in the venous anastomosis leads to an additional irritation of the venous wall.

Single-needle dialysis should only be used under exceptional circumstances.

Literature

Breuch G, König J (2008) Die single-needle-dialyse. Spektrum der nephrologischen Pflege 7:13–23

Chow J, Rayment G, San Miguel S, Gilbert M (2011) A randomised controlled trial of buttonhole cannulation for the prevention of fistula access complications. J Ren Care 37:85–93

Delorme JM, Guidoin R, Canizales S, Charara J, How T, Marois Y, Batt M, Hallade P, Ricci M, Picetti C (1992) Vascular access for hemodialysis: pathologic features of surgically excised ePTFE grafts. Ann Vasc Surg 6:517–524

Dias TS, Moysés Neto M, da Costa JA (2008) Arteriovenous fistula puncture: an essential factor for hemodialysis efficiency. Ren Fail 30:870–876

Hashmi A, Cheema MQ, Moss AH (2010) Hemodialysis patients' experience with and attitudes toward the buttonhole technique for arteriovenous fistula cannulation. Clin Nephrol 74:346–350

Hsiao JF, Chou HH, Hsu LA, Wu LS, Yang CW, Hsu TS, Chang CJ (2010) Vascular changes at the puncture segments of arterivenous fistula for hemodialyis access. J Vasc Surg 52:669–673

Krönung G (1984a) Die Punktion der CIMINO-Fistel. Dial Jour 9:2–10

Krönung G (1984b) Plastic deformation of cimino fistula by repeated puncture. Dial Transplant 13:635–638

Labriola L, Crott R, Desmet C, André G, Jadoul M (2011) Infectious complications following conversion to buttonhole cannulation of arteriovenous fistulas: a quality improvement report. Am J Kidney Dis 57:442–448

Ludlow V (2010) Buttonhole cannulation in hemodialysis: improved outcomes and increased expense – is it worth it? CANNT J 20:29–37

Rostoker G, Griuncelli M, Loridon C, Bourlet T, Welsch K, Benmaadi A (2009) Improving the efficiency of short-term single-needle hemodialysis. Ren Fail 31: 261–266

Toma S, Shinzato T, Fukui H, Nakai S, Miwa M, Takai I, Maeda K (2003) A timesaving method to create a fixed puncture route for the buttonhole technique. Nephrol Dial Transplant 18:2118–2121

Trakarnvanich T, Chirananthavat T, Maneerat P, Chabsuwan S, Areeyakulnimit S (2007) Is single-needle hemodialysis still a good treatment in end-stage renal disease? Blood Purif 25:490–496

van Loon MM, Goovaerts T, Kessels AG, van der Sande FM, Tordoir JH (2010) Buttonhole needling of haemodialysis arteriovenous fistulae results in less complications and interventions compared to the rope-ladder technique. Nephrol Dial Transplant 25: 225–230

Verhallen AM, Kooistra MP, van Jaarsveld BC (2007) Cannulating in haemodialysis: rope-ladder or button-hole technique? Nephrol Dial Transplant 22: 2601–2604

Wilson B, Harwood L, Thompson B (2009) Impact of single-needle therapy in new chronic hemodialysis starts for individuals with arteriovenous fistulae. CANNT J 19:23–28

18 Monitoring of Vascular Accesses

An AV vascular access undergoes morphologic and functional changes. These may exert local or systemic influences on the whole organism and entail serious complications. Most complications are not unexpected but may be anticipated much earlier. Therefore continuous monitoring during dialysis treatment is advisable. For this purpose no undue extra effort is necessary.

18.1 History

The patient should explicitly be asked for the following complaints and be examined for the following abnormalities:

- Pain of the extremity distal to the AV anastomosis (reduced peripheral perfusion?)
- Edema of the shunt extremity (venous congestion?)
- Exercise-induced dyspnoea or palpitations (cardiac strain due to shunt flow?)
- Fatigue/vertigo with AV accesses of the upper extremity (occlusion of the subclavian artery with subclavian steal syndrome?)
- Signs of pathologic recirculation/ineffective dialysis

18.2 Inspection

The inspection of a vascular access and its surroundings does not require any relevant additional time. The following particularities are of special interest:

- Edema (lymphatic? venous congestion? perigraft seroma?)
- Inflammatory erythema (infection?)
- Dilated veins central to the AV access (central venous stenosis?)
- Bright red reticular veins (retrograde venous arterialization?)
- Pallor distal to the AV anastomosis (reduced peripheral perfusion? capillary refill?)
- Aneurysms
- State of puncture sites

18.3 Palpation

Palpation allows for statements on:

- Function of an AV access
- Vascular morphology

Palpation helps evaluate:

- Character of the thrill
- Pulsatility
- Pressure

Based on these findings, the flow rate, the arterial inflow, and the venous outflow may be determined qualitatively.

The thrill originates in the anastomosis and in the adjacent segment of the AV vessel. It is caused by high frequency vorteces. Pressure changes are transmitted along the vascular wall. The thrill occurs when there is inflow of blood under high pressure (artery) into a wide-lumen low pressure vessel (vein or prosthesis). The higher the absolute blood pressure and the pressure gradients, the more pronounced the thrill.

H. Scholz, *Arteriovenous Access Surgery*,
DOI 10.1007/978-3-642-41139-7_18, © Springer-Verlag Berlin Heidelberg New York 2015

There is also a superposition of the pulsatile flow. Frequency and amplitude influence the thrill. The intensity of the thrill decreases with the distance from the AV anastomosis. Often the thrill is also transmitted into the feeding artery. This phenomenon can be observed distally more often than proximally. The following palpation technique has proven useful: The long fingers II–IV are gently placed side by side on the vessel. Thus a two-dimensional impression of the flow character may be gained.

18.3.1 Findings on Palpation for Flow Evaluation

Optimal Flow Characteristics

Conditions: sufficient inflow and outflow.

Palpation (Fig. 18.1a): strong, pulse-synchronous thrill.

Insufficient Arterial Inflow

Conditions: insufficient arterial inflow, low venous outflow resistance:

- Central arterial stenosis?
- Narrow feeding artery?
- Narrow anastomosis?
- Hypotension?

Palpation (Fig. 18.1b): attenuated, exclusively systolic thrill with low pulsatility

Insufficient Venous Outflow

Conditions: sufficient arterial inflow, high venous outflow resistance:

- Stenosis of the efferent vein?
- Central venous stenosis?
- Stenosis of the venous anastomosis with AV prosthetic grafts?

Palpation (Fig. 18.1c): strong pulsation with discrete systolic thrill

Stenosis Along the AV Access

Conditions: sufficient arterial inflow, low venous outflow resistance, stenosis of the AV vessel.

Palpation:

- Upstream from the stenosis: strong pulsations with low systolic thrill
- Stenosis: strong pulsation without thrill
- Downstream from the stenosis: strong pulse-synchronous thrill with attenuated pulse (Fig. 18.2)

Narrow AV Access Vein or Graft

Conditions: sufficient arterial inflow and narrow lumen of the AV vessel over a long segment.

Palpation: pulsation with only discrete thrill.

18.3.2 Clinical Tests Using Palpation

The following screening tests are most valid with wide lumen and superficial AV fistulas.

Arterial Inflow

After the (temporary) occlusion of the arterial anastomosis by manual compression and emptying the AV vessel in the central direction with the other hand, keep compressing he vein to avoid backflow. Upon the sudden release of the inflow, the time needed for refilling is determined. With a high inflow the vessel will fill immediately.

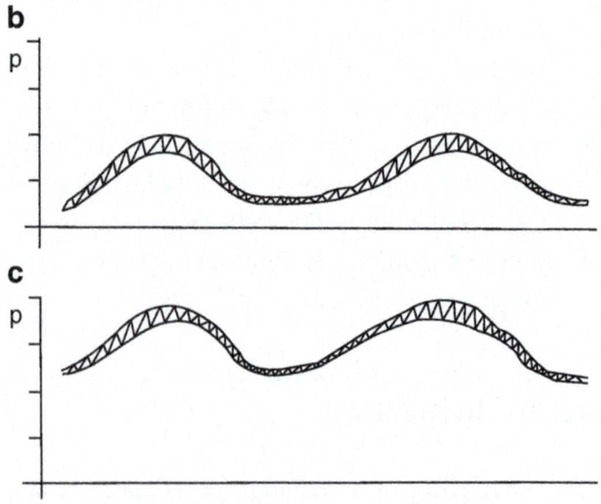

Fig. 18.1 Findings on palpation. (**a**) Optimal flow characteristics. (**b**) Low arterial inflow. (**c**) Disturbed venous outflow

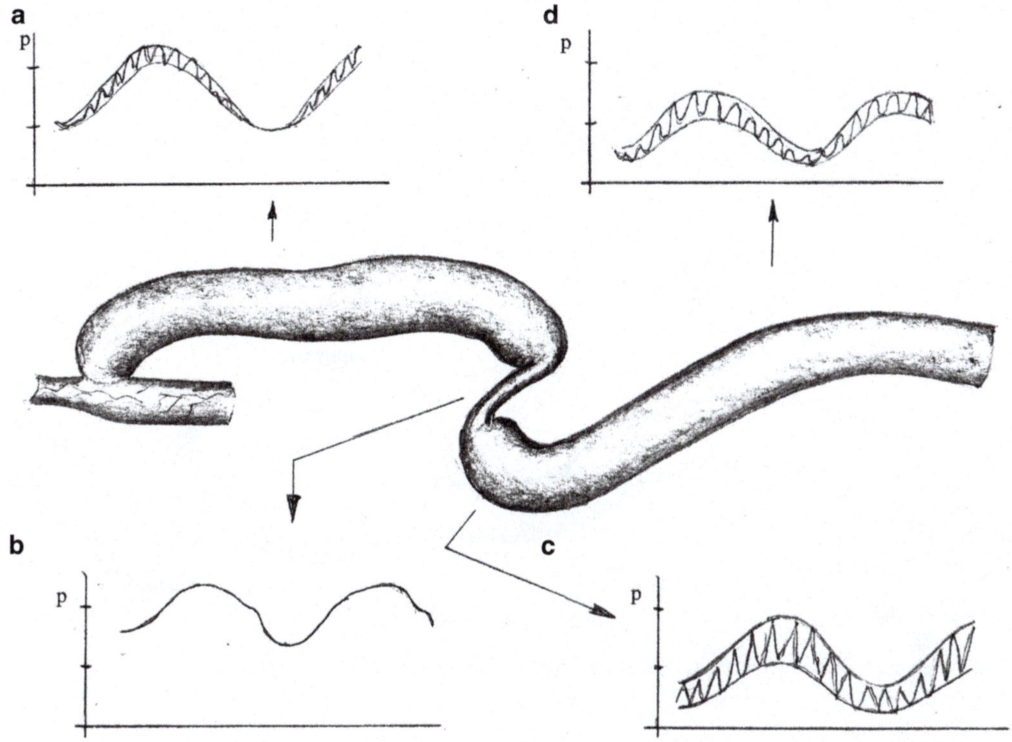

Fig. 18.2 Findings on palpation with stenosis in the AV vessel. (**a**) Pulsations with only slight systolic thrill. (**b**) Strong pulsations without thrill. (**c**) Strong thrill in sync with the pulsations. (**d**) Decrease of the thrill with increasing distance

Venous Resistance

There are two options:

- After the occlusion of the arterial inflow by manual compression, the other hand feels the pressure needed to empty the vein in the central direction. Unless there is an obstructed outflow path, hardly any resistance can be felt.
- For upper extremity access the arm of the supine patient is raised. With an unimpaired venous outflow path and an arterial inflow that is not too high, there will be a pulse-synchronous collapse of the AV vessel during diastole.

Estimation of the Flow Rate

The procedure is the same as described above with temporary occlusion of the arterial inflow and manual emptying of the vein. Additionally, you need to estimate the volume of the emptied vascular segment. The flow rate can then be derived from the time that is required until it is full again. This only works if the venous outflow is not obstructed. Furthermore, the current blood pressure has to be taken into account. This method ideally allows for approximations which are within 30 % of the results of duplex sonography studies.

18.3.3 Evaluation of Vascular Morphology

With a superficial path the vascular morphology of the AV access may well be assessed by its palpation. The intravascular pressure can be evaluated by the wall tension.

According to LaPlace's law,

$$T = p \times r$$

The wall tension T is proportional to the radius r and the pressure p. In an arterialized vein with a

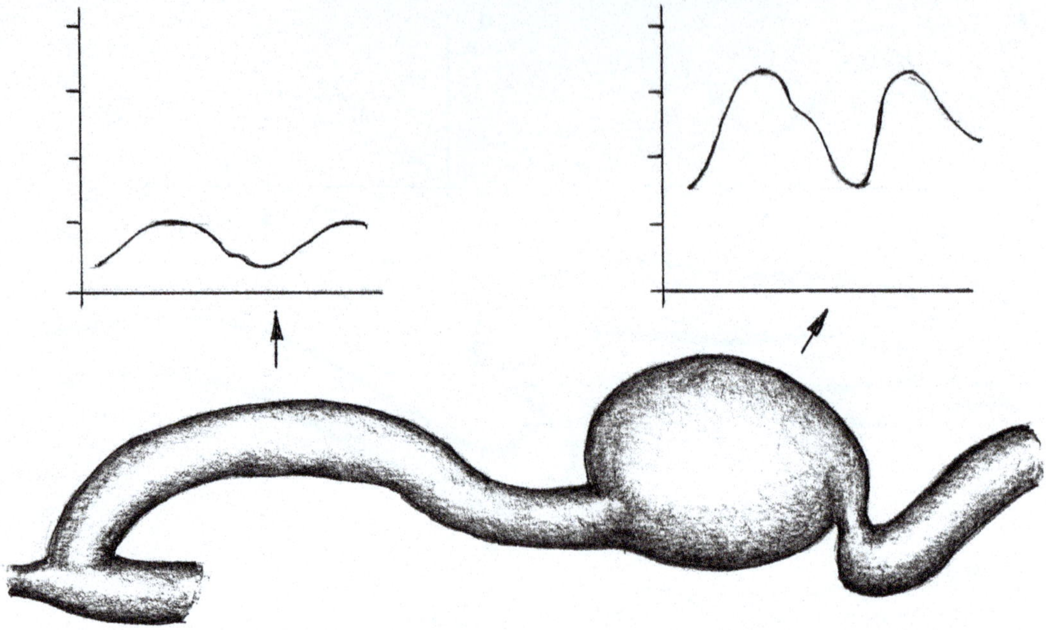

Fig. 18.3 Perceived pressure. Different impression on palpation for same intraluminal pressure

7-mm diameter that also has a 28-mm aneurysm, the tension of the aneurysmatic wall is four times higher than that of the nonaneurysmatic segment. Therefore the palpation of the aneurysmatic segment alone might make you suspect a much higher intraluminal pressure also in the non-aneurymatic part if you were not aware of LaPlace's law (Fig. 18.3). Thus you might erroneously think of a downstream stenosis.

18.4 Auscultation

Turbulence of the blood entering the venous low pressure system causes bruits. They are the acoustic equivalent of the palpable thrill. The faster the blood flow the higher the frequency and the sound volume.

- A pulse-synchronous bruit is typical for *a well-functioning AV access*. Frequency and pulsatility decrease with the distance from the anastomosis (Fig. 18.4).
- *Stenoses* cause early systolic, loud, high frequency bruits.
- A soft, less pulsatile bruit characterizes *a low flow* caused by a low arterial inflow or a high venous outflow resistance.

Should palpation prove unsatisfactory due to a low flow or a deep position of the vessel, auscultation may still provide useful information.

18.5 Tests During Dialysis

For optimal dialysis the concentration gradient of the substances which need to be eliminated should be high. This can only be achieved if enough blood enters the dialyzer and is returned to the venous system. If the blood which is returned from the dialyzer mixes with the arterial blood that still has to enter the dialyzer, there is recirculation. Detoxification may be insufficient. The most frequent cause of recirculation is a malfunction of the AV access due to a reduced shunt flow, so that a portion of the already purified blood is drawn into the dialyzer again. Different parameters, which can be registered during dialysis, indicate this difficulty.

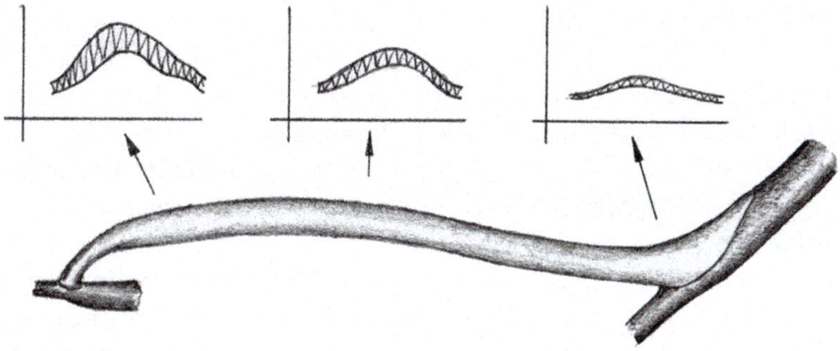

Fig. 18.4 Findings on auscultation depending on the distance to the arterial anastomosis. Sound volume and pulsatility decrease

18.5.1 Pressure Surveillance During Dialysis

During dialysis the "arterial" and "venous" pressure are continuously monitored in the machine. The "arterial" pressure means the pressure in the system leading to the dialyzer. The knowledge of these readings can be used as shown below:

- A decrease of the *"arterial" pressure* results from a reduced arterial inflow into the AV access which may lead to recirculation.
- An increase of the *"venous" pressure* is caused by an impaired venous drainage, which may also cause recirculation.

18.5.2 Elimination of Urea

The determination of the concentration of urea before and after dialysis and the (dimensionless) $K \times t/V$ allow for an evaluation of the effectiveness of dialysis (Daugirdas 1993; Gotch 2000). K denotes the urea clearance by dialysis (mL/min), t the length of dialysis (min), and V the volume of distribution of urea (mL). Thus it may also indicate the malfunction of a dialysis access (e.g., recirculation with an insufficient shunt flow).

18.5.3 Determination of Recirculation

Some dialyzers directly state recirculation with only small aberrations (thermosensor).

18.6 Further Investigations

With all unclear pathological findings the flow in the AV access should be evaluated by duplex ultrasonography and additional angiography if indicated. We recommend ultrasound investigations twice a year so as to:

- Recognize a critical decline in flow to initiate further investigations and therapy in time.
- Recognize high flow with resultant cardiac excess strain to initiate flow reduction in time.

18.6.1 Duplex Sonography

Flow Measurements

Whirls/turbulence may lead to faulty flow readings over the AV access. The most exact readings can be seen by examining the artery proximal and distal to the anastomosis. Frequently the distal artery also contributes to the flow in the access.

Evaluation of Freshly-Implanted ePTFE Prostheses

The wall of an ePTFE prosthesis shows a nodulous fibrillary structure with air-filled gaps, which fill with fluid within 2–3 days. As the air in the gaps impedes sound wave transmission, ultrasound examinations are not reliable during the first 2 postoperative days. The occlusion of a shunt may then be wrongly assumed.

18.6.2 Angiography

To avoid misinterpretations and to achieve best results, the following rules should be observed.

Position of the Arm During Angiography

- The arm abduction angle should be at least 45°. If the arm touches the thorax wall, especially in obese patients, axillary veins may be compressed. Artificial stenoses might then be seen on the images.
- The forearm should be in a supine position (external rotation). This facilitates the topographic evaluation without venous superpositions.

Injection into the AV Access

If you suspect a stenosis of the outflow path, it can only be safely visualized by a contrast medium injection directly into the AV access. An injection into a neighboring vein or a peripheral vein will not be sufficient.

Paying Attention to the Respiratory Phase

During expiration a flow of contrast medium into the side branches of the axillary and subclavian veins may frequently be observed. During inspiration this can be followed by a fast, centrally-directed outflow. If only the expiration images are examined, a non-existing stenosis might be wrongly diagnosed. A large enough number of images (two per second) is required.

Arterial Imaging

The compression of the AV access central to the injection site allows for a depiction of the AV anastomosis as well as the arterial periphery. With a sufficiently high flow of the contrast medium, the afferent artery may also be shown.

18.7 Documentation

All our patients receive a “shunt brochure” as a handout with a sketch of their individual access and important findings. Additional information is stored in the in-house data management system.

Literature

Besarab A, Asif A, Roy-Chaudhury P, Spergel LM, Ravani P (2007) The native arteriovenous fistula in 2007 surveillance and monitoring. J Nephrol 20:656–667

Daugirdas JT (1993) Second generation logarithmic estimates of single-pool variable volume Kt/V: an analysis of error. J Am Soc Nephrol 4:1205–1213

Gotch FA (2000) Kt/V is the best dialysis dose parameter. Blood Purif 18:276–285

Henry ML (2006) Routine surveillance in vascular access for hemodialysis. Eur J Vasc Endovasc Surg 32:545–548

19 Histopathology of AV Vascular Accesses

19.1 Introduction

Stenosis, thrombosis, and aneurysmatic dilatation are the most frequent postoperative complications in vascular access surgery. Microscopic analysis of resected specimens or small biopsies can help explain the exact etiology of these complications (Janzen 2005, 2010).

The surgeon should communicate whether the histopathological specimen consists of:

- The wall of the native vein.
- The wall of the arterialized vein which has been dissected for the creation of the original vascular access.
- The wall of a vein which had not been touched previously for its in situ arterialization.
- The hypertrophic wall of a vein at a puncture site.
- The hypertrophic and dilated wall of a vein which has not been exposed during former surgery (Krönung 2008).

Exact specifications of the site from which the specimen has been taken, type of prosthesis, and the patient's history may help the vascular pathologist find the diagnosis. As for light microscopy, the arterialized vein of a fistula shows an irregular fibrosis of the tunica media, a newly-formed respectively double internal elastic membrane, and hypertrophy/hyperplasia of the smooth muscle cells of the tunica media (Figs. 19.1 and 19.2). In rare cases myocytic hyperplasia is a precursor of fibromuscular dysplasia in the tunica media.

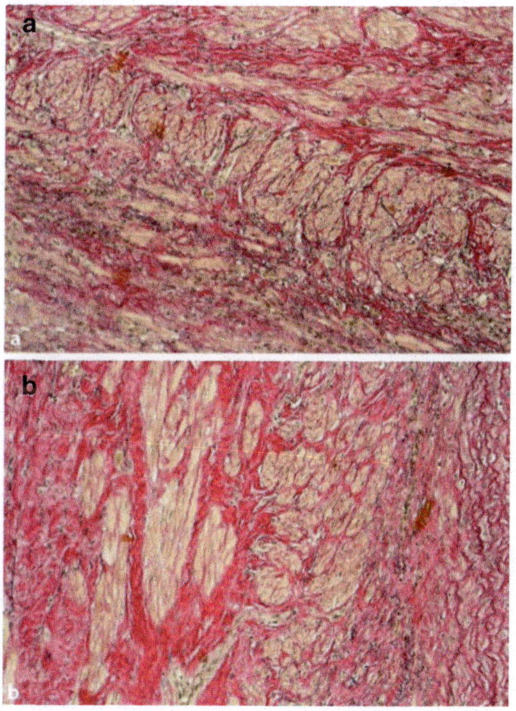

Fig. 19.1 Arterialized vein of a cephalic fistula with myocytic hyperplasia/hypertrophy. (**a**) With irregular media fibrosis. (**b**) Elastica van Gieson (EVG) stain, ×200

19.2 Stenosis

The histomorphologic spectrum of the underlying changes of fistulas is heterogenous. Non-atherosclerotic causes dominate. In clinical jargon, stenosis is generally referred to as neointima. However, an exact histopathologic analysis shows

H. Scholz, *Arteriovenous Access Surgery*,
DOI 10.1007/978-3-642-41139-7_19, © Springer-Verlag Berlin Heidelberg New York 2015

a far more detailed picture. The intraoperative finding of an "inflammatory" shrinking (Fig. 19.3), for instance, does not describe a genuine inflammatory process, but mostly an intimal hyperplasia. This can be divided into three subtypes – neointimal, fibrotic, and combined intimal hyperplasia (Figs. 19.4, 19.5, and 19.6) (Janzen and Mickley 2006).

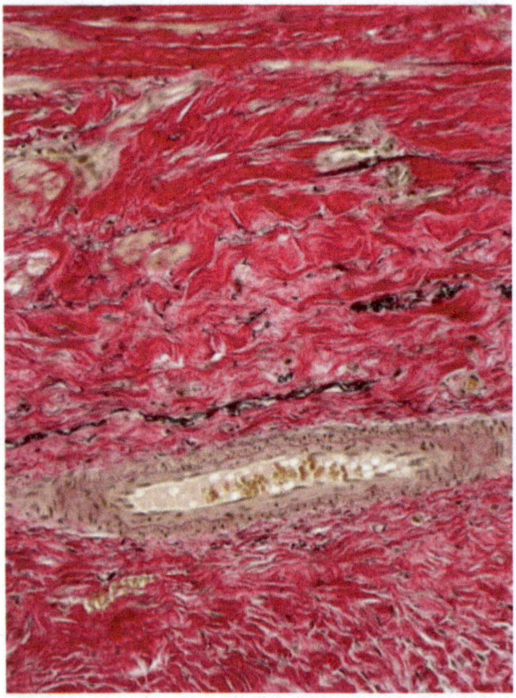

Fig. 19.2 Newly-formed internal elastic membrane (*black in the middle*) in arterialized fistula vein, EVG stain, ×200

The pathologic alterations are located in the subendothelial stratum of the tunica intima. Therefore we prefer subendothelial intimal hyperplasia (SIH) to intimal hyperplasia (IH). SIH is one of the main causes for stenosis formation.

The neointimal SIH consists of myofibroblasts arranged in a star-shaped pattern, fibroblasts, fibrocytes, and a pale eosinophilic matrix. Overlying endothelium shows enlarged nuclei as a sign of increased metabolic activity. Their development mainly seems to be favored by local hemodynamic factors such as altered wall shear stress and oscillating forces (Haruguchi and Teraoka 2003; Sivanesan et al. 1999). Specific immune markers (calponin, actin, smooth muscle actin, desmin, vimentin, etc.) help distinguish between the different cell types of the neointima (Fig. 19.7). In IH increased cell proliferation and apoptosis (oncoprotein bcl-2), raised growth factors, an overexpression of Bax proteins/Bax mRNA, and a significant correlation between the extent of a stenosis and bcl-2-positive areas can be seen (Rekhter et al. 1993; Hayakawa et al. 1999; Weiss et al. 2001). Furthermore, arterial as well as venous forms of IH have been postulated. Kim et al. (2004) assumed a different biological behavior of vascular smooth muscle cells. Others claim that the following criteria have to be fulfilled for a venous IH:

- Migration and proliferation of vascular smooth muscle cells and myofibroblasts
- Initiation of angiogenesis
- Foreign body reaction in vascular prosthetic grafts

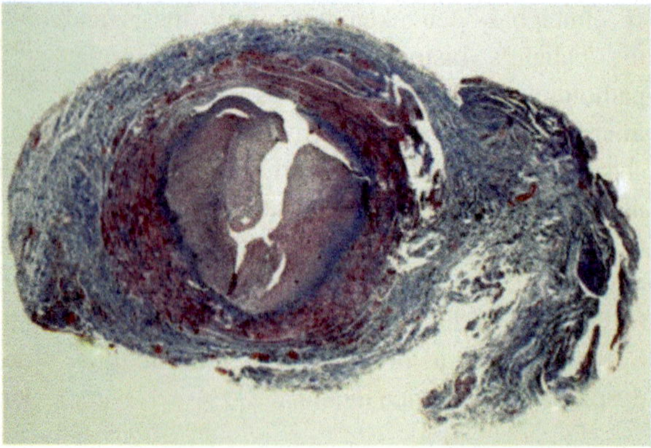

Fig. 19.3 Shrunk fistula vein, MTC stain, ×200

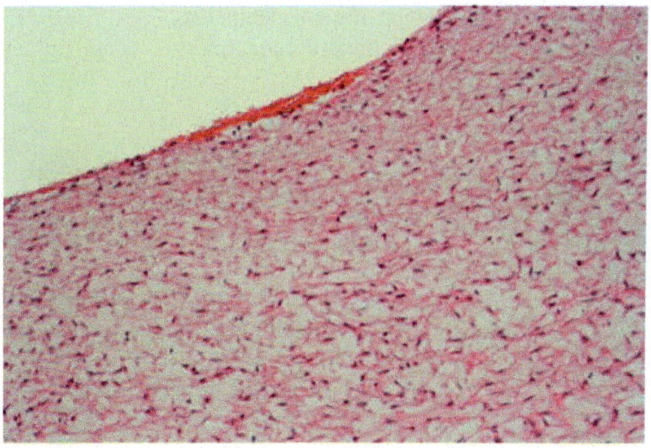

Fig. 19.4 Neointimal type of subendothelial intimal hyperplasia, H&E stain, ×100

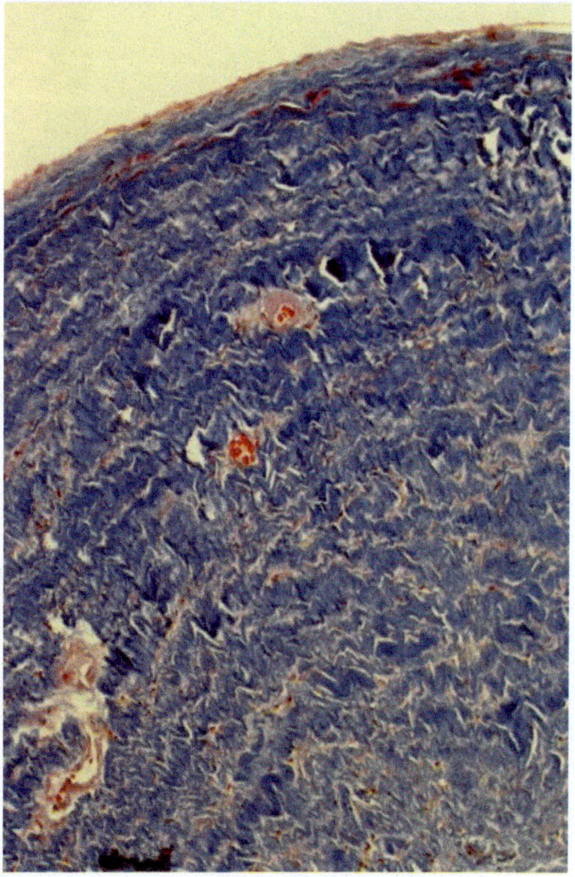

Fig. 19.5 Fibrotic type of subendothelial intimal hyperplasia, MTC stain, ×100

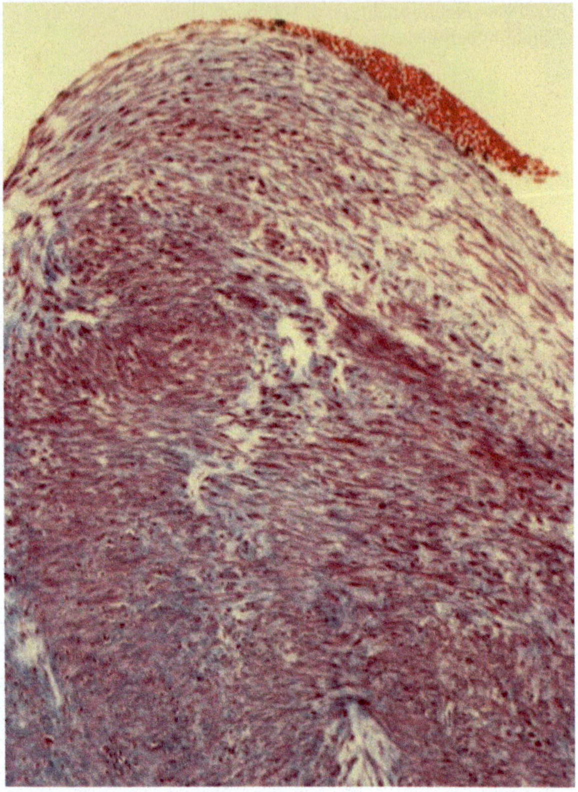

Fig. 19.6 Combined type of a subendothelial intimal hyperplasia (neointimal-fibrotic mixed type), EVG stain, ×100

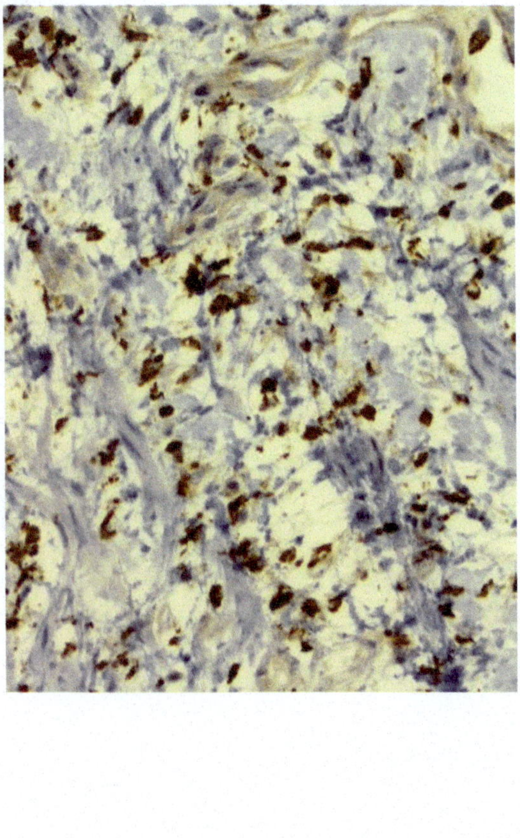

Fig. 19.7 Neointima with calponin expression of myofibroblasts, ×200

- Accumulation of extracellular matrix proteins (Roy-Chaudhury et al. 2003; 2007)

In my experience there are light microscopically identical pictures of arterial and venous SIH (Fig. 19.8). The neointimal SIH can easily be distinguished from the fibrotic SIH. There are, however, also smooth transitions between these two entities so that most likely neointimal SIH is a preliminary stage of fibrotic SIH. The latter is histomorphologically characterized by a lower cell count and the presence of collagen subtypes I, III, and IV. Remarkably there is no atherosclerosis whatsoever in the shrunken fistula veins (Janzen and Mickley 2006, 2007).

19.3 Aneurysmatic Dilatation

Several factors influence aneurysmatic dilatation. Repeated punctures for hemodialysis weaken the walls of fistulas or grafts (Figs. 19.9, 19.10, 19.11, 19.12, and 19.13), but the intravascular fistula pressure is also an important factor. Should the internal elastic lamina membrane rupture due to an increase in pressure, this event will accelerate the formation of an aneurysm (Fig. 19.14). Puncture trauma also causes false aneurysms (pseudoaneurysms) of the native fistula or the graft. There blood collects in the neighboring fibrolipomatous soft tissue (Figs. 19.15, 19.16, and 19.17) (Janzen et al. 2007).

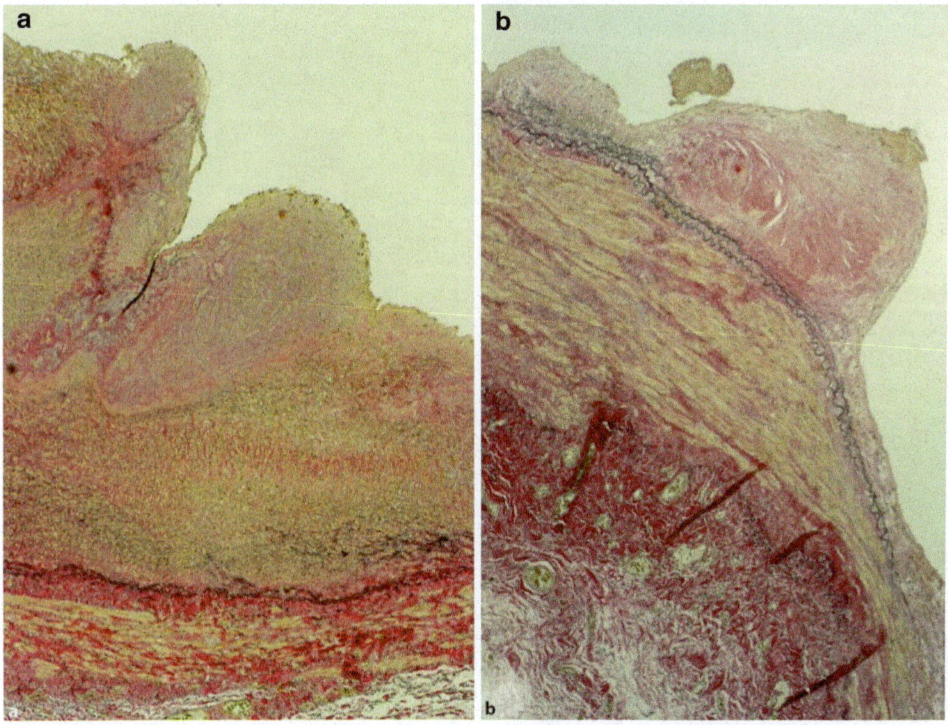

Fig. 19.8 Fibrotic subendothelial intima hyperplasia in the (**a**) arterial and (**b**) venous anastomosis, EVG stain, ×40

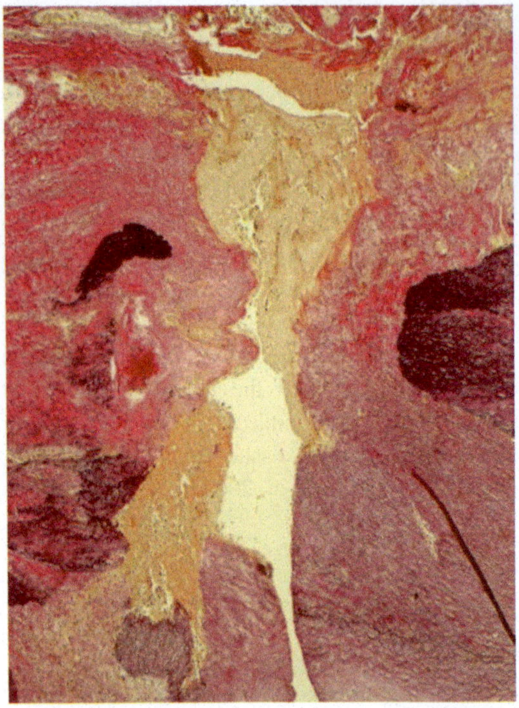

Fig. 19.9 Acute puncture trauma with fibrin precipitates, EVG stain, ×100

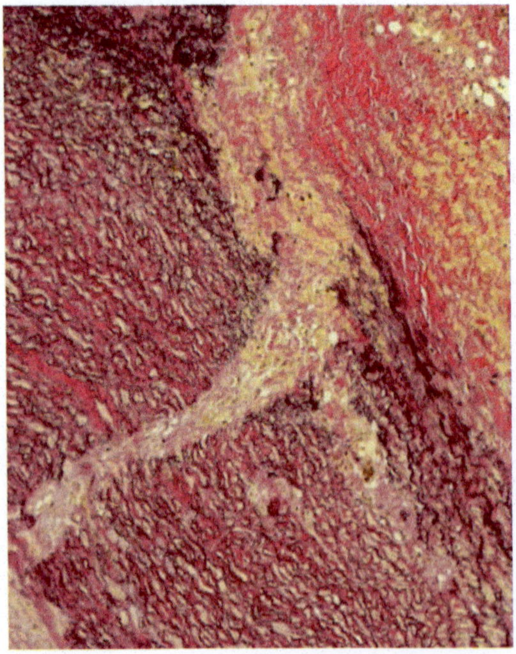

Fig. 19.10 Connective tissue repair of a needlestick tract in the tunica media, EVG stain, ×100

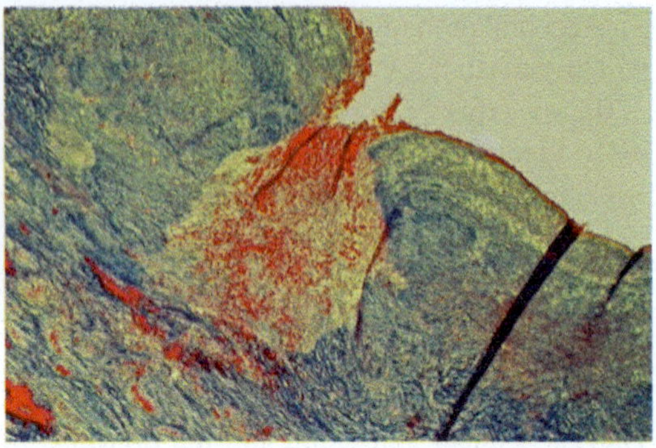

Fig. 19.11 Puncture site with granulation tissue, MTC stain, ×200

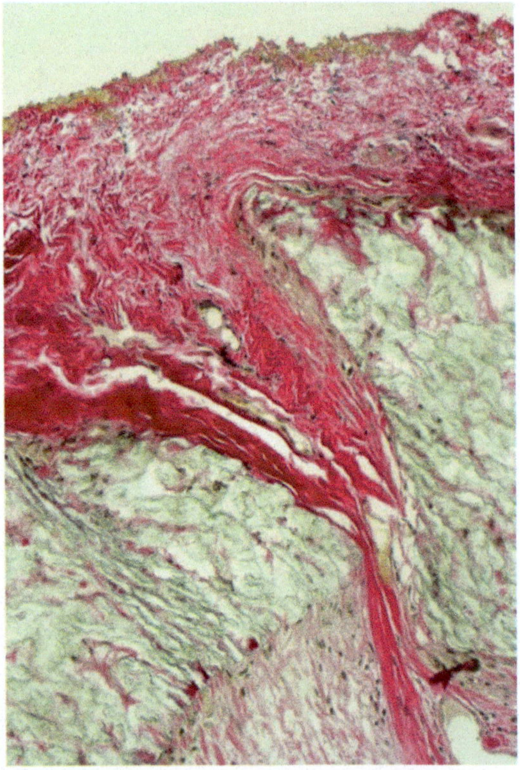

Fig. 19.12 Connective tissue repair of a needlestick tract in the graft wall, EVG stain, ×200

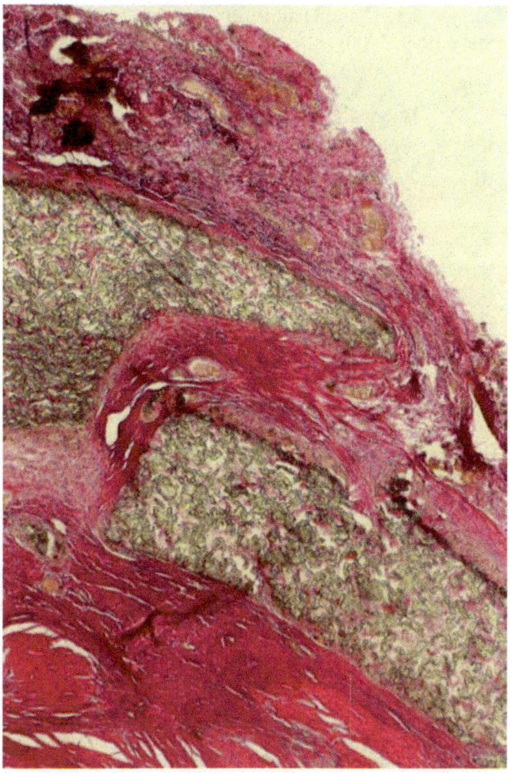

Fig. 19.13 Scarred graft defect with sclerosis, EVG stain, ×200

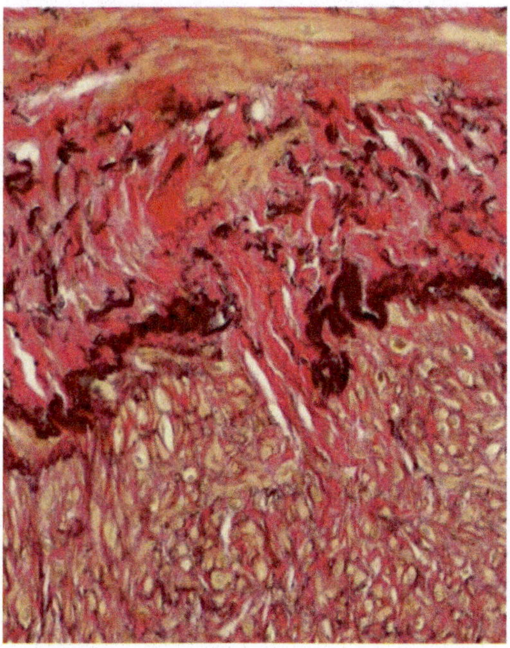

Fig. 19.14 Destroyed elastic internal membrane as starting point of aneurysmogenesis, EVG stain, ×200

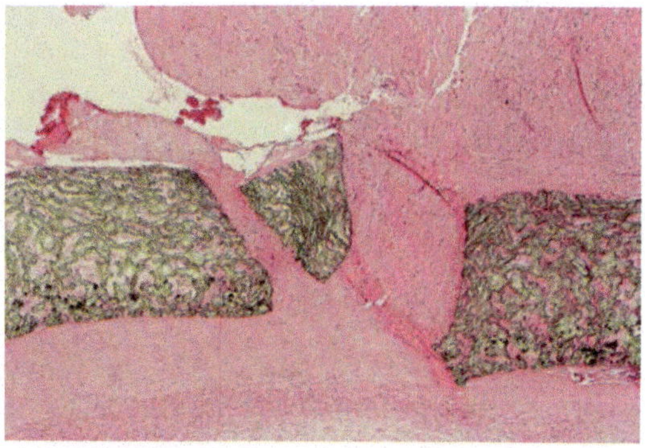

Fig. 19.15 Early stage of false aneurysm (spurious aneurysm), EVG stain, ×200

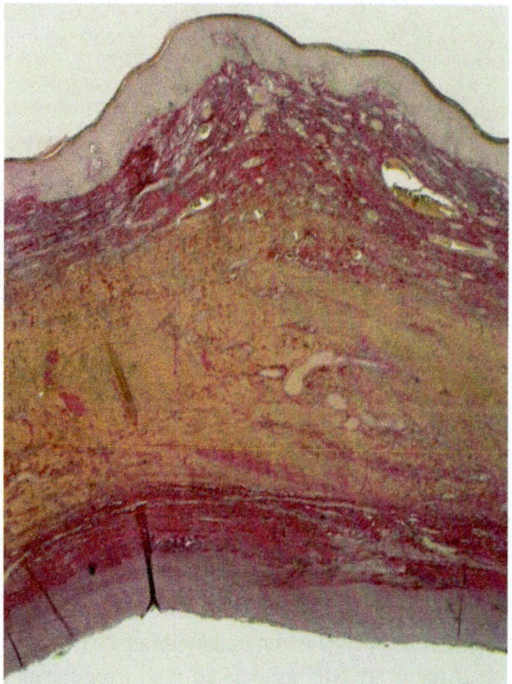

Fig. 19.16 Spurious aneurysm (*bottom*) ante perforationem, EVG stain, ×40

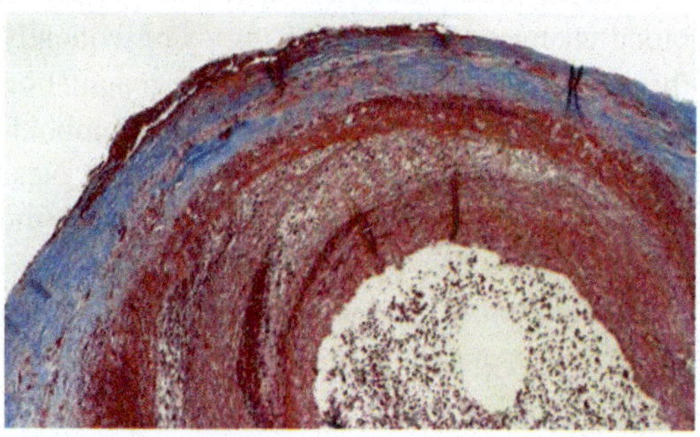

Fig. 19.17 Spurious aneurysm with white (separation) thrombus, MTC stain, ×40

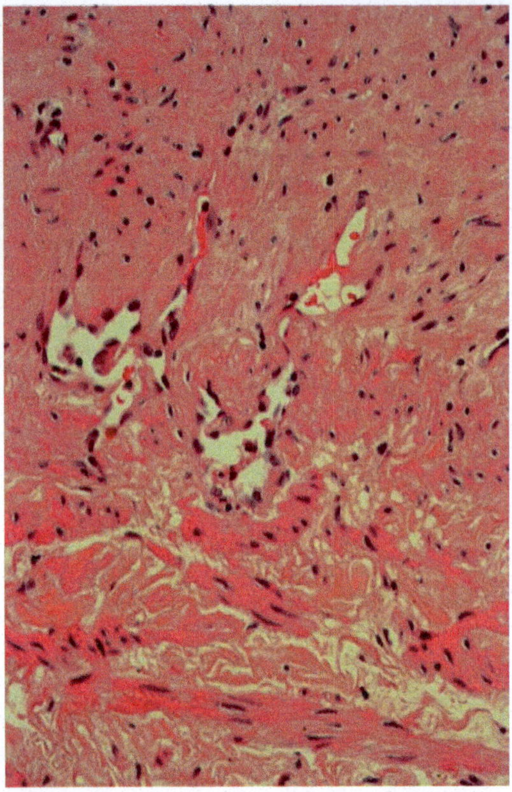

Fig. 19.18 Recanalizations of a mixed fistula thrombosis, H&E stain, ×200

Risk factors for aneurysm formation comprise the destruction of the vasa vasorum during dissection or the complete isolation of the vessel from the periadventitial tissue. The compression of the vascular wall by fibrosis also impairs the nutritive supply (Janzen and Widmer 2011).

If there are SIH-associated wall irregularities in AV accesses with aneurysmatic dilatations, the decelerated blood stream (Virchow's triad) will lead to the deposition of thrombocytes at the endothelium. Furthermore, the flow pattern of the blood changes (laminar/swirling). Consequently thrombocytes agglutinate, and fibrin coagulation starts through thrombocyte or tissue thrombokinases. The coagulation process continues. Near the vessel wall there is a parallel layering of the blood. Microscopic investigations of these specimens show mixed thrombi in most cases, which are both separation and agglutinative thrombi (Fig. 19.18).

Table 19.1 Classification of atherosclerotic lesions (Stary 1999, 2000)

Type	
I	Isolated macrophage foam cells
II	Multiple foam cell layers
III	*Preatheroma*, intermediate lesion
IV	*Atheroma*
V	*Fibroatheroma*
VI	Fissured, ulcerated, hemorrhagic, thrombotic lesion
VII	Calcific lesion
VIII	Fibrotic lesion

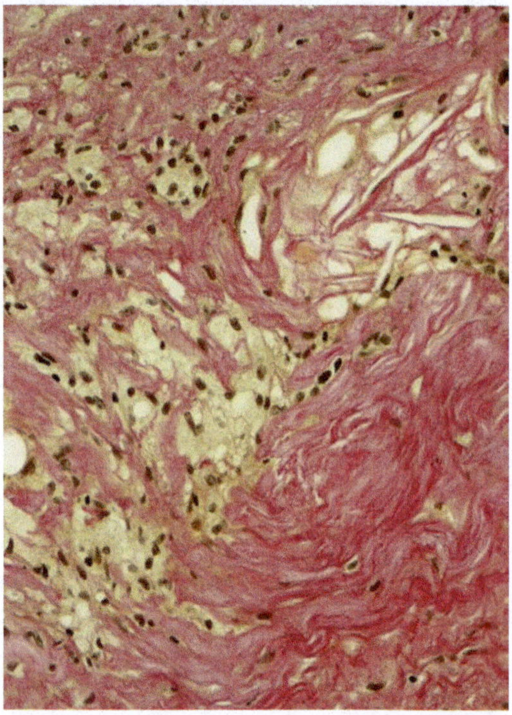

Fig. 19.19 Atherosclerosis of the vein of an AV fistula, Stary type II: foam cells and cholesterol clefts, EVG stain, ×200

19.4 Atherosclerosis

Atherosclerosis is a disease of the tunica intima. According to Stary, there are eight histopathological types (Table 19.1). In the vast majority of cases, the types I–IV occur in fistulas. Complex atherosclerotic changes with ruptures of the

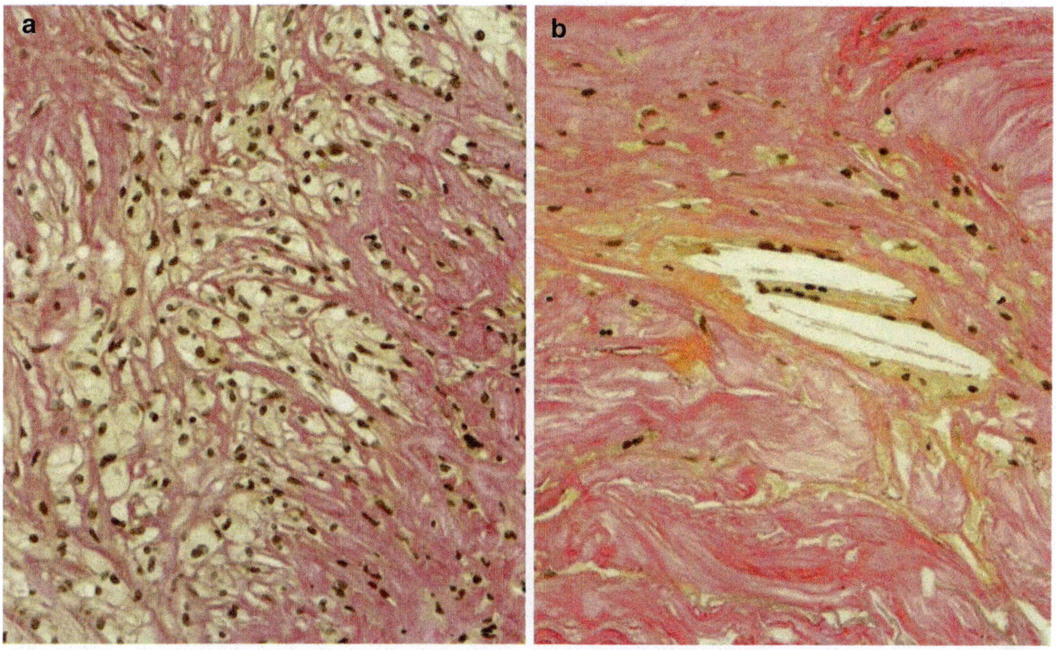

Fig. 19.20 Atherosclerosis of the vein of an AV fistula, Stary type II: (**a**) foam cells and (**b**) cholesterol clefts, EVG stain, ×200

cover can hardly be observed. Atherosclerosis concerns arterial as well as venous fistula segments (venous atherosclerosis) (Stehbens and Karmody 1975) and does not differ from "common" atherosclerosis.

Lipid-storing macrophages (foam cells) in the tunica intima characterize early atherosclerotic damage (Stary types I, II). In order to confirm specifically the presence of isolated foam cells the monoclonal antibody CD68 proves useful. Type III (preatheroma) shows extracellular lipid deposits and calcifications. Stary type IV describes atheromatous plaques with intact fibrous caps. A necrotic lipid core is found in the center of the atheroma (Figs. 19.19, 19.20, 19.21, and 19.22).

19.5 Calcification/Ossification

Degenerative fistula or graft changes like calcification or ossification have to be distinguished from atherosclerosis. The etiology of calcification is complex. Apart from dystrophic and metastatic forms due to the underlying renal disease, there is also atherosclerosis-associated and Moenckeberg calcification. Histomorphologically, initial stages of calcification show bluish violet amorphous granulations, which fuse to bolt-shaped or compact structures (Janzen and Vuong 2001). Newer findings suggest the inhibitory effect of the matrix G1a protein. Ossification is situated close to calcium deposits. Occasionally there may also be hematopoietic bone marrow in the fistula wall (Fig. 19.23).

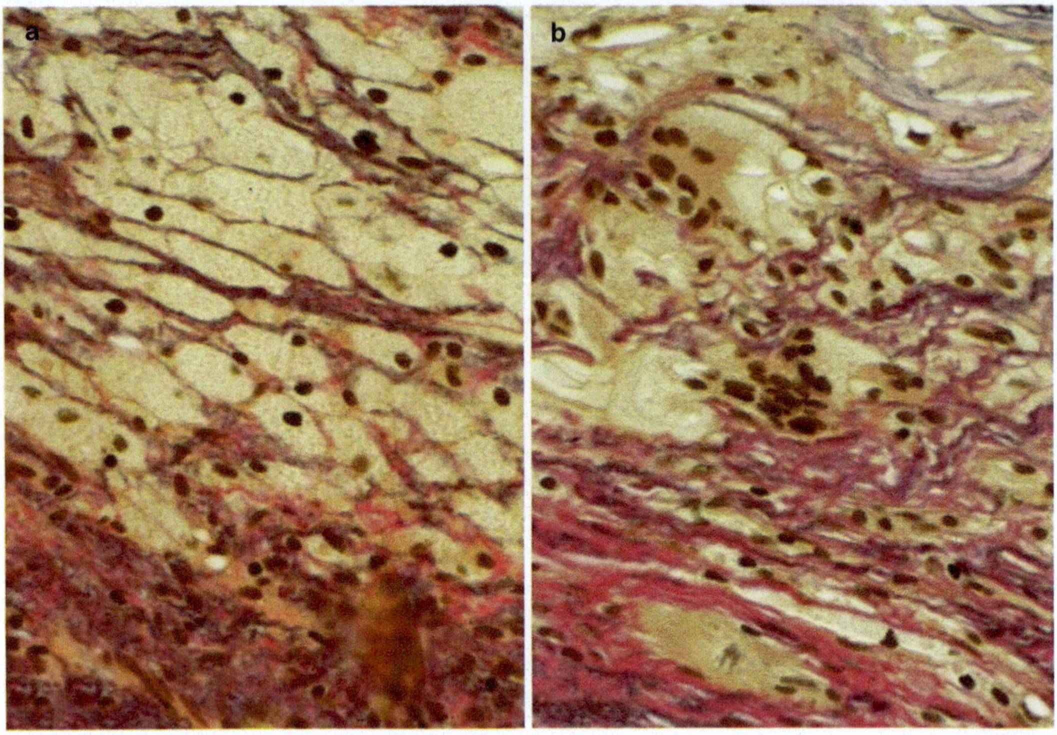

Fig. 19.21 Atherosclerosis of the vein of an AV fistula, Stary type III: (**a**) preatheroma and (**b**) multinucleated giant cells, EVG stain, ×400

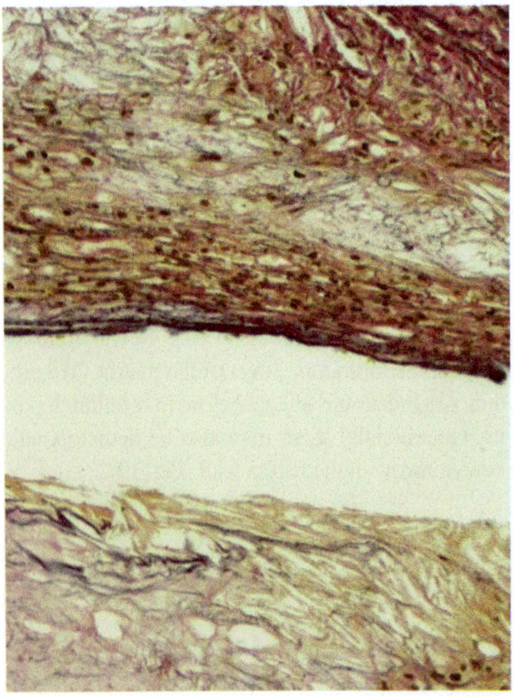

Fig. 19.22 Atherosclerosis of the vein of an AV fistula, Stary type IV: atheroma with intact fibrous cap, EVG stain, ×100

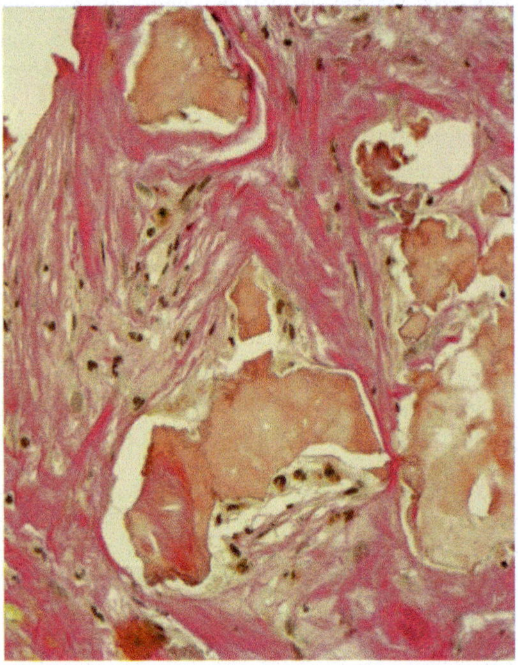

Fig. 19.23 Ossification of the vein of an AV fistula, EVG stain, ×100

Literature

Haruguchi H, Teraoka S (2003) Intimal hyperplasia and hemodynamic factors in arterial bypass and arteriovenous grafts: a review. J Artif Organs 6:227–235
Hayakawa Y, Takemura G, Misao J, Kanoh M, Ohno M, Ohashi H, Takatsu H, Ito H, Fukuda K, Fujiwara T, Minatoguchi S, Fujiwara H (1999) Apoptosis and overexpression of bax mRNA in smooth muscle cells within intimal hyperplasia of human radial arteries: analysis with arteriovenous fistulas used for hemodialysis. Arterioscler Thromb Vasc Biol 9:2066–2077
Janzen J (2005) Macroscopic findings of insufficient arterio-venous fistulae in hemodialysis patients. Invited lecture, 4th International congress of the Vascular Access Society, Berlin
Janzen J (2010) Histological findings in failing fistulas. Invited lecture, Course of Vascular Access Society, Bern
Janzen J, Widmer MK, Mickley V (2007) Basic pathology of hemodialysis arterio-venous fistulae. In: Poster presentation, 5th International congress of the Vascular Access Society, Nizza
Janzen J, Mickley V (2006) Histologie der Hämodialysefistel. Perfusion 19:305–309
Janzen J, Mickley V (2007) Insufficient arterio-venous fistulae in hemodialysis patients. Blood Purif 25:151–154
Janzen J, Vuong PN (2001) Arterial calcifications: morphological aspects and their pathological implications. Z Kardiol 90:Suppl. 3,III/6 – III/11
Janzen J, Widmer MK (2011) Aneurysmogenesis in autologous shunts. In: Poster presentation, 7th International congress of the Vascular Access Society, Istanbul
Kim SJ, Masaki T, Leypoldt JK, Kamerath CD, Mohammad SF, Cheung AK (2004) Arterial and venous smooth-muscle cells differ in their responses to antiproliferative drugs. J Lab Clin Med 144:156–162
Krönung G. Dialyseshunts (2008) Dialyse Aktuell, 12 (Sonderdruck):13–15
Rekhter M, Nicholls S, Ferguson M, Gordon D (1993) Cell proliferation in human arteriovenous fistulas used for hemodialysis. Arterioscler Thromb Vasc Biol 13:609–617
Roy-Chaudhury P, Munda R, Edwards J, Kelly BS (2003) Hemodialysis vascular access dysfunction from clinical stenosis to specific cell types. J Nephrol 16:277–285
Roy-Chaudhury P, Arend L, Zhang J, Krishnamothy M, Wang Y, Banerjee R, Samaha A, Munda R (2007) Neointimal hyperplasia in early arteriovenous fistula failure. Am J Kidney Dis 50:782–790
Schurgers LJ, Aebert H, Vermeer C, Bultmann B, Janzen J (2004) Oral anticoagulant treatment: friend or foe in cardiovascular disease? Blood 104:3231–3232
Sivanesan S, How TV, Black RA, Bakran A (1999) Flow patterns in the radiocephalic arteriovenous fistula: an in vitro study. J Biomech 32:915–925
Stary HC (1999) Atlas of atherosclerosis: progression, and regression. Parthenon Publishing Group, New York
Stary HC (2000) Natural history and histological classification of atherosclerotic lesions. Arterioscler Thromb Vasc Biol 20:1177–1178
Stehbens WE, Karmody AM (1975) Venous atherosclerosis associated with arteriovenous fistulas for hemodialysis. Arch Surg 110:176–180
Weiss MF, Scivittaro V, Anderson JM (2001) Oxidative stress and increased expression of growth factors in lesions of failed hemodialysis access. Am J Kidney Dis 37:970–980

20 Short Introduction to Fluid Dynamics: Relevant Aspects for Hemodynamics

The mechanics of solid bodies is fundamentally different from the mechanics of liquids and gases. The latter is called fluid mechanics. Flowing gases and liquids are summarized as *fluids* (Prandtl et al. 1990; Tipler and Mosca 2009). An accurate definition of the word fluid involves motion: "Fluid is free to change in form" (Munson et al. 1994).

Hemodynamics deals with the physical basics of blood flow. As opposed to other real flows, blood flow is characterized by its pulsatility and its flow-dependent viscosity.

20.1 Principles of Fluid Mechanics

For the description of some essential laws of fluid mechanics, the understanding of the following terms is necessary:

- Stationary and non-stationary flow
- Streamline, pathline, and streakline
- Stagnation point
- Reynolds number, laminar and turbulent flow
- Dead water zone

If the flow is not time dependent, it is called stationary. Then the same unchanging flow pattern may be found at any moment in time. Conversely, a time-dependent flow with continuously changing flow patterns is called non-stationary. Therefore the pulsatile flow in the blood circulation is non-stationary.

Flow velocity denotes the change of position per time unit. It is a vector. Therefore it needs a magnitude, a direction, and a starting point (e.g., the coordinates of a fluid particle). A single vector characterizes the velocity of a single point mass (an infinitely small fluid particle). If the starting points of the vectors of a flow pattern are connected in such a way that the vectors become curve tangents, the resulting lines are called *streamlines*. Streamlines help illustrate flow patterns (cf. Fig. 4.17). They do not kink, and they do not intersect. At a given point there cannot be two velocities at the same time (Bohl 1994; Prandtl et al. 1990). Zero velocity streamlines at the stagnation point constitute an exception (see below), as they may intersect and branch out. Imagine numerous swimming tea lights on a water surface. If you took a photo after an exposure time which is just long enough to change the light points into lines, they would be streamlines.

With stationary flows, streamlines are the same as pathlines. With nonstationary flows, however, this is not the case: Streamlines depict the momentarily simultaneously existing velocity directions, whereas pathlines show the velocity directions of a particle over a course of time. In our thought experiment with the tea lights, you would have to have a very long exposure time in order to obtain the pathline of a single tea light.

Streaklines are a third type of lines. They are the curves of all particles that pass the very same topographical point over the course of time. In an experiment streaklines may be visualized by injecting dye at a certain point (in the thought experiment: a chain of tea lights) (Smits and Lim

H. Scholz, *Arteriovenous Access Surgery*,
DOI 10.1007/978-3-642-41139-7_20, © Springer-Verlag Berlin Heidelberg New York 2015

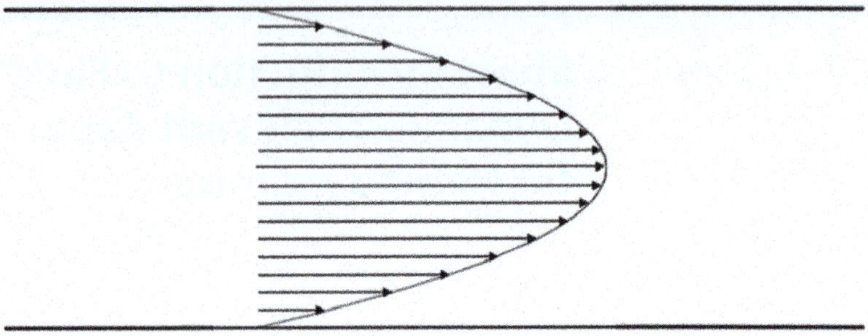

Fig. 20.1 Parabolic velocity profile of the laminar flow in a pipe

2000). Then all particles which pass this point will be colored (e.g., Fig. 4.5). If you place a static solid body into a flow, the streamline that meets the body will divide according to the solid body's shape and flow around it. The front branch point is called *stagnation point.*

At this point the whole kinetic energy of the fluid is completely transformed into pressure, and the flow comes to a standstill (Gersten 1991; Prandtl et al. 1990). The pressure at the stagnation point is called stagnation pressure (cf. Bernoulli's law, Chap. 20.2). Likewise you can also find stagnation points when the flow hits a wall (cf. Fig. 4.9a).

In order to compare flows in geometrically similar structures, dimensionless quantities are used. The most important is named after Osborne Reynolds (1842–1912). For the flow in pipes it is

$$\text{Reynolds number } Re = \rho \frac{\bar{v} d}{\eta}$$

with $\bar{v}$ – mean velocity, d – diameter of the pipe, ρ – density, and η – dynamic viscosity.

A *laminar* flow is a stratified flow. Between neighboring layers there is no exchange of fluid particles perpendicular to the flow direction. A laminar flow of a real fluid in a pipe (blood vessel) has a parabolic velocity profile (Fig. 20.1). The velocity reaches its maximum in the center of the pipe and drops to zero at the walls (no slip condition, cf. Chap. 20.4); the change from a laminar flow into a *turbulent* flow occurs at the critical *Reynolds number* of Re= 2,300 (Gersten 1991; Opitz and Pfeiffer 1984; Zamir 2000). Other authors do not see such a strict cut off. Below Re=2,000 there is a laminar flow, and above Re = 3,000 the flow is turbulent. In between, the flow pattern is unstable and can swing from one state to the other (Tipler and Mosca 2009). The *turbulent* flow is characterized by random oscillations which are superimposed upon the basic flow. There is an intensive exchange of fluid particles between the different layers, which mix even more with increasing Reynolds numbers. The velocity profile flattens in the center of the tube, and is almost evened out with high Reynolds numbers. Apart from the zones near the wall, it is almost constant over the entire cross section. Except for the conditions at systolic peak velocity in the ascending aorta, the in vivo Reynolds numbers in the human circulation are below the critical region (Opitz and Pfeiffer 1984; Prandtl et al. 1990).

During an experiment, Reynolds directed a thin line of dye into a flow. With a laminar flow the dye stays together within a thin compact fluctuating line. In a turbulent flow the line dissolves quickly over the whole cross section.

A *dead water zone* is not or hardly perfused. Such regions develop behind the regions of flow separation (cf. Chap. 20.3). The basic flow is significantly slowed. Depending on the Reynolds number, regular vortices or a turbulent flow form. The dead water region is separated from the laminar main stream by a divisive line. In the dead water zone the flow is much less harmonious than in the main stream and can stagnate completely under extreme conditions (e.g., in certain regions behind a closed mechanical heart valve). In the dead water zone there are especially long interactions between the flow and the vascular wall. These regions are predestined for thrombus formation or the lining of the wall with "pseudointima" (cf. Chap. 4.1, Heise et al. 2011).

20.2 Continuity Equation

If you determine the velocities of the particles which flow through an arbitrary area A, then the average of these velocities can help establish the volume of the flow that passes the area A during the time interval Δt:

$$\Delta V = \bar{v} A \Delta t.$$

The division of both sides of this equation by Δt yields the volume over time, the *volume flow*, which is most often referred to as flow rate or simply flow Q. In medicine the common measuring unit is $Q = [\text{mL/min}]$.

With flowing incompressible fluids without air or other gas inclusions in an impermeable pipe, it seems obvious that the same amount of fluid which enters the pipe during a given interval of time must also leave the pipe during the same time. Fluid is neither added nor lost. If the cross section is constant, then

$$Q = \bar{v} A = \text{constant}.$$

This equation is called the *continuity equation* and describes the conservation of mass. Transferred to a vessel with changing cross sections (Fig. 20.2a) this means that the flow rate in the different areas A1 and A2 is constant. If the cross section changes, the mean flow velocity also has to change. Further considerations can be found in Chap. 20.4.

20.3 Bernoulli's Equation

In a stagnant fluid the pressure which a fluid column exerts on its base depends on its height:

$$p = \rho g h$$

with p – hydrostatic pressure, ρ – density, g – gravity, and h – height.

The pressure is the same for all points of a certain height (constant over the whole cross section) and increases proportionally with height.

A pressure p_0 which is exerted on the surface of a non-flowing fluid (e.g., via a piston) leads to a uniform increase in pressure everywhere in the

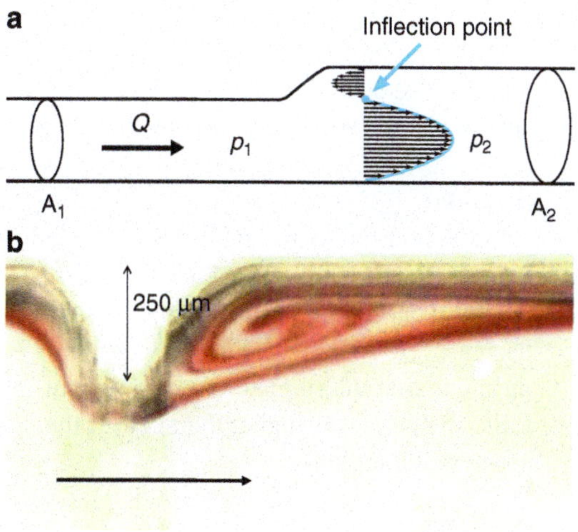

Fig. 20.2 (**a**) As the pipe diameter increases, there will be flow separation. The mark shows the inflection point of the velocity profile (zero velocity). (**b**) Further downstream a vortex will form (microscopic photo of a reproduced vascular wall in the pulsatile flow model; the *arrow* indicates the flow direction)

fluid (Pascal's principle). Then the total pressure p_G is

$$p_G = \rho g h + p_0.$$

With flowing fluids, an additional pressure component has to be taken into account: the dynamic pressure or *stagnation pressure*. It depends on the velocity v:

$$p_d = \frac{1}{2} \rho v^2.$$

Example: Dynamic Pressure on the Floor of the Venous Anastomosis

The density of the model fluid is $\rho = 1.1\ \text{g/cm}^3$ (Chap. 4.2). Figure 4.11a shows the approximate velocity at the stagnation point: $v = 0.75$ m/s. Supposing that the flow hits the venous wall at this speed (conversion factors $1\ \text{N} = 1\ \text{kg} \times \text{m/s}^2$ and $1\ \text{Pa} = 1\ \text{N/m}^2$), the resulting dynamic pressure is

$$p_d = \frac{1}{2} \times 1{,}100\ \text{kg/m}^3 \times \left(0.75\ \text{m/s}^2\right)$$
$$= 309.4\ \text{Pa}.$$

The pressure maximum in Fig. 4.13 is 322 Pa. The accordance is quite good considering that, at a supposed velocity of 0.77 m/s, the calculated dynamic pressure is 326 Pa.

To estimate this value the pressure is converted into mmHg: $p = 322$ Pa $= 2.4$ mmHg. At the venous anastomosis the pressure decreases by 10 mmHg (Fig. 4.13a, b). This means that at the stagnation point the pulsatile stress is 24 % higher than in the other anastomotic regions.

The pressure equation of the Swiss mathematician and physicist Daniel Bernoulli (1700–1782) is a basic equation of fluid mechanics. It says that the combination of pressure, geodesic height, and flow velocity assumes the same value for each point of the flowline. The equation is also fundamentally important to the fluid mechanics of stationary, incompressible, and non-viscous flows. Its integrated form is

$$p_1 + \rho g h_1 + \frac{1}{2}\rho v_1^2 = p_2 + \rho g h_2 + \frac{1}{2}\rho v_2^2 = \text{constant}.$$

With incompressible flow pressure does not result in the compaction of the fluid but in a change in its motion. There is no internal friction in non-viscous fluids.

Regarding a purely horizontal flow, $\rho g h$ is dropped, which makes comprehension easier. The simpler form of the equation for this special case is

$$p + \frac{1}{2}\rho v^2 = \text{constant}.$$

This form of the Bernoulli equation clearly shows the way the pressure changes with a changing cross section. If the cross section diminishes, the velocity must increase as the same amount of fluid must pass (continuity equation). As a consequence the static pressure drops in this place. The pressure drop can be so pronounced that a suction effect may occur. As this phenomenon seems contradictory at first, it is called hydrodynamic paradoxon.

An easily-performed experiment with rattling spoons visualizes how this can happen. The facing convex sides of two vertically-held spoons lightly touch a water jet which passes between them. As the spoons diminish the space for the water, its velocity must increase. The pressure drops till it is lower than the pressure of the surrounding air. Suction makes the spoons hit each other. The falling following water drives the spoons apart, and a new cycle starts. The resulting rattle shows that you can hold the Bernoulli equation in your hands.

Irrespective of the limitations mentioned above, the Bernoulli equation offers very good solutions to a multitude of problems. It can explain the action of a nebulizer, the curved trajectory of a baseball (Tipler and Mosca 2009), how a sail boat can sail into the wind (Seemannschaft 2003), why it is possible to measure the pressure with a tube in the flow (Venturi effect; Munson et al. 1994; Bohl 1994), and why cavitation occurs behind high speed marine propeller blades.

20.4 Flow Separation and Secondary Flow

Flow separation is crucial when examining different anastomotic designs. The following example explains the flow separation from a wall (Fig. 20.2a). Imagine a pipe with a laminar flow, whose diameter suddenly changes. The total flow Q is constant ($Q = Q_1 = Q_2$, *continuity equation*). As the area A_1 is smaller than A_2, the mean velocity v_1 must be higher than v_2 because $v = Q/A$. According to Bernoulli's principle, the mean pressure p_2 must be higher than p_1. This does not mean, however, that the pressure p_2 of the wide pipe segment has to be higher than p_1 in every place. In fact there is a pressure distribution that can be described by complex equations (Prandtl et al. 1990). They also show that in the center of a tube, the pressure decreases along the flow direction, and that the velocity profile is curved convexly. Near the wall downstream from the widening of the pipe there is a pressure increase in the flow direction. The velocity profile is curved concavely. The inflection point of the profiles (transition from a convex to a concave curve) is exactly the point where a pressure reversal occurs. At this point, particles close to the wall begin to stand still, and to flow backwards with increasing pressure reversal. As fluid continues to arrive, the retrogradely flowing layers increase and push the oncoming orthograde fluid away from the wall. The separation zone then dissolves while vortices form (Fig. 20.2b).

Flow separation also occurs in a flow which follows a curve. Consider a curve in a pipe with a circular cross section. At the transition from the straight to the curved path, the central stream tends to continue straight onwards because of its higher velocity (principle of inertia). As an immediate result the flow separates from the inside of the curve (Fig. 20.3b) and forms a vortex.

Figure 20.4a shows a further flow phenomenon of the cross section in position AB (cf. Fig. 20.3b) – the formation of a secondary flow. The fast-moving flow portions from the central stream displace the slower peripheral flow at the outer side of the curve. The particles from these layers flow along the circumference to the inside of the curve while displacing the particles flowing ahead of them. In accordance with the continuity equation, the backflow occurs back to the outer wall of the curve along the symmetry plane. The velocity of this movement is comparatively slower than the velocity in the main flow direction (21 cm/s vs 68 cm/s in Fig. 20.3a). These flows are called secondary

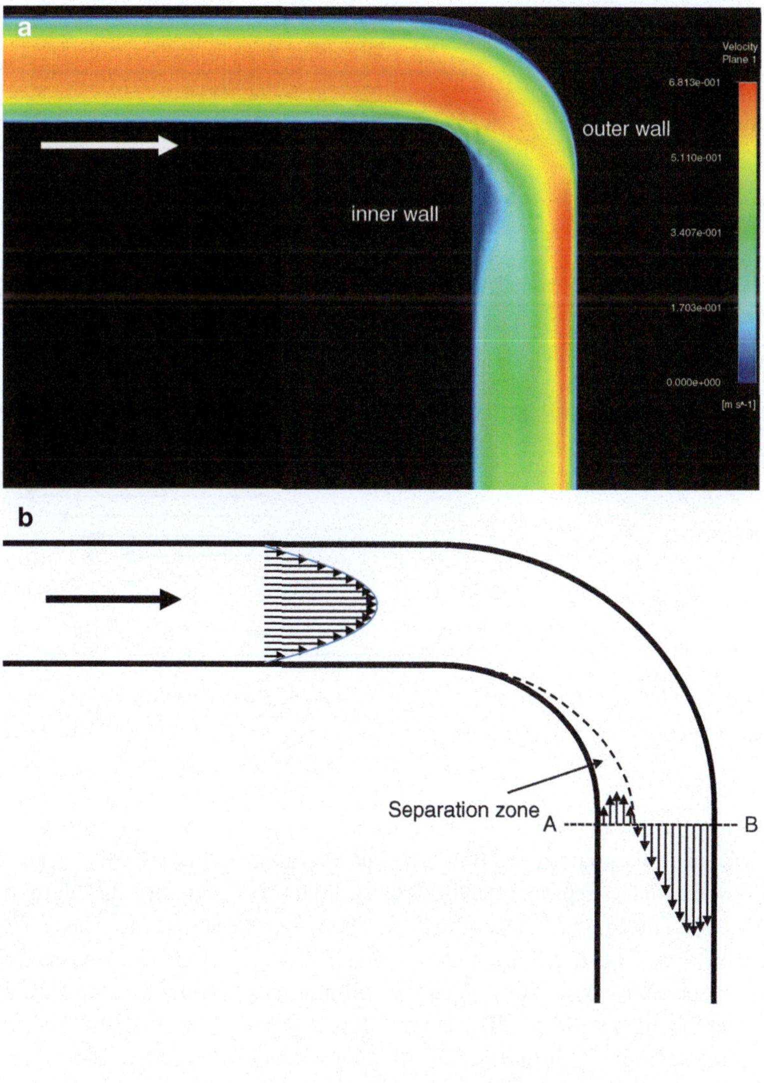

Fig. 20.3 Flow in a curve. (**a**) The *arrow* indicates the flow direction. (**b**) Behind the curve there will be flow separation

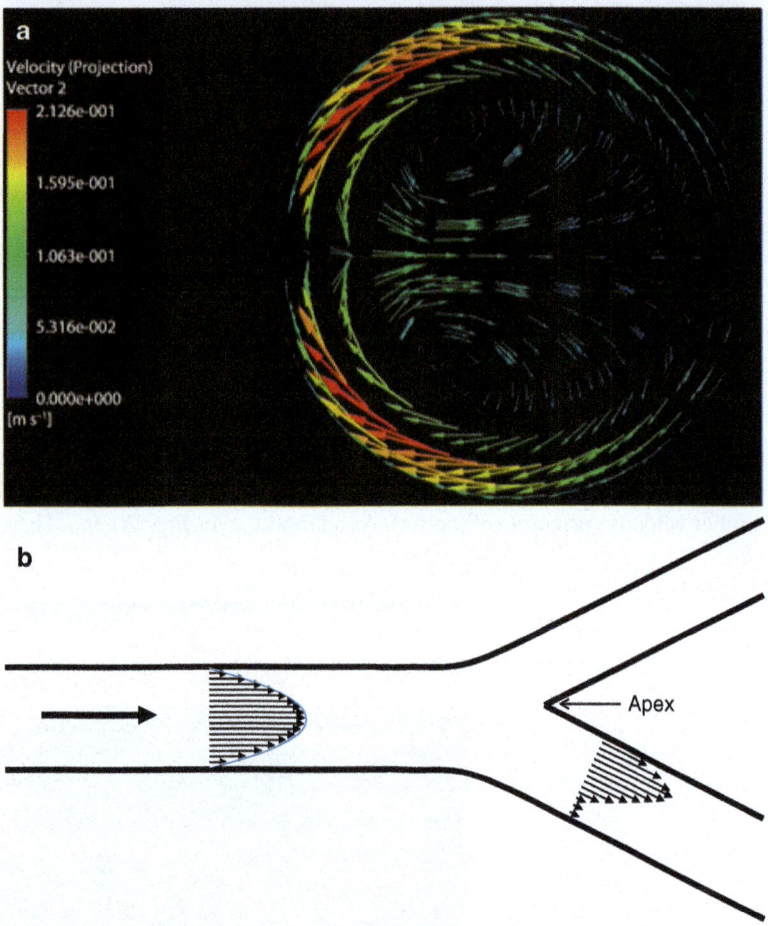

Fig. 20.4 (**a**) Secondary flow in the cross section (line AB in Fig. 20.3). (**b**) Secondary flow also forms in bifurcations

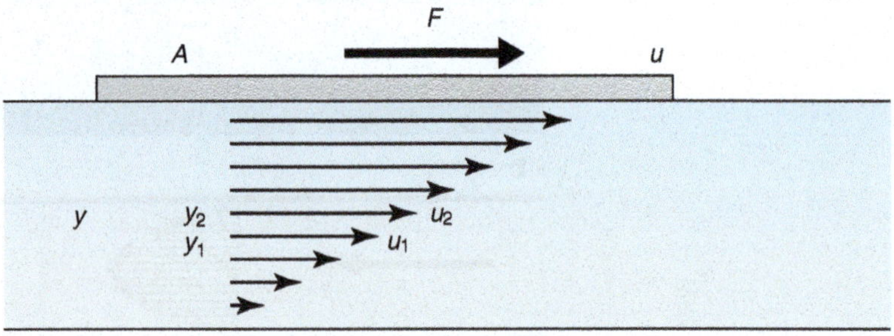

$$\text{Shear stress } \tau = \frac{F}{A} = \eta \times \frac{u_2 - u_1}{y_2 - y_1} = \eta \times \frac{\Delta u}{\Delta y}$$

Fig. 20.5 Shear flow between two parallel boards. Force F moves a board A over a real fluid

flows. They can only be found in planes perpendicular to the main flow. Together with the main flow they lead to spiral trajectories of the fluid particles (Gersten 1991; Munson et al. 1994; Fung 1997; Prandtl et al. 1990).

Secondary flows also occur in bifurcations (van Steenhoven 1993). The central flow divides at the apex. As an immediate result, high velocities occur at the insides of the bifurcation (Fig. 20.4b). The flow pattern resembles the velocity distribution behind a curve. In bifurcations retrograde flow in the separation zone (Fig. 20.3) is less frequent but possible (Li 2004). Here, too, the slower layers near the wall are displaced from the inner sides of the bifurcation, leading to secondary flows.

20.5 Viscosity, Shear Rate, and Shear Stress

The drop in pressure in the direction of flowing real liquids cannot be sufficiently explained by Bernoulli's principle because it neglects the viscosity of a real fluid. Viscosity, which leads to internal friction of the flow, is a characteristic of liquids and gases. The flow resistance which has to be overcome originates from the forces between the molecules of a fluid (*cohesion*) and between the fluid and the boundary surfaces (*adhesion*). Figure 20.5 shows a real fluid between two boards. Board *A* moves relative to the base board (velocity *u*). This movement requires a certain force *F* which increases the more the board adheres. Imagine thin liquid layers. The layers directly bordering on the boards have the same speed as the boards (zero at the base board and *u* at the moving board). This phenomenon is called *no-slip condition* (Li 2004; Zamir 2000). Each of the thin liquid layers sticks to the neighboring layer and diminishes (coming from the base) or increases (coming from the moveable board) its velocity. Consequently a linear velocity profile develops between the boards.

The most common symbol for velocity is *v*. However, in a three-dimensional coordinate system with the axes *x*, *y*, and *z*, the corresponding velocity components are called *u*, *v*, and *w*, respectively.

The ratio between force and area is called *shear stress*:

$$\tau = \frac{F}{A}$$

Its unit is the same as for pressure (Pa). The velocity gradient $\Delta u/\Delta y$ (if nonlinear: $\mathrm{d}u/\mathrm{d}y$) is called *shear rate* $\dot{\gamma}$ ($1/\mathrm{s} = \mathrm{s}^{-1}$). With a laminar, parabolic velocity gradient, the shear rate is minimal in the center of the flow, as there the neighboring velocities differ only slightly (Fig. 20.1). The shear rate increases from the pipe center to the walls. The correlation between shear stress and shear rate is expressed by Newton's friction law:

$$\tau = \eta \frac{\mathrm{d}u}{\mathrm{d}y} = \eta \dot{\gamma}.$$

The factor η is the dynamic viscosity (unit Pa×s) and it characterizes the cohesion of the liquid layers. A fundamental consequence of viscosity is that nowhere in the flow does an abrupt, step-like change of velocity exist. Increasing temperatures lead to the expansion of the fluid. The mean distance between the molecules also increases along with the amplitude of the thermal motion. The mean attraction between molecules diminishes. Both phenomena lead to a drop of viscosity with rising temperatures. Conversely, in gases the viscosity increases with rising temperatures for similar reasons. Thus gases and liquids not only differ because of their different compressibility, but also because of their diametrically-opposed temperature dependance as far as viscosity is concerned.

Fluids whose viscosity is independent of their flow velocity are called Newtonian fluids. The particularities of blood viscosity are discussed in Chap. 20.7.

20.6 Hagen–Poiseuille's law and Peripheral Resistance

When taking friction into account, the Bernoulli equation has to be completed with another term (Sumner 1996):

$$p_1 + \rho g h_1 + \frac{1}{2}\rho v_1^2 = p_2 + \rho g h_2 + \frac{1}{2}\rho v_2^2 + \Delta p$$

In reality, the pressure along the stream line is not constant. The kinetic energy is partially transformed into heat due to the internal friction. The resulting drop in pressure is expressed by Δp. The pressure upstream (index 1) is higher than downstream (index 2). *This difference in pressures makes the fluid move.* Blood circulation results from pressure differences between the individual vascular segments. Analagous to Ohm's law, the blood flow *Q* (= flow rate) is determined by the pressure gradient Δp and the flow resistance *R*:

$$Q = \frac{\Delta p}{R}.$$

For a straight pipe with a circular cross section and a stationary flow of a fluid with a constant viscosity, the resistance R can be calculated as follows according to the Hagen–Poiseuille law:

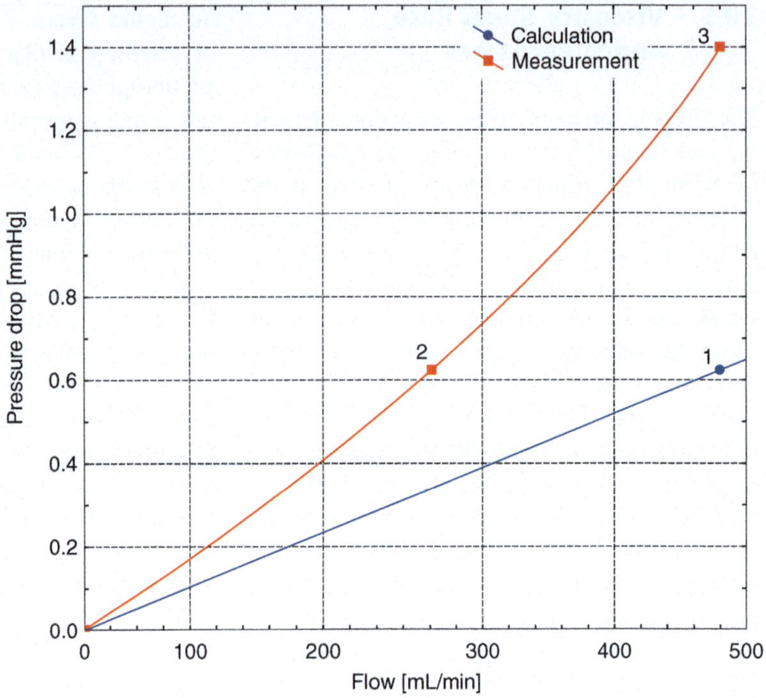

Fig. 20.6 Deviation of the real flow resistance from Hagen–Poiseuille's law (Modified after Sumner 1995). The resistance was calculated from the pressure and flow values in the original ($R = \Delta p/Q$). 1: 481 mL/min, 0.624 mmHg, 1.23 mPRU, 2: 263 mL/min, 0.624 mmHg, 2.37 mPRU, 3: 481 mL/min, 1.4 mmHg, 2.93 mPRU. 4: 0-0-0. Thus Hagen–Poiseuille's law yielded $\Delta p = 0.00123 \times Q$, and the function for the measured values $\Delta p = 0.00172 \times Q + 2.467 \times 10^{-6} \times Q^2$

$$R = \frac{8\eta L}{\pi r^4}$$

where L is the length and r is the radius of the pipe. The dependence of the resistance on the fourth power of the radius is essential. If the radius of a pipe is halved, there is a 16-fold increase in pressure for a given flow rate. This means that a 16 times higher pressure is needed to pump the same amount of fluid through the pipe per unit of time. This relation explains the crucial role of changing vascular diameters when regulating blood flow. Furthermore, a pathologic stenosis of the arteries considerably reduces the downstream blood flow.

Strictly speaking the Hagen–Poiseuille law is not valid for the blood circulation. The flow is pulsatile and therefore non-stationary. Blood viscosity is dependent on velocity (cf. Chap. 20.7). Nevertheless the Hagen–Poiseuille law offers a good approximation to clinical conditions. Thus it is possible to estimate the flow resistance of a prosthesis.

In the vascular system, energy losses are caused by:

- Resistance of the blood against pulsatile accelerations (inertia)
- Radial acceleration and secondary flows in each curve of the vasculature
- Pressure loss caused by vortices at stenoses and dilatations
- Pressure loss and secondary flows in bifurcations (Sumner 1996; Schmidt and Thews 2000)

To estimate the degree of error when using Hagen–Poisseuille's law in order to determine the real resistance, have a look at Fig. 20.6 (modified after Sumner 1995; pressure and flow values were taken from the original graph and the shown functions were calculated). In an animal experiment, the resistance of a single artery ($l = 9.45$ cm, $r = 2.8$ mm) was determined while slowly increasing the flow by successively releasing an upstream occlusion device. The pressure drop along the arterial segment was measured (uninterrupted line). At the same time the resistance was calculated according to Hagen–Poisseuille's law (interrupted line). The higher the flow rate was, the more the calculated resistance differed from the measurement results. At the upper limit of the range the experimentally determined resistance was 2.4 times higher than the calculated one. Note that this experiment only registered the differences caused by the blood's inertia against its acceleration.

Analogous to the experiment above, intraoperative measurements of flow and pressure at the entrance of a vascular segment may help determine its resistance including capillaries and venous drainage. This resistance is called peripheral resistance. All influences which lead to the pressure loss mentioned above are included. Its importance is discussed in the literature (Adeberg 2009; Heise et al. 1999, 2001, 2003; Krüger 1998; Krueger et al. 2000).

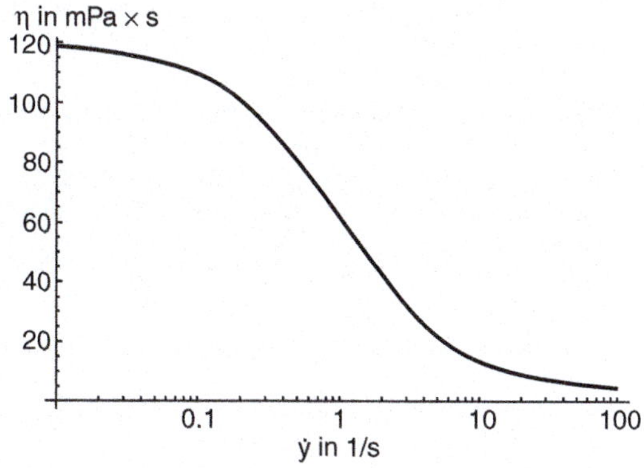

Fig. 20.7 Cross's three parameter function concerning the dependency of blood viscosity η on shear rate γ

20.7 Blood Viscosity

Blood is a cell suspension in a colloidal protein solution. Its viscosity is determined by different factors:

- Plasma viscosity
- Hematocrite
- Diameter of the perfused vessels
- Flow velocity

Fluids whose viscosity is velocity-dependent are called *non-Newtonian* fluids. Blood is a so-called shear-thinning fluid (Lerche et al. 1993). This means that a rise in shear rate leads to a drop in viscosity. Then the ratio of shear stress and shear rate (= viscosity) is not a constant that characterizes a fluid. This ratio is also called "apparent viscosity" (Ulbrecht and Mitschka 1967). For blood several mathematical models describe this dependence (Cho and Kensey 1991; Heethaar 1993; Lerche et al. 1993). Crosse's three-parameter function was used for our numerical simulations (Cross 1965; Cho and Kensey 1991).

From the graph of this function you can derive the flow characteristics of blood (Fig. 20.7). At low shear rates, viscosity is mainly determined by the reversible "rouleau" (stack) formation of erythrocytes. It reaches as high as 100 mPa×s. Aggregation can occur with extremely low flows (under shock) or in poorly perfused regions (ramifications, dilatations) and dead water zones (Liepsch 1989).

Increasing shear rates cause hemodynamic disaggregation (structural viscosity) with ensuing increasingly solitary erythrocytes. Above shear rates of 50 s^{-1} viscosity remains almost constant due to the deformation of erythrocyte aggregates. Arterial shear rates are almost always above 50 s^{-1} except for axial flow.

The aggregation of erythrocytes in axial flow has provoked controversional discussions. Some authors (Prandtl et al. 1990; Ghista et al. 1979; Heethaar 1993) characterize the central flow by rouleau formation of erythrocytes. It shows a constant velocity (plug flow). The parabolic velocity profile then is flattened in the center of the pipe. Others think that, due to the high speed in the arteries (10–100 cm/s, Schmidt and Thews 2000), the time is insufficient for this aggregation (up to several seconds, Lerche et al. 1993). The specifically heavier erythrocytes are drawn into the faster axial flow and are arranged along their longitudinal axes within the flow (Schmidt and Thews 2000; Opitz and Pfeiffer 1984; Tipler and Mosca 2009).

Literature

Adeberg P (2009) Auswirkungen der intravenösen Gabe von Iloprost und Alprostadil auf den intraoperativ gemessenen peripheren arteriellen Widerstand während femoro-distaler Rekonstruktionen. Dissertation, Medizinische Fakultät Charité – Universitätsmedizin Berlin

Affeld K, Kertscher U (2011) Vorlesungsskript: Strömungsmechanik in der Medizin – Biofluidmechanik. www.charite.de/biofluidmechanik/downloads/SkriptBiofluidmechanik1.pdf

Bohl W (1994) Technische Strömungslehre. Vogel Buchverlag, Würzburg
Cho YI, Kensey KR (1991) Effects of the non-Newtonian viscosity of blood on flows in a diseased arterial vessel. Part 1: Steady flows. Biorheology 28:241–242
Cross MM (1965) Rheology of non-Newtonian fluids: a new equation for pseudoplastic systems. J Colloid Sci 20:417–437
Davies AH, Magee TR, Baird RN, Horrocks M (1993) Intraoperative measurement of vascular graft resistance as a predictor of early outcome. Br J Surg 80:854–857
Fung YC (1997) Biomechanics: circulation, 2nd edn. Springer, New York
Gersten K (1991) Einführung in die Strömungsmechanik. Verlag Vieweg, Braunschweig
Ghista DN, Van Vollenhoven E, Yang WJ, Reul H (1979) Blood: rheology, hemolysis, gas and surface interactions, vol 3, Advances in cardiovascular physics. S. Karger, Basel
Heethaar RM (1993) Viscosity of media. In: Strackee J, Westerhof N (eds) The physics of heart and circulation. Institute of Physics Publishing, Bristol/Philadelphia, pp 273–293
Heise M, Krüger U, Settmacher U, Sklenar S, Neuhaus P, Scholz H (1999) A new method of intraoperative hydraulic impedance measurement provides valuable prognostic information about infrainguinal graft patency. J Vasc Surg 30:301–308
Heise M, Krüger U, Pfitzmann R, Neuhaus P, Scholz H, Settmacher U (2001) The influence of intraarterial prostaglandin E(1) on vascular hydraulic impedance and infrainguinal graft patency. Eur J Vasc Endovasc Surg 22:219–225
Heise M, Krüger U, Rückert R, Rad F, Scholz H, Neuhaus P, Settmacher U (2003) Correlation between angiographic runoff and intraoperative hydraulic impedance with regard to graft patency. Ann Vasc Surg 17:509–515
Heise M, Husmann I, Grüneberg AK, Knobel A, Kirschner P, Heidenhain C (2011) Comparison of straight and Venaflo-type cuffed arteriovenous ePTFE grafts in an animal study. J Vasc Surg 53:1661–1667
Krueger U, Scholz H, Heise M, Adeberg P, Petzold M, Zanow J, Karrenberg R (2000) Effect of intravenous iloprost and alprostadil (PGE1) on peripheral resistance during femoro-distal reconstructions. Int Angiol 19:358–365
Krüger U (1998) Hämodynamische Optimierung von Gefäßprothesen – dargestellt am Beispiel distaler End-zu-Seit Anastomosen am Unterschenkel. Verlag Dr. Köster, Berlin
Lerche D, Koch B, Vlatos G (1993) Das Fließverhalten des Stoffsystems Blut. Rheology 93:105–112
Li JK-J (2004) Dynamics of the vascular system, series on bioengineering and biomedical engineering, vol 1. World Scientific Publishing Co. Pte. Ltd, Singapore
Liepsch D (1989) Pulsierende Strömung von nicht-Newtonschen Fluiden in starren und elastischen Modellen der menschlichen Arterien. Hamostaseologie 9:82–107
Munson BR, Young DF, Okiishi TH (1994) Fundamentals of fluid mechanics. Wiley, New York
Opitz H, Pfeiffer C (1984) Das kardiovaskuläre System. Georg Thieme Verlag, Leipzig
Prandtl L, Oswatitsch K, Wieghardt K (1990) Führer durch die Strömungslehre. Verlag Vieweg, Braunschweig
Schmidt RF, Thews G (2000) Physiologie des Menschen. Springer, Berlin
Seemannschaft (2003) Handbuch für den Yachtsport. Hrsg. Deutscher Hochseesportverband "Hansa" e. V., Verlag Delius, Klasing & Co. KG, Bielefeld
Smits AJ, Lim TT (2000) Flow visualization. Techniques and examples. Imperial College Press, London
Sumner DS (1995) Essential hemodynamic principles. In: Rutherford R (ed) Vascular surgery, 4th edn. W.B. Saunders Company, Philadelphia, pp 18–44
Sumner DS (1996) Hemodynamics and rheology of vascular disease: applications to diagnosis and treatment. In: Haimovici H (ed) Haimovici's vascular surgery. Blackwell Science, Inc, Cambridge, pp S104–S123
Tipler PA, Mosca G (2009) Physik. Spektrum Akademischer Verlag, Heidelberg
Ulbrecht J, Mitschka P (1967) Nicht-Newtonsche Flüssigkeiten. Deutscher Verlag für Grundstoffindustrie, Leipzig
van Steenhoven AA (1993) Velocity profiles in large arteries. In: Strackee J, Westerhof N (eds) The physics of heart and circulation. Institute of Physics Publishing, Bristol/Philadelphia, pp S295–S319
Zamir M (2000) The physics of pulsatile flow, Biological Physics Series. Springer, Berlin/Heidelberg/New York

Our Methods

21

For the hemodynamic investigations we used two different methods: experimental flow investigations in a pulsatile flow system and numerical simulation. Experimental and numerical flow investigations are used when analytical and formula-based considerations alone do not lead to the solution of a flow-related problem. This also applies to the hemodynamic investigations presented here due to their complex geometries. The two methods do not compete but complement each other.

21.1 Experimental Flow Investigations

21.1.1 Creation of the Anastomotic Models for Flow Visualization

For the investigations, transparent silicone models were created using two different techniques.

1. The *first method* involved a four step procedure:
   (a) *Wax originals*: Idealized original size models of the regions to be examined were created from dental wax. Liquid wax was poured into unilaterally-closed and fixated silicone pipes. After opening the pipes, the resulting wax rods were attached to each other using wires. We manually modeled the anastomotic regions.
   (b) *Silicone molds (negative of the wax originals):* The wax models served to form two-piece gray silicone molds. The wax originals were suspended in frames. Repeatedly applying a release agent, the molds were partially filled with silicone. After curing, the second half of the mold was finished.
   (c) *Metal cast*: A metal alloy (melting at 70 °C, bismuth-containing) was used for casting. Subsequent grinding and polishing yielded smooth surfaces, which did not impair the optical properties of the future silicone models.
   (d) *Transparent silicone models*: The metal blanks were fixed in another mold and covered with a release agent. All air inclusions were removed from the two components of the transparent silicone before the molds were cast. After curing, the metal alloy was removed by heating in a water bath.
2. The *second method* began with the manual shaping of a metal model. Then the transparent silicone model was created. We used this method if only single models (instead of series) were needed. A detailed description of method 1 is listed in Huhle (2002) and Petzold (2001). Method 2 is described in Reddemann (2010).

21.1.2 Pulsatile Flow System

The pulsatile flow system that we developed is characterized by the maintenance of constant

H. Scholz, *Arteriovenous Access Surgery*,
DOI 10.1007/978-3-642-41139-7_21, © Springer-Verlag Berlin Heidelberg New York 2015

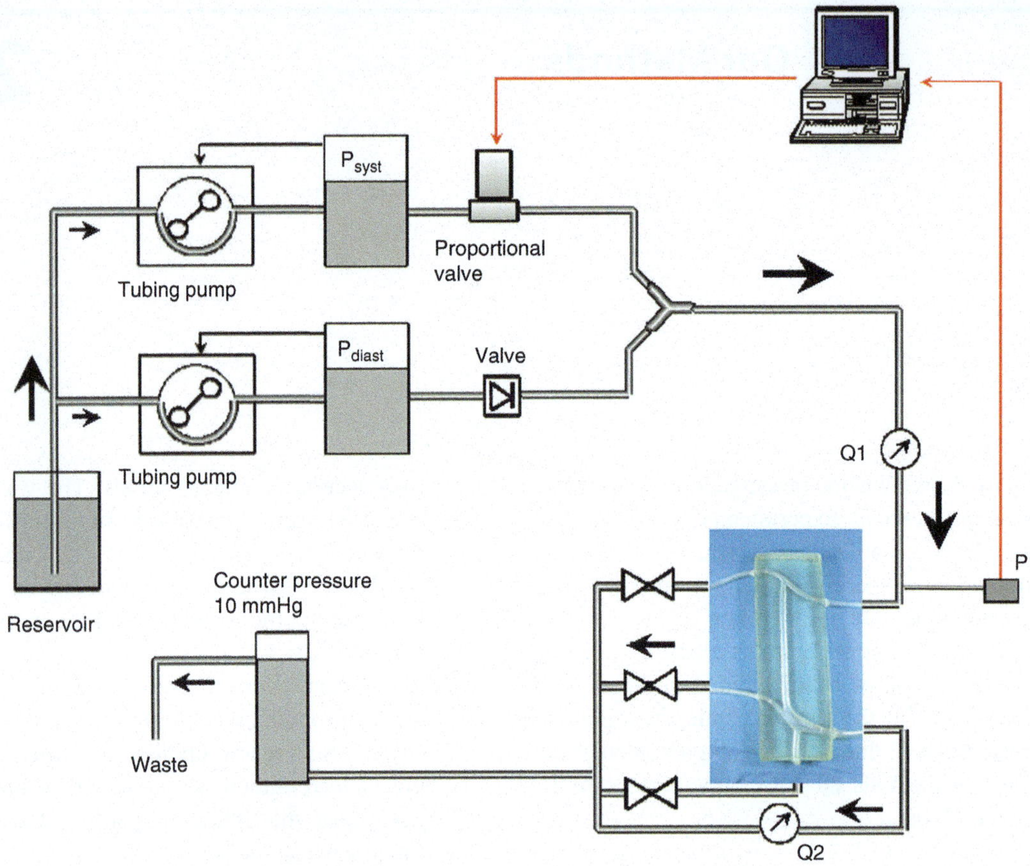

Fig. 21.1 Simplified pulsatile flow system. The video camera looked down at the model

pressure irrespective of flow rate (Figs. 21.1 and 21.2). Two pressure reservoirs for the systolic (p_{syst}) and diastolic (p_{diast}) pressures, respectively, form its basis. The pressure for each is regulated separately within the range 0–290 mmHg. Two pressure-controlled peristaltic pumps operating at variable speeds filled the pressure reservoirs dependent on the total flow rate.

The diastolic pressure continuously prevailed at the outflow of the pulsatile flow system. During systole a solenoid valve opened and directed the systolic pressure to the outflow. This proportional valve, whose control voltage supply determined the displacement of a piston and thus the amplitude of the outflow pressure, was controlled by a personal computer. The typical pressure curve copied former intraoperative pressure readings, and was compared to the current pressure at the inflow of the model. This deviation generated the control signal. The diastolic reservoir was separated from the systolic pressure by a unidirectional valve. Corresponding to the constant preselected pulse rate of 60 min^{-1}, the duration of each pulse cycle was 1 s.

For higher flow rates (Chap. 20), blood viscosity is almost that of a Newtonian fluid. Therefore, with higher shear rates, blood can be replaced by Newtonian fluids in the model flow system (Li 2004; Affeld and Kertscher 2011).We chose a water–glycerin mix (57.5 %/42.5 %), whose viscosity was equivalent to whole blood. For the exact adjustment of its viscosity (3.60 mPa×s at 25 °C) we used a capillary viscometer. For constant conditions the model fluid was tempered to 25 °C. At this temperature heat loss was small. Temperature control took place directly upstream from the arterial inflow. The density of the water–glycerin mix was 1.11 g/cm^3.

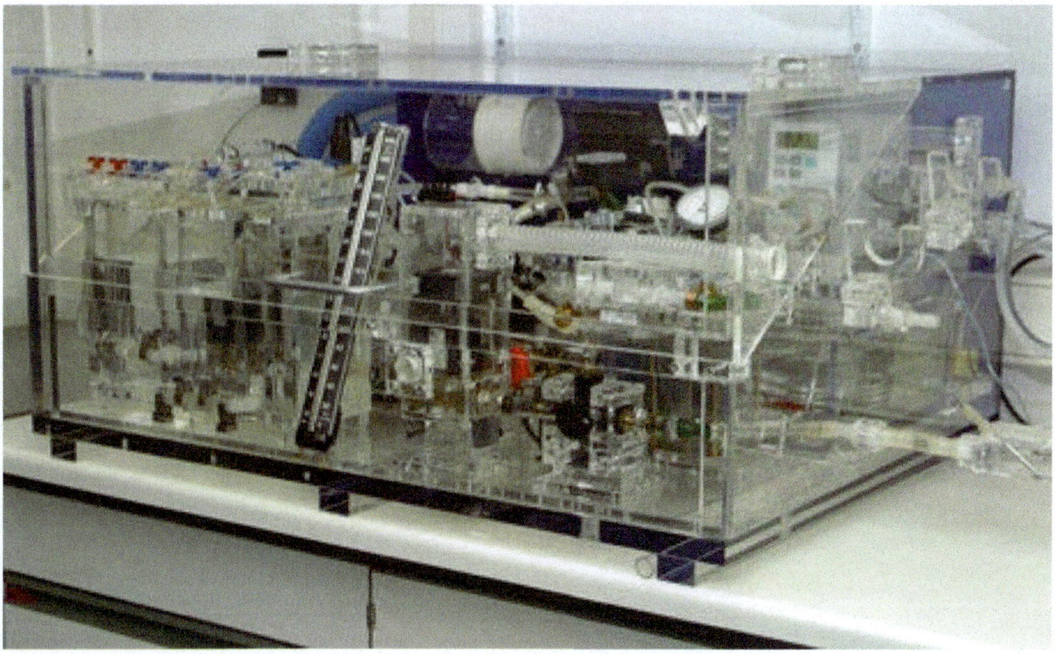

Fig. 21.2 Pulsatile flow system

We could record up to four flow rates simultaneously by using two two-channel flow meters. These gauges also allowed for pressure monitoring. The proximal outflow resistance was realized by a static counterpressure of 10 mmHg (equivalent to central venous pressure).

21.1.3 Visualization of the Flow Patterns

We used two methods to visualize the flow, of which only one method is depicted here:

1. Dye injection into the afferent pipe. The site of the injection was far enough upstream to warrant a velocity of the dye in the anastomosis that was equivalent to the model fluid. To achieve an even distribution of the dye with the flow, the intense silk paint was mixed with the model fluid before injection to ensure that its density did not differ from that of the colorless model fluid. This was checked with a hydrometer.
2. Microspheres in laser slit light (e.g., Fig. 21.3). A defined amount of microspheres (glass spheres, mean diameter 10 µm) was injected into the model fluid. A continous wave Nd:YVO4 laser beam (wave length 532 nm, output 20 mW, slit 0.1 mm) was optically transformed by a slit. Due to their identical density, the microspheres follow the model fluid flow without delay and reflect the laser light. The setting allowed for scanning all levels of the model.

With both methods, a digital video camera mounted above the anastomotic model recorded the flow patterns.

Apart from the visualization of the flow in transparent models (Figs. 4.9, 4.15, 4.19, 4.22a, 17.12b, and 20.2b), the flow system also provides for extensive investigations of hemodynamic readings (cf. Chap. 11).

21.2 Computational Fluid Dynamics

As well as flow model investigations, we also carried out investigations based on computational fluid dynamics for two reasons:

1. Experimental flow investigations are laborious. The production costs for a model

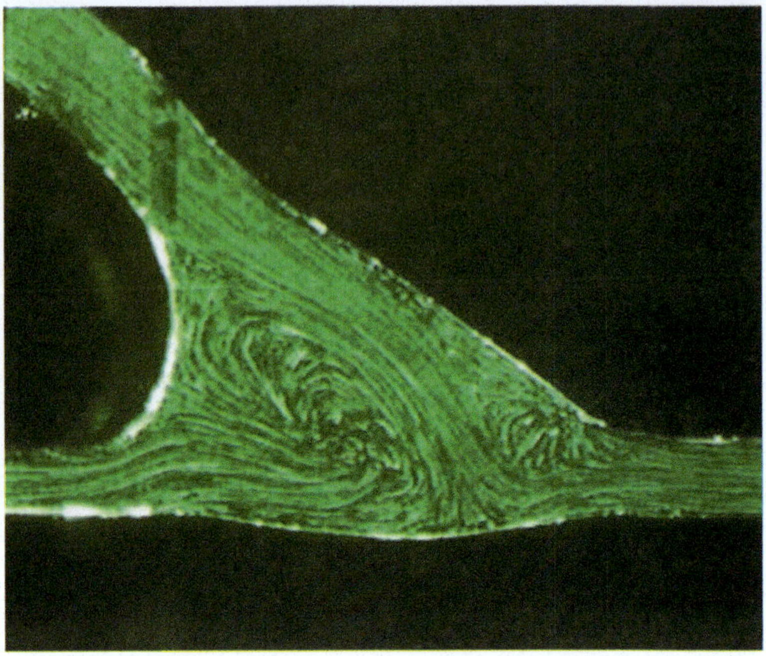

Fig. 21.3 Example for visualizing with the help of microspheres in laser slit light

(time and material) are considerable. Small changes of the geometry of a model require the time-consuming production of a new silicone model. Computer models, however, can be created much faster.

2. The limited resolution of conventional video cameras means that certain areas cannot be fully or closely examined. Also, fluid particles which move at a speed of 50 cm/s have already travelled 2 cm between two video images if the camera records only 25 images per second. High-speed camera systems are expensive. Numerical simulations may provide much more complex data as to the geometrical and time resolution, and other complex physical magnitudes which characterize a flow.

In summary, a combination of numerical and experimental investigations offers the chance of an economical validation while producing additional study parameters (Patankar 1980; Grieber et al. 1995; Kleinstreuer 2006).

Computational fluid dynamics (CFD) is an established method of fluid mechanics. Its aim is to solve flow-related problems using numerical methods. The basic equations of fluid mechanics are partial differential equations, which cannot be solved numerically. The path to their solution involves the so-called discretization of the anastomotic models, i.e., the transformation of a continous problem to a problem that is only considered for a definite number of points. In this context this means that the regions under investigation will be covered by virtual close mesh grid cells (finite volume method).

Due to discretization, only the inflow and outflow of these cells is calculated. The corresponding system of differential equations is numerically soluble. Each grid cell is observed in relation to its neighboring cells. The continuity principle requires that no mass is lost, which means that the same total volume that leaves a cell has to enter the neighboring cells (Fig. 21.4a–c).

With the given initial conditions, the differential equations for the whole region are solved iteratively. If the boundary conditions have been chosen correctly, and if the mesh structure is fine enough, the calculated result will be close to reality.

The idealized original-sized anastomotic forms are constructed in a computer simulation and an unstructured grid of tetrahedrons is generated. To enhance the precision of wall shear stress calculations, we refined the grid close to the wall with five layers of triangular prisms. Depending on the problem, each computerized model is then subdivided into $0.2–1.5 \times 10^6$ control volumes (cf. Fig. 21.5).

For the anastomotic and vascular wall regions, the no-slip condition was set as the boundary condition. Inflow and outflow conditions were set in analogy to the experimental investigations. In each case the systolic Reynolds number was below the critical threshold of 2,300. For the fluid the Cross model (Cross 1965) defined non-Newtonian characteristics. To avoid mistakes due to less than fully-developed flows, we considered two full cycles for the calculations. All results presented here are exclusively based on the second cycle.

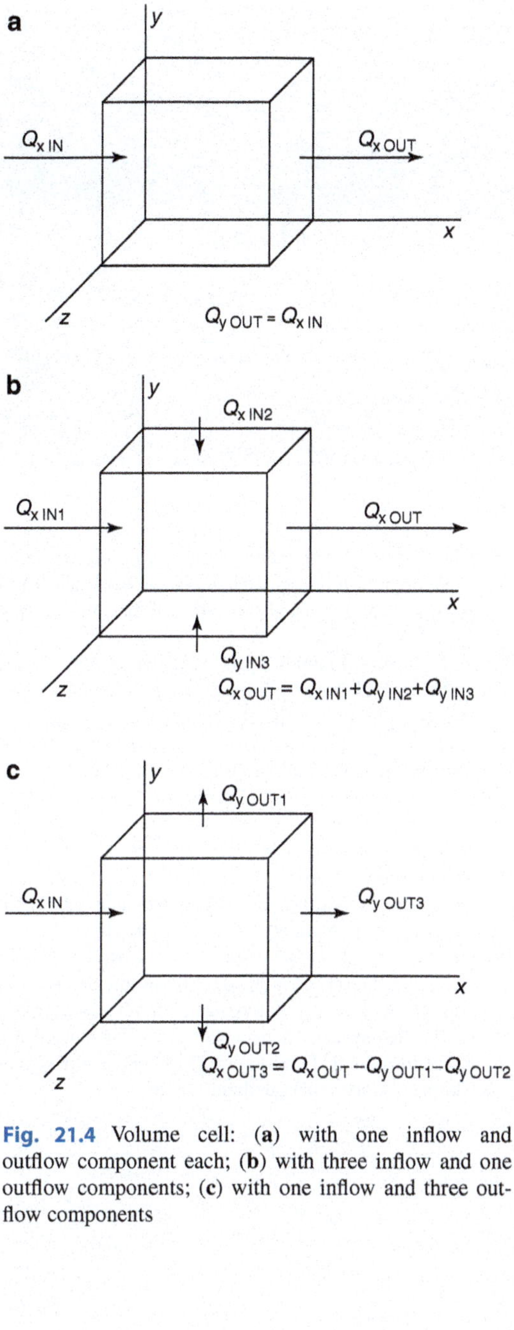

Fig. 21.4 Volume cell: (**a**) with one inflow and outflow component each; (**b**) with three inflow and one outflow components; (**c**) with one inflow and three outflow components

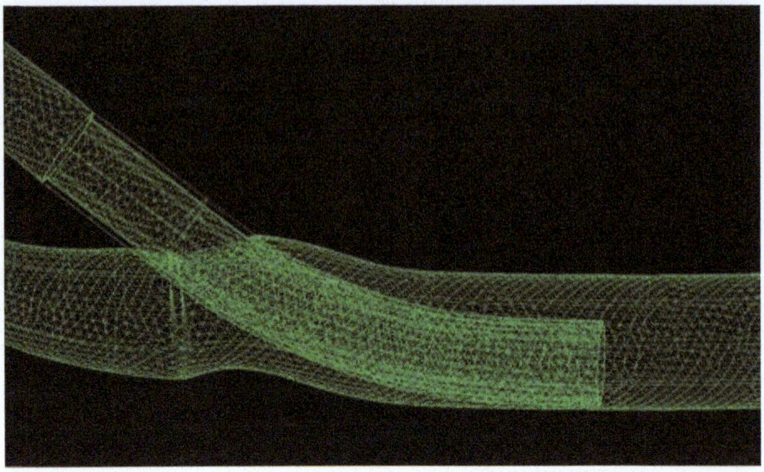

Fig. 21.5 Example of a fine grid. There is a straight covered stent in the venous anastomosis

Literature

Affeld K, Kertscher U (2011) Vorlesungsskript: Strömungsmechanik in der Medizin – Biofluidmechanik. www.charite.de/biofluidmechanik/downloads/SkriptBiofluidmechanik1.pdf. Zugegriffen: 25 Jan 2012

Cross MM (1965) Rheology of non-Newtonian fluids: A new equation for pseudoplastic systems. J Coll Sci 20: 417–437

Grieber M, Dornseifer T, Neunhoeffer T (1995) Numerische Simulation in der Strömungsmechanik. Vieweg, Braunschweig, Wiesbaden

Huhle A (2002) Die Flussdynamik in der arteriellen Anastomose arterio-venöser Interponate in Abhängigkeit von der Anastomosenmetrik und der arteriellen Speisung. Dissertation, Medizinischen Fakultät Charité der Humboldt-Universität zu Berlin

Kleinstreuer C (2006) Biofluid dynamics: principles and selected applications. Taylor Francis Inc, Boca Raton

Krüger U (1998) Hämodynamische Optimierung von Gefäßprothesen - dargestellt am Beispiel distaler End-zu-Seit Anastomosen am Unterschenkel. Verlag Dr. Köster, Berlin

Li JK-J (2004) Dynamics of the vascular system (Series on bioengineering and biomedical engineering, Vol 1). World Scientific Publishing, Singapore

Patankar SV (1980) Numerical heat transfer and fluid flow. Hemisphere Publishing Corp, New York

Petzold K (2001) Experimentelle und klinische Untersuchungen zur Beeinflussung der subendothelialen Intimahyperplasie im Bereich der venösen Anastomose gerader arteriovenöser Interponate am Oberarm. Dissertation, Medizinischen Fakultät Charité der Humboldt-Universität zu Berlin

Reddemann P (2010) Der Einfluss der Lokalisation der arteriellen Anastomose und des Flussminutenvolumens von arterio-venösen Gefäßzugängen auf den peripheren Perfusionsdruck bei in vitro Untersuchungen am Kreislaufmodell. Dissertation, Medizinische Fakultät Charité – Universitätsmedizin Berlin

Appendix

List of Suppliers

Product	Company
Prosthesis	Atrium Europe B.V. Rendementsweg 20B2 3641 SL Mijdrecht, The Netherlands
Patch prothesis	Bard Limited Forest House Brighton Road Crawley, West Sussex RH 11 9BP England
PUR patch	B.Braun Melsungen AG Postfach 1120, 34209 Melsungen Germany
Schwartz clamp	Fehling Instruments GmbH&Co.KG Hanauer Landstr. 7 a, 63791 Karlstein Germany
Prosthesis development	JOTEC GmbH Lotzenäcker 23, 72379 Hechingen Germany
Flow meter	Medistim ASA – Headquarters Økernveien 94 0579, Oslo Norway
Microspheres	LaVision GmbH Anna-Vandenhoeck-Ring 19, 37081 Göttingen Germany
Multilayer impermeable graft	Vascutek Newmains Avenue Inchinnan Renfrewshire PA4 9RR Scotland UK

H. Scholz, *Arteriovenous Access Surgery*,
DOI 10.1007/978-3-642-41139-7, © Springer-Verlag Berlin Heidelberg New York 2015

Glossary

Angle of the anastomosis Angle between (a) feeding artery and vein of the fistula or (b) feeding artery and shunt prothesis, (c) or shunt prothesis and efferent vein.

Arterial phase In single-needle dialysis, during this phase blood coming from the patient is pumped into the dialysis machine.

AV fistula AV access with direct arterialization of the fistula's vein.

AV shunt AV access with arterialization of the vein via an interposition graft.

Back flow Flow portion which runs in the reverse direction to the main flow.

Collectors/precollectors In the lymphatic system, lymph capillaries drain into precollectors, which in turn merge into collectors.

Dead water region A region without or with hardly any flow.

DRIL "Distal revascularization interval ligation" (therapy for insufficient peripheral perfusion).

Fibrin sealing Selective coating of the exterior wall of an ePTFE prosthesis to prevent perigraft seromas.

Flow Laminar flow: movement of the fluid particles on trajectories parallel to the pipe axis without any noteworthy transverse exchange. Turbulent flow: superposition of transverse movements on the main flow leading to continous mixture of fluid particles between the different layers.

Fluid Term used for both gases and liquids.

Inflow radius The radius of the curved segment near the anastomosis with interposition grafts.

Inflow resistance Resistance in the vein of an AV fistula or in the graft of an AV shunt.

Newtonian fluid Fluid in which viscosity is independent of flow velocity.

Non-Newtonian fluid Fluid in which viscosity changes with flow velocity.

No-slip condition Adherence of the fluid to the wall. If the wall does not move, the fluid velocity will also be zero.

Oscillation Reversal of flow direction within the same cardiac cycle.

Outflow resistance Resistance in the efferent vein of an AV access.

PAI Proximalization of cardiac inflow (therapy for insufficent peripheral perfusion).

Patch anastomosis Bulbous anastomosis between shunt prosthesis and efferent vein.

Patch prosthesis Specially designed shunt prosthesis whose bulbous venous anastomosis allows for a harmonious outflow.

Patch size Design of the venous end of a patch prothesis adapted to the venous diameter.

Perfusion pressure Pressure difference which maintains tissue perfusion.

Permanent catheter Wide lumen venous catheter implanted as a long-term dialysis access.

PRU Peripheral resistance unit, 1 PRU = 1 mmHg/(mL/min).

PTA Percutaneous transluminal angioplasty.

PTFE (ePTFE) Polytetrafluoroethylene, extended polytetrafluoroethylene.

Pulsatile flow system Model for the experimental investigation of the flow in selected regions in analogy with the human circulatory system.

Recirculation (a) Quality measurement for the efficacy of hemodialysis. (b) In hemodynamics the same as backflow.

Reynolds number Dimensionless number that characterizes the flow (laminar or turbulent).

Scribner/Buselmeier shunts Partially extracorporal arteriovenous shunt for connection to the dialyzer (obsolete).

Secondary flow Additional flow with comparatively low velocity that runs in a plane perpendicular to the main flow; occurs downstream from curves and in bifurcations.

Shear In general the deformation of a substance without volume changes by two opposing parallel forces.

Shear rate Change of velocity perpendicular to the flow.

SIH Subendothelial intimal hyperplasia.

Stagnation point Point where local flow velocity is zero (e.g., in front of an obstacle). The kinetic energy is completely transformed into pressure.

Steal effect Steal of arterial blood without relevant clinical symptoms.

Steal syndrome Steal of arterial blood with relevant clinical symptoms.

Stream line Runs tangentially to the starting points of velocity vectors.

Symmetry plane Plane that divides an object into two identical mirrored planes.

Transit-time method Method to determine intraoperative flow based on the time difference needed for an ultrasound signal to return with/against the blood flow.

Venous floor Venous wall opposite the anastomotic suture line.

Viscosity Internal friction of a flowing fluid.

Vortex Streamlines form concentric circles. This spinning occurs if there are major differences in flow velocity.

Wall shear stress Force exerted on a wall segment. The direction of the force is tangential to the wall.

Wash out phenomenon Complete flushing of a vascular space without a dead water zone.

Femoral Arterioarterial Graft

Institution

for: ❑ ***dialysis unit*** ❑ ***patient***

Femoral arterioarterial grafts

patient

On ______(date)______ an arterioarterial femoral graft was placed using a ____mm ePTFE prothesis.

Punctures should not start before the ____ postoperative week.

This kind of graft was chosen due to

- ❑ occlusion of all central veins
- ❑ just one central vein patent
- ❑ chronic decompensated heart failure
- ❑ insufficient peripheral perfusion
- ❑ other: ______________________

comments: ______________________

Veins still available for central catheters are:

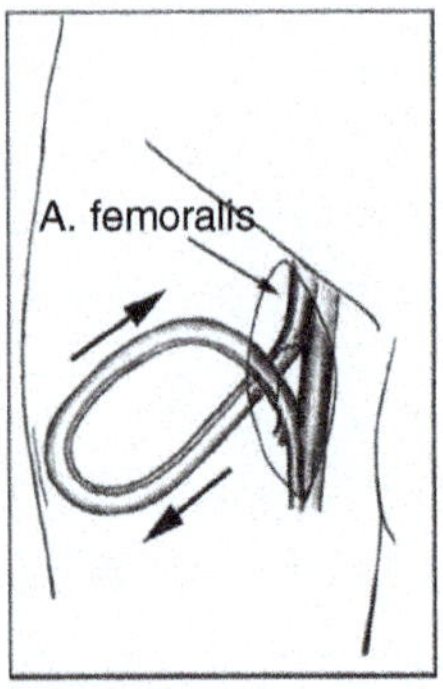

Physiology of arterioarterial grafts

As the graft has been placed into the course of the artery, the pulsatile arterial flow persists. Therefore the graft has **no** influence on heart rate and peripheral perfusion.

Unlike with arteriovenous grafts, the arterial pressure persists over the whole graft. There will be no thrill.
Please note that only drugs meant for arterial injection may be added to the dialyzate.

Please make sure

1. not to use material sterilized with ethylene oxide.
2. to flush the dialysis filter sufficiently for complete deaeration.
3. to administer only drugs meant for intraarterial application.
4. to use isoosmolar infusions only.

Recommendations for puncture:

1. Puncture in the direction of the flow .
2. Aperture of the cannula should face the the graft.
3. Long compression after dialysis (up to 40 minutes).
4. Apply air-permeable dressing.
5. Rope ladder punctures using the whole loop.

We recommend the administration of oral anticoagulants (INR 2,5 –3,5). If this is contraindicated, consider clopidogrel.

Please contact with your questions:

vascular surgery:
office:
ward:
fax:

nephrology:
ward:
dialysis unit:
fax:

Subclavian Arterioarterial Graft

Institution

for: ❑ ***dialysis unit*** ❑ ***patient***

Subclavian arterioarterial grafts

patient

On ___(date)___ an arterioarterial subclavian graft was placed using a __ mm ePTFE prothesis,

Punctures should not start before the___ postoperative week.

This kind of graft was chosen due to
- ❑ occlusion of all central veins
- ❑ just one central vein patent
- ❑ chronic decompensated heart failure
- ❑ insufficient peripheral perfusion
- ❑ other: __________

comments: __________

Veins still available for central catheters are: __________

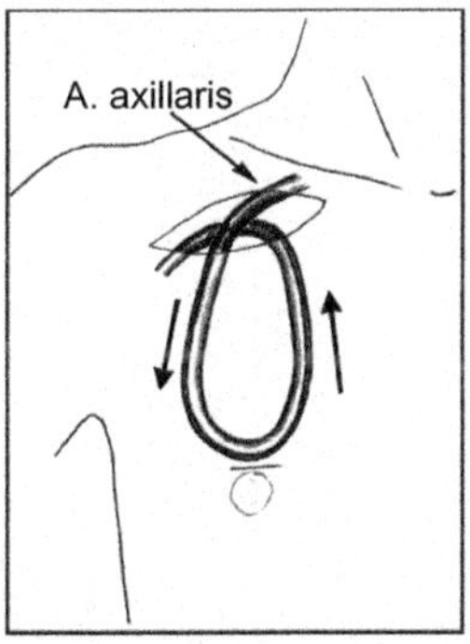

Physiology of arterioarterial grafts

As the graft has been placed into the course of the artery, the pulsatile arterial flow persists. Therefore the graft has **no** influence on heart rate and peripheral perfusion.

Unlike with arteriovenous grafts, the arterial pressure persists over the whole puncturable graft. There will be no thrill. Please note that only drugs meant for arterial injection may be added to the dialyzate.

Please make sure
1. not to use material sterilized with ethylene oxide.
2. to flush the dialysis filter sufficiently for complete deaeration.
3. to administer only drugs meant for intraarterial application.
4. to use isoosmolar infusions only.

Recommendations for puncture:
1. Puncture in the direction of the flow.
2. Aperture of the cannula should face the graft.
3. Long compression after dialysis (up to 40 minutes).
4. Apply air-permeable dressing.
5. Rope ladder punctures using the whole loop.

We recommend the administration of oral anticoagulants (INR 2,5 – 3,5).If this is contraindicated, consider clopidogrel.

Please contact with your questions

vascular surgery:
office:
ward:
fax:

nephrology:
ward:
dialysis unit:
fax:

Index

A

Acetylsalicylic acid, 182
Anastomosis
  laterolateral, 11, 37, 51–52
  laterotrminal, 11, 12, 16, 33, 35, 37, 38, 51, 57, 83, 153, 157, 169
  patch, 63–71, 75, 78, 82, 202
  terminolateral, 35, 45, 59, 63–67, 69, 71–73, 99, 108, 202
Anastomotic angle, 12, 62, 68–71
Anastomotic region, 12, 58–59, 66, 73, 78, 228, 235
Anatomy
  axillary artery and vein, 44
  basilic vein in the forearm, 48, 49
  cubital fossa, 35–36
Aneurysms
  prosthesis, 29
  puncture, 26, 107, 108, 110–112, 114–118, 218
  spurious, 219
  thrombus, 122, 219
Angiography, 3, 5, 26, 99, 111, 195, 211, 212
Anticoagulation, 23, 192, 195
Arterialization (retrograde venous), 11, 34, 136, 207
Artery, 3, 11, 57, 107, 123, 139, 142, 145, 175, 185, 187, 190, 207, 232
  dilatation, 190, 191, 197
AV access
  amputees, 192
  arterial reconstruction, 175–183
  cardiac insufficiency, 145–172
  cardiac strain, 145–172
  diabetics, 146, 172, 191
  histopathology, 213–232
  hypercoagulopathy, 192
  hypotension, 192, 195, 208
  IV drug abuse, 23–25, 193
  malignancy, 192
  prophylaxis of infections, 185
AV fistula
  anastomosis, 11–14, 16, 18–25, 27–30, 32–35, 37, 38, 40–45
  anastomotic angle, 12
  aneurysm, 23, 26–30, 41–43, 51–52
  basilic fistula in the upper arm, 19–21
  cephalic and basilic veins in the cubital fossa, 35
  cubital fossa and upper arm, 35–53
  deep position, 31, 43
  distal basilic fistula, 19–21
  distal cephalic fistula in the forearm, 19, 23
  forearm, 90
  great saphenous vein, 52–54
  insufficient arterial inflow, 32
  insufficient peripheral perfusion, 3
  median antebrachial vein, 16, 21–22, 35, 38, 39, 47, 50, 51
  pathophysiology, 12
  proximal basilic fistula, 20–21
  proximal cephalic fistula, 19
  reconstruction, 28, 29, 32, 33, 38, 41–44, 49–50, 52, 53
  reconstruction of the basilic vein, 49–50
  reconstruction of the cephalic vein in the cubital fossa, 41–42
  reconstruction of the cephalic vein in the forearm, 41–42
  reconstruction of the cephalic vein in the shoulder and central regions, 43–45
  reconstruction of the cephalic vein in the upper arm, 42–43
  renal transplants, 189–190
  rotational error, 14–15, 22
  side branches, 22, 30, 35, 51
  snuff box fistula, 16
  spasm, 12, 13
  stenosis, 13, 22, 25–29, 41
  stenosis of the feeding artery, 32
  superficialization of the basilic vein in the forearm, 48
  superficialization of the basilic vein in the upper arm, 44–46
  thrombosis, 15, 22–25
  transposition of the cephalic vein, 43, 44
AV shunt
  arterial anastomosis, 57, 61, 62, 70, 74, 75, 78, 82, 83, 85, 91, 112, 113
  caliber changes, 61, 78
  crossover shunt, 102
  design and length, 62–63
  femoral graft, 102
  first puncture, 110
  forearm, 90
  hemodynamics, 59–76, 85

H. Scholz, *Arteriovenous Access Surgery*,
DOI 10.1007/978-3-642-41139-7, © Springer-Verlag Berlin Heidelberg New York 2015

AV shunt (*cont.*)
infections, 76, 78, 91, 101
looped graft, 76, 79, 100
narrow segment, 61, 62, 75, 78, 81, 83
patch anastomosis, 63–69, 71, 75, 78
pathophysiology, 57–58
position of the anastomoses, 59, 81, 96, 97, 100–102
pressure curve, 61
puncturable segment, 57–58
reconstruction, 87, 92, 93, 101
stenosis, 57, 71–73, 81, 87, 91, 92, 96, 98, 101
straight graft, 63, 75, 78, 81, 83–86, 88–90
subclavian graft, 70, 99
subclavianjugular graft, 99–102
subcutaneous tunnel, 78–81, 85, 91, 96, 101
suture techniques, 83
thrombosis, 58, 74–76, 83, 85, 91
tissue proliferation, 58–59
upper arm, 86–92
venous anastomosis, 57, 58, 63–73, 81–86, 91, 95, 96, 101, 102
venous side branch, 63, 69, 75, 82

B

Bernoulli's principle, 228, 231

C

Calciphylaxis, 125
Cardiac strain, 2, 31, 145–172, 183, 207
Catheter
central venous, 2, 3, 7–9
permanent, 2, 8–9
temporary, 2, 7–9, 116, 119
variants, 2, 9
Catheter exit site, 9
Catheter materials
polyurethane, 8
silicone, 8
Chemotherapy, 12, 22, 23, 25, 137
Coagulation, 2, 3, 7, 22, 58, 74, 76, 192, 195, 220
bipolar, 3
Computational flow dynamics, 237–240
Cosmetics, 27, 41
anticoagulants
Cubital fossa, 3, 12, 21, 26, 33–54, 90, 126, 148, 152, 155, 157, 160, 168, 169, 187
arterialization of the cephalic vein, 34, 38–45, 50–51

D

Dila(ta)tion, 12, 13, 25, 31, 32, 45, 49, 53, 57, 64, 82, 83, 117, 145–148, 152, 155, 157, 172, 182–183, 190, 191, 197, 198, 213, 217–220, 232, 233
aneurysmatic, 12, 117, 213, 217–220
Distal revascularization and interval ligation (DRIL), 159, 164–171
Double lumen catheters, 8, 9
DRIL. *See* Distal revascularization and interval ligation (DRIL)
Duplex sonography, 3, 5, 25, 26, 30–32, 91, 147, 158, 159, 172, 176, 209, 211
respiration-dependent flow, 3

E

Elongation, 12, 42
ePTFE prosthesis, 33, 40, 57, 59, 64, 78, 103, 141, 178, 181, 182, 197–198, 211
fibrin sealing, 77

F

Fibrin sealing, 77–78, 141–144
Filtration, 77, 82, 141–143, 188
Flow reduction
narrow segment, 61, 75, 149–153, 157–159
suture, 152–156
Fluid, 64, 65, 68, 77, 135, 141–143, 160, 163, 185, 201, 211, 225–233, 236–239
Fluid mechanics
Bernoulli's principle, 228, 231
dead water, 225, 226
dynamic pressure, 227, 228
flow pattern, 225, 226
fluid, 225–226, 228, 238
Hagen–Poisseuille equation, 232
Reynold's number, 225, 226
turbulence, 75, 147, 210, 211

H

Hematocrit (HCT), 75
Hemodynamics, 1, 2, 12, 25, 58–76, 78, 82, 137, 192, 195, 197, 201–204, 225–233, 235, 237
Heparin solution, 9, 12, 82, 83, 113
High flow catheter, 8
Hypercoagulability, 22, 93, 111, 112, 118, 192, 195

I

Immobilization, postoperative, 4
Incisions
longitudinal, 4, 16–19, 21, 22, 24, 27, 28, 30–34, 37, 39–42, 45, 46, 48, 49, 51, 53, 85, 86, 89, 91, 99, 113, 118, 121–123, 180, 186, 187
transverse, 17, 23, 44, 91, 101, 108, 111, 122, 180, 186, 187
Infection
AV fistula, 122–124
incision film, 79, 96
prevention, 76–77, 122
prosthesis, 125–130
Inflow radius, 63, 70–71, 76, 95, 96
Inflow resistance, 12, 57, 74, 145, 146, 150, 159–162, 171, 172

Interposition graft
arterioarterial, 2, 3, 99, 107–110, 148, 169, 172, 192, 195
indication, 32, 33, 39, 41, 44, 88, 93, 99, 100
length, 62, 75
looped, 75, 76, 79–81, 86–87, 90, 100, 116, 118, 119, 121
physiology, 107
reconstruction, 87
spurious aneurysm, 219
stenosis, 41, 44, 61, 86, 87, 96, 98
straight, 61, 77, 78
thrombectomy, 25, 118
thrombosis, 63, 75, 91
Intravenous (IV) drugs, 22, 25, 193

K
Kinking, 9, 12–15, 22, 25, 27, 31, 38, 44, 82, 85, 86, 99, 152, 181

L
Laplace's equation, 208
Life expectancy, 1, 9, 27, 57, 138
Longitudinal incision, 4, 16–19, 21, 22, 24, 27, 28, 30–34, 37, 39–42, 45, 46, 48, 49, 51, 53, 85, 86, 89, 91, 99, 113, 118, 121–123, 180, 186, 187
Lymph edema
chronic, 133, 186
postoperative, 185–186
prevention, 186
venous congestion, 186

M
Magnifying glasses, 5
Micro instruments
Schwartz clamp, 5
Yasargil clip, 5
Minimal perfusion, peripheral, 191
Minimum blood flow, 2
Monitoring
angiography, 212
duplex sonography, 211
pressure surveillance, 211
recirculation, 211
urea elimination, 211

N
Narrow segment, 61, 62, 75, 78, 81, 83, 149–151, 155, 159
Necklace shunt, 100
Newtonian fluid, 160, 231, 236
Numerical simulation
static pressure, 66, 227, 228
velocity vectors, 65–66
wall shear stress, 66–69, 71–73, 204, 213, 238

O
Obesity, 2, 191
One armedness, 3
Oscillation, 12, 59, 62, 65, 67, 75, 226

P
PAI. *See* Proximalization of arterial inflow (PAI)
Partial thrombosis, 27
Patch anastomosis, 63–71, 75, 78, 202
Patch plasty, 25, 41, 42, 86, 91, 98, 102, 138, 139
Patch prosthesis
patch anastomosis, 63
patch size, 63, 82
radius, 63
side branch, 63
trimming, 67, 82–83
Pathophysiology, 12, 57, 131–132, 136, 137, 141, 145–146, 185, 197–198
Percutaneous transluminal angioplasty (PTA), 3, 25, 32, 41, 42, 86, 99, 102, 133–135
Perineurium, 4, 5, 188
Peripheral resistance unit (PRU), 159
Prophylaxis of thrombosis, 9
Prosthetic graft
false aneurysm, 114–115
stenosis, 111, 112, 118, 119
thrombectomy, 111–115, 118
thrombosis, 111–114
Proximalization
cubital fossa, 126, 148, 152, 160, 168, 169, 187
forearm fistula, 168, 169
infraaxillary, 168, 169, 180
procedure, 148
Proximalization of arterial inflow (PAI), 159–168, 171
PRU. *See* Peripheral resistance unit (PRU)
PTA. *See* Percutaneous transluminal angioplasty (PTA)
Pulsatile flow system, 61, 62, 64–65, 67–69, 71, 149–152, 159, 202, 235–237
flow, 202, 208, 225, 227
proximalization, 237
Pulsatility, 75, 207, 208, 210, 211, 225
Puncture
bleeding, 111, 138
wall structure, 114
Puncture technique, 1, 121, 197–204

R
Reconstruction AV fistula
interposition graft, 24, 25, 33–35, 39–42, 44
transposition of the distal cephalic vein, 32
Residual thrombi, 118
Risk of rupture, 27, 114

S
Secondary flow, 59, 65, 70, 228–230, 232
Septic focus, 2, 3, 29, 51, 53, 125
Shear, 12, 59, 65–67, 69, 71, 73–75, 204, 214, 230, 231, 233, 238

Shear rate, 65, 73, 74, 231, 233, 236
Side branch, 22, 25, 26, 30–31, 35, 51, 63, 68, 69, 75, 82, 85, 95, 131, 133, 189, 212
SIH. *See* Subendothelial intimal hyperplasia (SIH)
Single-lumen catheters, 8, 9
Single-needle dialysis, 201–204
Snuff box fistula, 16–17
Spasm, 12–13, 193
Steal syndrome, 145, 166, 207
Stenosis
  arterial, 208
  AV anastomosis, 32, 132–135, 175
Subendothelial intimal hyperplasia (SIH), 58, 61, 69, 73, 74, 214–217, 220
Suture technique, 83

T

Thrill, 12, 57, 59, 65, 110, 111, 175, 201, 207–210
Thrombogenicity, 7, 23, 57, 74, 75
Thrombosis, 7, 9, 12–16, 22–23, 27, 58, 63, 74–76, 83, 85, 91, 107, 108, 110–112, 123, 131, 138, 156–158, 171, 172, 183, 191, 192, 195, 213, 220
  prophylaxis, 9
Tissue proliferation, 22, 25, 58, 59, 96, 110, 118, 149, 157, 197

U

Urgency, 2, 32

V

Valve insufficiency, 30
Vascular prosthesis, 76
Vein
  aneurysm, 13, 23, 26–30, 41–42, 51–52, 58, 98, 100, 101, 108, 110, 111, 114–117, 126, 197, 210, 217, 219
  dilatation, 12, 31, 49, 64, 155, 190
  kinking, 9, 12–15, 22, 25, 26, 31, 38, 44, 82, 85, 86, 99, 152, 181
  side branch, 22, 25, 26, 30–31, 35, 51, 63, 68, 69, 75, 82, 95, 131, 133, 189, 212
  venous trunk, 31
Venograms, 143, 144
Venous congestion, 131–136, 138, 185
  retrograde venous arterialization, 131, 136, 207

W

Wash out effect, 65, 67, 75

The manufacturer's authorised representative in the EU is Springer
Nature Customer Service Centre GmbH, Europaplatz 3, 69115 Heidelberg,
Germany. If you have any concerns regarding our products, please
contact ProductSafety@springernature.com

Printed and bound by CPI Group (UK) Ltd, Croydon, CR0 4YY
22/09/2026
02221056-0007